Infant and Young Child Feeding

Challenges to Implementing a Global Strategy

Edited by

Fiona Dykes
Ph.D., M.A., R.M., A.D.M., Cert. Ed.
Director, Maternal and Infant Nutrition and Nurture Unit (MAINN)
School of Public Health and Clinical Sciences
University of Central Lancashire
Preston, UK

Victoria Hall Moran
Ph.D., M.Med.Sci., B.Sc.
Maternal and Infant Nutrition and Nurture Unit (MAINN)
School of Public Health and Clinical Sciences
University of Central Lancashire
Preston, UK

D1395923

WILEY-BLACKWELL
A John Wiley & Sons, Ltd., Publication

This edition first published 2009
© 2009 Blackwell Publishing Ltd

Blackwell Publishing was acquired by John Wiley & Sons in February 2007. Blackwell's publishing programme has been merged with Wiley's global Scientific, Technical, and Medical business to form Wiley-Blackwell.

Registered office
John Wiley & Sons Ltd, The Atrium, Southern Gate, Chichester, West Sussex, PO19 8SQ, United Kingdom

Editorial office
9600 Garsington Road, Oxford, OX4 2DQ, United Kingdom
2121 State Avenue, Ames, Iowa 50014-8300, USA

For details of our global editorial offices, for customer services and for information about how to apply for permission to reuse the copyright material in this book please see our website at http://www.wiley.com/wiley-blackwell.

Library of Congress Cataloging-in-Publication Data
Infant and young child feeding : challenges to implementing a global strategy / edited by Fiona Dykes, Victoria Hall Moran.
       p. ; cm.
   Includes bibliographical references and index.
   ISBN 978-1-4051-8721-3 (pbk. : alk. paper) 1. Infants–Nutrition. 2. Breastfeeding.
3. World health. I. Dykes, Fiona. II. Moran, Victoria Hall.
   [DNLM: 1. World Health Organization. 2. Breast Feeding. 3. Guidelines as Topic.
4. Health Promotion. 5. Maternal Nutritional Physiological Phenomena. 6. Nutrition Policy.
7. World Health.   WS 125 I43 2009]
   RJ216.I495 2009
   362.198'92–dc22

                                                                                    2009021835

A catalogue record for this book is available from the British Library.

Set in 10/12.5pt Sabon by Graphicraft Limited, Hong Kong
Printed and bound in Great Britain

1   2009

Contents

Contributor biographies

James Akre has academic and practical experience in sociology, public and international affairs, and public health, with an early focus on economic and social development and the welfare of populations in low-income rural environments. His community development and international public health nutrition career spans four decades, including more than 30 years' working in three agencies of the United Nations system, dealing with labour and social issues and public health. He has worked and travelled extensively in Africa, Asia, the Caribbean and Europe, including a cumulative seven years resident in Cameroon, Haiti and Turkey. Although formally retired, from his base in Geneva, Switzerland, he continues to research, publish and present on international public health nutrition policy and the sociocultural dimensions of child feeding and the health of mothers and children. He serves as a member of the Board of Directors of the International Board of Lactation Consultant Examiners (IBLCE), the Editorial Board of the *International Breastfeeding Journal*, and the Scientific Committee of La Leche League France.

Andy Bilson is Professor of Social Work Research at University of Central Lancashire and a fellow of the Cybernetics Society. His work has a focus on organisational change and children's rights. He has carried out research and consultancy for a range of organisations including the Economic and Social Research Council, UNICEF, World Bank, Save the Children and governments, particularly in Europe and Central Asia. Andy has published widely on both social work and systemic approaches to organisational change and was the editor of *Evidence Based Practice in Social Work* and co-author of *Social Work Management and Practice: Systems Principles*. He is currently undertaking research with Fiona Dykes and others into the implementation of the Baby-Friendly Hospital Initiative in the UK and Australia and writing a book on social work leadership and management.

Anne Marie Coufopoulos is a Senior Lecturer in Health in the Department of Health a Applied Social Science at Liverpool Hope University and also a Registered Dietician. Anne has a particular focus upon the impact of poverty on nutrition, especially among homeless women and children. Anne is currently involved in collaborative public health nutrition research projects in the north-west of England, including the evaluation of a community food initiative. Anne is actively involved in the promotion of homeless women and children's nutrition and health, through training staff working with this group in Liverpool, UK.

Fiona Dykes is Professor of Maternal and Infant Health and Director of the Maternal and Infant Nutrition and Nurture Unit (MAINN), School of Public Health and Clinical Sciences, University of Central Lancashire. She is also Adjunct Professor at University of Western Sydney. Fiona has a particular focus upon the global, sociocultural and political influences on infant and young child feeding practices. Fiona is topic editor (breastfeeding) for the international journal, *Maternal and Child Nutrition*, published by Wiley-Blackwell. Fiona has worked on WHO, UNICEF, Government (Department of Health), the National Health Service, the National Institute of Health and Clinical Excellence (NICE), TrusTECH Service Innovation (UK), and British Council funded projects. She is currently involved in projects in Africa, Australia, European Union and Pakistan. In addition to co-editing this book, Fiona is single author of *Breastfeeding in Hospital: Mothers, Midwives and the Production Line*, published by Routledge, and co-editor of *Maternal and Infant Nutrition and Nurture: Controversies and Challenges*, published by Quay Books.

Renée Flacking is a researcher at the Department of Women's and Children's Health, Uppsala University, Sweden. She is neonatal nurse and employed as a Practise Developer at the Department of Paediatrics, Falun Hospital, Sweden. In 2007, Renée completed her Ph.D. 'Breastfeeding and becoming a mother – influences and experiences of mothers of preterm infants'. Her main research areas are breastfeeding and parenting in families with preterm infants, focusing on emotional, relational and sociocultural aspects. Her research has included large epidemiological studies on breastfeeding, interventions to support mothers and fathers when their infants are admitted to neonatal units and qualitative studies on issues related to breastfeeding and to health. At present, Renée is conducting an ethnographic study in Sweden and England on breastfeeding and relationality in mothers of preterm infants at neonatal units.

Kevin D. Frick is trained as a health economist and is an Associate Professor at the Johns Hopkins Bloomberg School of Public Health in the Department of Health Policy and Management and has joint appointments in the Departments of International Health, Ophthalmology, and Economics and the School of Nursing. His participation in collaborative economic evaluations has included an evaluation of a community health nurse and peer counsellor-based intervention to encourage low income mothers who had already decided to breastfeed to continue longer. At present, he is working with a student analysing the interaction of different drug regimens for human immunodeficiency virus (HIV)-positive mothers and uninfected children in resource-poor environments in which breastfeeding is the only option for infant nutrition. He has taught extensively about both cost-effectiveness and economic analysis and has developed a framework for understanding how the two fit together in understanding health behaviours, healthcare utilisation, and health policy.

Danielle Groleau is Associate Professor at the Division of Social and Transcultural Psychiatry, McGill University where she teaches two courses on qualitative methodologies. She is also Associate Researcher at the Jewish General hospital in Montréal, Canada. As a FRSQ Fellow, Danielle also conducts qualitative and multidisciplinary research (medical anthropology, public health, transcultural psychiatry) in reproductive health with a focus on psychocultural barriers to breastfeeding in vulnerable populations (poverty, migration, prematurity, HIV) and sociosomatic problems (hyperemesis gravidarum, insufficient breast milk, depression). She is part of the editorial board of the *Journal of Transcultural Psychiatry* published by SAGE and has done some consulting work for WHO, Pan American Health Organization (PAHO), the Québec Ministry of Health, with Tibetan refugees in India, and for several projects in Brazil. She is currently co-leading the evaluation of the implementation of the Québec breastfeeding policy, and developing research on breastfeeding and HIV in Burundi and Brazil, and on breastfeeding and prematurity in Montréal.

Allan Frederick Hackett graduated from Leeds University in 1974 with a degree in Agricultural Science and then qualified as a State Registered Dietician but rapidly moved into research on the causes of post-surgical malnutrition in the Department of Surgery at Leeds. Allan then moved to the Dental School at Newcastle upon Tyne and conducted the world's first longitudinal study of diet and dental caries working with Professors Neil Jenkins and Andrew Rugg-Gunn. Allan then completed his Ph.D. in the Department of Child Health at Newcastle working on the role of diet in the management of children with diabetes mellitus. After working with a paediatric epidemiologist, Allan took up a lecturing post at Liverpool Polytechnic. Allan was made a Reader in Community Nutrition in 1993 and most of his research has focused on children's eating habits and childhood obesity and how to improve them.

Julia Keenan is a researcher at the Leeds Social Sciences Institute, University of Leeds, UK. She is a social and cultural geographer with interests in health, risk and governmentality perspectives, the new genetics and parenting cultures. In 2006, she gained her Ph.D. from the University of Sheffield: 'The governance of health through risk: sickle cell and thalassaemia in Sheffield'. Julia then carried forward her interests in health, embodiment and governance to explore women's food/feeding choices for themselves and their infants/young children and families on the project entitled 'Changing habits? Food, family and transitions to motherhood'. This was undertaken as part of a larger interdisciplinary Leverhulme Trust funded research programme called 'Changing families, changing food'. She is currently working on family life and alcohol consumption exploring the intergenerational transmission of drinking practices funded by the Joseph Rowntree Foundation.

Victoria Hall Moran is a Senior Lecturer in the Maternal and Infant Nutrition and Nurture Unit (MAINN), University of Central Lancashire and Editor-in-Chief of *Maternal & Child Nutrition* (Wiley-Blackwell). Victoria's research interests include the evaluation of breastfeeding experiences and support needs and nutritional intake and status indicators during pregnancy and lactation. Victoria has worked on WHO, government (Department of Health) and British Council funded projects. She is currently involved in the European Union EURRECA Network of Excellence project, which aims to address the problem of national variations in micronutrient recommendations. Victoria is also co-editor of *Maternal and Infant Nutrition and Nurture: Controversies and Challenges*, published by Quay Books.

Naoko Hashimoto is a Japanese midwife and independent researcher in Japan, and Research Associate at Thames Valley University (TVU), London, in the UK. Naoko has experience of working in obstetrics and postnatal unit in a general hospital in Tokyo, and is currently working in an urban community in Tokyo, mainly doing postnatal visits and breastfeeding support. Naoko completed her Ph.D. in Midwifery at TVU in 2006 on a narrative/ethnographic study of Japanese women's experience of breastfeeding in the current Japanese social context. Naoko's research interest is based on her everyday practice as a midwife, and her focus is to fill the theory–practice gap in breastfeeding and also to develop a theoretical framework of understanding breastfeeding practice through cross-cultural dialogues.

Christine McCourt is Professor of Anthropology and Health in the Faculty of Health and Human Sciences, Thames Valley University London, where she is also Director of the Centre for Research in Midwifery and Childbirth (CeMaC). She joined the centre after several years working on health policy at Brunel University, where she taught within medical anthropology and social policy, having previously worked and studied at the London School of Economics. Her degree and Ph.D. were in Anthropology and her key interest at doctoral level was in applying anthropological theory and methodology to studying 'Western' healthcare. Since then her main work has been on maternity and women's health, with particular interests in institutions and service change and reform, on women's experiences of childbirth, transition to motherhood and maternity care and in the culture and organisation of maternity care. She had published and presented widely in these areas. She is a member of the International Congress of Midwives Research Standing Committee and Managing Editor of the international applied anthropology journal *Anthropology in Action*.

Charo Rodríguez joined McGill University in June 2003. As of June 2008, she holds the position of Associate Professor in the area of Health Services and Policy Research of the McGill Department of Family Medicine. After seven years of clinical practice as general practitioner in Alicante (Spain), she developed her master's studies in Public Health (Management option) at the Valencia Institute of Public Health. Charo also holds a Ph.D. degree in Public Health (Health Organization option) with distinction from the University of Montreal. Charo has spearheaded a research agenda in healthcare organisations with a particular focus on organisational discourse. This research agenda, for which she was awarded 'Chercheur Junior 1' by the 'Fonds de recherche en santé du Québec' (FRSQ) in 2004, and 'Chercheur Junior 2' in 2008, comprises five main axes, namely information technology, identity, inter-organisational collaboration, shared decision making and qualitative research synthesis. Charo has been a member of the editorial board of the *Management Information Quarterly* journal. Among others, she has published in journals such as *Administration and Society*, the *Journal of Interprofessional Care*, *International Journal of Integrated Care*, *Health Care Management Review*, *Healthcare Policy*, and the *Journal of Health Services and Policy*.

Helen Stapleton is a Lecturer at the University of Sheffield with a background in midwifery and herbal medicine. Her research interests include qualitative methodologies, the social context of sexuality and reproduction, the health and wellbeing of children, young people and families and parenting cultures. Helen's empirical research covers a broad range of areas including organisational cultures, food and eating practices, transitions to motherhood, eating disorders, adolescent sexual health services and obesity in children/young people. She is a member of various professional organisations and a board member for the Centre for the Study of Childhood and Youth, University of Sheffield.

Lucy Thairu is a postdoctoral scholar at the Stanford University Medical School. She obtained a bachelor's degree in Biochemistry from Nantes University in France, and a master's and a Ph.D. in nutrition from Cornell University. Her research focuses on breast milk HIV transmission in sub-Saharan Africa using qualitative research techniques. In her research, she draws upon her unique experience growing up and working in Africa to elicit sensitive information from interviewees. In addition to research, Thairu serves as a consultant for UNICEF and WHO. She also coordinates the World Wide AIDS Coalition, a non-profit organisation that provides laboratory diagnostics in Ghana, Burkina Faso and Zimbabwe.

Anthony F. Williams is Reader in Child Nutrition at St George's, University of London and a Consultant in Neonatal Paediatrics at St George's Hospital. He trained in medicine at University College London and Westminster Medical School, qualifying in 1975. His interest in nutrition developed while training as a paediatrician in London, Leicester and Liverpool. In 1980, he became a Research Fellow in Oxford and worked on human lactation, particularly the nutritional requirements of very low birth weight babies. After gaining a D.Phil., he completed his paediatric training in Bristol and was appointed at St George's in 1987. He is adviser to a number of governmental and non-governmental organisations, both within the UK and abroad. In 2003 he was awarded an honorary Fellowship of UNICEF to recognise his contribution to establishing the Baby-Friendly Initiative in the UK.

Foreword

Ultimately, we owe the existence of the *Global Strategy for Infant and Young Child Feeding* (World Health Organization (WHO) 2003) to the wisdom of the men and women who set up the United Nations (UN) charter and assigned specific responsibilities to its agencies. The WHO was given the mandate to oversee and set standards for the health of the world's population. From that initial charge to a global strategy for infant and young child feeding is a very long journey involving the dedication, skill and commitment of tens of thousands of people. This book will take its place, along with all of the work that has preceded it, and all the work that will follow, as one step in this vital journey.

Establishing standards is, itself, a complex undertaking. In most areas of health, including nutrition, available information is usually inadequate to provide definitive guidance, and as the requirements for what constitutes evidence have tightened, honouring the UN mandate has almost always involved WHO in developing and sponsoring new research efforts. For example, for many years WHO accepted the growth standards developed by the USA (the National Institutes of Health standards), albeit, only after considerable debate and review of a large body of data. However, when the validity of applying standards based on a predominantly formula-fed population to breastfed children became increasingly questionable, WHO spearheaded a major international study to develop new standards.

It is a logical step from establishing standards to articulating a global strategy to guide the implementation of policy. In the area of breastfeeding, and more recently in complementary feeding, the UN agencies have played a major role in bringing together the technical information that serves as a basis for policy making. This undertaking has been even more complex than the already daunting challenges that face efforts to achieve consensus on standards. Political concerns play a major role, along with differing perspectives that have their origins in basic social and cultural traditions.

Establishing a global strategy for infant feeding took an enormous amount of effort and required negotiation and compromise on conflicting issues that are dear to the heart of many of the participants in the effort. Arriving at the statement that was adopted by the World Health Assembly in 2003 was a major achievement. Impressive as this is, it is not the end point. From the perspective of improving the health and wellbeing of infants, mothers and their families, the existence of a well-articulated global strategy is just the beginning. As difficult as it has been to establish a global strategy, the biggest challenges are in implementing it.

Implementing the infant and young child feeding strategy rests on many shoulders – ministries and departments of health, other governmental agencies and departments, international agencies, bilateral aid agencies, national and international non-governmental organisations and private sector groups of many different types. Compared with establishing standards and developing a global strategy, the challenges of implementation make the former efforts look positively easy. The primary reason that implementation of a global strategy for any health issues is so difficult can be summed up in a single word: context. A global strategy is, by definition, couched in generic terms. Implementation always occurs within a context of cultural, social, historical, and political and policy conditions that determine what can be done and how to do it.

A number of agencies have recognised the significance of the challenges that have to be faced in the translation of any global, generic health strategy to specific contexts. WHO, in particular, has been aware of the importance of context (perhaps because of its governing structure). However, as a biomedically oriented institution it has often lacked the resources to address the challenges of facilitating translation of generic strategies and principles in the contexts of 'the real world'.

In response to these challenges a number of approaches have been developed. One approach is to provide technical assistance in the form of external consultants, whose contributions vary from short-term visits to longer-term involvement. Another approach is to set up short-term training courses or workshops at country or regional levels, in which participants are introduced to tools, techniques and skills that are intended to assist them to engage in the process of translation of recommendations to specific conditions and situations.

With respect to translation to specific contexts, an important initiative of the WHO programme addressed to acute respiratory infections in children was to invest in the development of guidelines to conduct Focused Ethnographic Studies (ARI Programme 1993). These were developed to assist national programmes to obtain vital information on how families perceived and managed respiratory infections in children, their views about when and where to seek care and other related matters. Designed to be feasible within the economic and time constraints of national programmes, they also included information about larger issues of the local context, such as economic, social and situational constraints to the utilisation of services (Gove & Pelto 1994). This was an important step because it attempted to bridge the gap between specific context-related questions and generic treatment guidelines.

Yet another approach to assisting national programmes with implementing a global strategy is the creation of implementation guidelines. For example, the WHO Programme for Control of Diarrheal Diseases (CDD) in the 1980s and 1990s devoted substantial resources to assisting programmes to translate generic guidelines into implementable programmes through the development of programme managers' materials, training materials, counselling aides, and communication guidelines (see e.g. Division for the Control of Diarrhoeal and Respiratory Infections 1995).

When 'Integrated Management of Childhood Illness' (IMCI) replaced disease-specific child health programmes in WHO, the concept of 'local adaptation' of management guidelines continued to be part of the implementation strategy (Division of Child Health and Development 1997). The concept was most fully developed for the nutrition counselling component, for which a protocol to obtain information to contextualise feeding recommendations (breastfeeding and complementary feeding) was created and tested (Santos *et al.* 2001).

Apart from the IMCI adaptation guide, there have been a number of important efforts to develop tools to assess local context for use by programmes that are explicitly charged with promoting breastfeeding and young child feeding, most notably, Designing by Dialog (Dickin *et al.* 1997) and the Pan American Health Organization (PAHO)-initiated effort known as PROPAN.

Shifting from international agencies to the larger public health and public nutrition community, we find that for breastfeeding the recognition of the importance of context has considerable time depth. In fact, beginning more than 40 years ago there is a rich, if relatively small, empirical and theoretical literature illustrating the multiple dimensions of contextual issues in breastfeeding (see e.g. Raphael 1973; Butz 1977; Leslie 1988; Mead & Newton 1978; Pelto 1981; Van Esterik 1981; Van Esterik & Greiner 1989). The importance of context has also been consistently highlighted in the wide-ranging work on clinical management and support of Baby-Friendly Hospitals spear-headed by Felicity Savage King and Elisabet Helsing (Helsing & King 1982).

Until the publication of this volume, however, there has not been a significant effort to rigorously review and illustrate the relationships of context to the explicit challenge of implementing a global strategy for infant feeding. Thus, this book is a milestone. Conceptually it represents a significant step in the chain from the evidence base for best practice recommendations to the implementation of programmes that help to make best practice a social and behavioural reality. Wisely, the editors have included a broad range of topics thereby ensuring that readers of this important collection of original chapters will appreciate the complexity of the issues that are involved in the challenges of moving from best practice recommendations and an explicit infant and young child feeding strategy to real programmes in real places. Their selection of topics draws attention to the fact that implementation of the global strategy involves multiple dimensions and multiple challenges – economic, behavioural, psychological and cultural, as well as biological.

In the following sections I briefly review several different dimensions that are covered in the chapters in this volume.

A primary dimension that affects implementation across all contexts is the *macro-level to micro-level* dimension. Typically edited volumes tend to focus attention on just one level: the macro-level of policy, or the intermediate level of service delivery and programmes, or the micro-level of families, mother–infant dyads or even only the individual levels of mothers or infants. Fortunately, for this volume the editors have commissioned chapters across the range, thus ensuring that this essential dimension does not go unnoticed. Some of the chapters are centred on one level and some of them cross levels.

In Chapter 10, Frick describes macro-level policy issues from an economic perspective, highlighting macro-level concerns that affect social strategies within a broader societal public health context. In Chapter 1, Akre uses the macro to micro level dimension to organise his review and presentation of proposals to address policy challenges for going to scale in the implementation of the global strategy. He examines how variations in cross-cultural and cross-national economic and policy assumptions affect what happens 'on the ground'. In Chapter 6, Thairu also includes a macro-micro dimension in her chapter. She examines the implications for national policy of shared micro-level (individual-level) beliefs. The studies in Japan (Chapter 4, Hashimoto & McCourt), Quebec (Chapter 5, Groleau & Rodriquez), and the UK (Chapter 7, Stapleton & Keenan, and Chapter 8 Coufopoulos & Hackett) provide insights about micro-level factors.

Biological concerns are another critical dimension that must be carefully considered in translating a global policy into specific contexts. Rather than beginning with the usual review of the well-described biology of breastfeeding, in Chapter 2, Bilson and Dykes start with concepts about the bio-cultural nature of cognition, drawing from the work of the biologist, Humberto Maturana. In their innovative chapter they go on to explore the implications for breastfeeding programmes of the 'intertwining of emotional and rational processes'. They challenge the common assumption of simple linearity and raise the possibility of reconceptualising not only local programmes but also the basic approach to implementation of a global strategy for infant and young child feeding.

Focusing still on the matter of biological variation, the editors have chosen to highlight another feature of biological variation – the fact that all babies are not born equally prepared to undertake breastfeeding. In Chapter 3, Flacking deals specifically with the challenge of prematurity within a specific cultural context. She reveals the insights that are to be gained from a sensitive analysis of the challenges of biologically based differences in a pro-breastfeeding culture. The implications extend well beyond the case study that provides the empirical basis for these insights.

Thairu is also concerned with the effects of biological differences in a pro-breastfeeding culture. Here the biological variation is the result of the tragedy of human immunodeficiency virus (HIV) infection, in which the management of breastfeeding and complementary feeding is severely compromised by the existence of this significant source of biological variation within a population.

Stepping back to place findings from specific contexts into a larger, bio-cultural framework, in Chapter 9 Williams presents a holistic discussion of how biological and social conditions of individuals and families affect maternal and infant nutrition.

Attention to cultural issues is essential for all countries as part of national strategic planning. Cultural beliefs and underlying values contribute significantly to infant feeding behaviours. No matter how well they are managed, programmes that are not built on an understanding of cultural patterns in the population and thereby fail to make use of the cultural factors that support breastfeeding and address the cultural issues that impede adoption of best practices are unlikely to achieve their goals. At the national level many, if not most, countries have to deal with the fact that their nation contains multiple ethnic groups, and that different approaches, language and programme content may be necessary. Urban–rural differences and urban migration also present challenges for programme implementation.

The importance of deeply embedded cultural values in the complex interactions of breastfeeding promotion is examined by Hashimoto and McCourt in relation to the challenges of modern urban life in Japan. They provide a compelling description and analysis of the implications of cultural and social dynamics for programme implementation. In Chapter 7, Stapleton and Keenan reveal the wealth of ideas and expectations that women bring to an antenatal education activity. They highlight the fact that beneficiaries of programmes, the 'users', do not arrive at the point of encounter with the delivery system as 'blank slates' to be filled with new, correct information. They are not passive recipients of the information that is being imparted. Planning and implementation of programme delivery has to be based on the locally documented reality of the ideas, beliefs and experiences that women bring to the encounter. As the authors show, it is also important to recognise the significance of intracultural diversity in those ideas, beliefs and experiences, and not assume that all women arrive with the same assumptions and conceptual structures.

The far-reaching effects of economic factors on household behaviours is another dimension that is highlighted in this volume. The challenges of maintaining exclusive breastfeeding in conditions of poverty in developing countries have been well described, but they have not been as readily understood when the focus is on women and children living in poverty in the midst of well-off nations. The study by Groleau and Rodríquez in Quebec highlights features of breastfeeding challenges among the poor living in a wealthy country. In this chapter the authors show how poverty affects breastfeeding for poor women who live within a larger context of wealth. Continuing the focus on poverty in the context of industrialised countries, Coufopoulos and Hackett hone in on its effects on two generations; in this case, homeless women and children in the UK. They effectively use the results of ethnographic interviews to bring a description of the reality of women's experiences to bear in their broad discussion of the challenges homelessness presents for two generations living in serious poverty.

In their concluding chapter the editors highlight the themes discussed above. They also introduce another critically important idea, which they call the 'rhetoric–reality gap'. They point out that for both breastfeeding and complementary feeding there is a great deal of evidence-based knowledge about best practices, which are embedded in the *Global Strategy* recommendations. But there is a large gap between that knowledge and the realities experienced by women and children throughout the world. This volume helps to shed light on the reasons for that gap and points to critical issues that need to be addressed in order to design effective programmes to close it.

Gretel H. Pelto

Gretel H. Pelto currently holds the title of Graduate Professor in the Division of Nutritional Sciences at Cornell University, having retired in 2007, but still active. She was trained as a medical anthropologist specialised in the social determinants of health. She was a member of the nutrition faculty at the University of Connecticut for more than two decades before moving to the WHO, where she was in charge of behavioural, programme-related research in the Department of Child and Adolescent Health. She joined the Cornell University faculty in 1999. Throughout her career her primary focus of research and programmatic activity has been infant and young child feeding, particularly concerned with how sociocultural factors and conditions affect household behaviours and responses to nutrition interventions and nutritional status outcomes for infants and children.

References

Acute Respiratory Control Programme (1993) *Manual for Focused Ethnographic Study of Acute Respiratory Infections*. WHO, Geneva.

Butz, W. (1977) Economic aspects of breast feeding. In: Mosley, W.H. (ed) *Nutrition and Human Reproduction*. Plenum, New York, pp. 231–255.

Dickin, K., Griffiths, M. & Piwoz, E. (1997) *Designing by Dialogue: Consultative Research to Improve Young Child Feeding*. The Support for Analysis and Research in Africa (SARA) Project, Health and Human Resources Analysis (HHRAA) Project Washington D.C., USAID.

Division of Child Health and Development (1997) *Integrated Management of Childhood Illness Adaptation Guide: Protocol for Identifying and Validating Local Terms for Childhood Illnesses*. WHO, Geneva.

Division for the Control of Diarrhoeal and Respiratory Infections (1995) *Guidelines on Using Ethnography to Improve Communication Between Families and Health Workers*. WHO, Geneva.

Gove, S. & Pelto, G.H. (1994) Focused ethnographic studies in the WHO Programme for the Control of Acute Respiratory Infections. *Medical Anthropology*, **15**: 409–424.

Helsing, E. & King, F.S. (1982) *Breastfeeding in Practice: A Manual for Health Workers*. Oxford University Press, Oxford.

Leslie, J. (1988) Women's work and child nutrition in the third world. In: Leslie, J. & Paolisso, M. (eds) *Women, Work and Child Welfare in the Third World*. Westview Press, Boulder, Colorado, pp. 19–58.

Mead, M. & Newton, N. (1978) Cultural patterning of perinatal behavior. In: Richardson, S.A. & Guttmacher, A.F. (eds) *Childbearing: Its Social and Psychological Aspects*. Wilkins and Williams, New York.

Pelto, G.H. (1981) Perspectives on infant feeding: decision-making and ecology. *Food and Nutrition Bulletin*, **3**: 16–29.

Raphael, D. (1973) The role of breast feeding in a bottle-oriented world. *Ecology of Food Nutrition*, **2**: 121–126.

Santos, I., Victora, C.G., Martines, J., Goncalves, H., Gigante, D.P., Valle, N.J., *et al.* (2001) Nutritional counseling increases weight gain among Brazilian children. *Journal of Nutrition*, **131**: 2866–2873.

Van Esterik, P. (1989) *Beyond the Breast-Bottle Controversy*. Rutgers University Press, New Brunswick, New Jersey.

Van Esterik, P. & Greiner, T. (1981) Breast-feeding and women's work: constraints and opportunities. *Studies in Family Planning*, **12**: 182–195.

WHO (2003) *Global Strategy for Infant and Young Child Feeding*. Fifty-fifth World Health Assembly. World Health Organization, Geneva.

1 From Grand Design to Change on the Ground: Going to Scale with a Global Feeding Strategy

James Akre

1.1 Introduction

In May 2002, the World Health Organization (WHO) adopted the *Global Strategy for Infant and Young Child Feeding* (WHO 2003a). This marked the culmination of a complex process, which included WHO's methodical consultation of the governments of its then entire membership of 191 governments, solicitation of inputs from an array of other interested parties (including health professional bodies, individual experts, non-governmental organisations, and commercial enterprises and their associations), extensive review of the scientific literature, and technical consultations on crucial topics such as the optimal duration of exclusive breast-feeding (WHO 2001a) and prevention of mother-to-child transmission of human immunodeficiency virus (HIV) (WHO 2001b).

As with any global WHO policy instrument, far from being a one-size-fits-all approach, governments were urged to adapt the *Global Strategy* to the specific circumstances of their nutrition and child health policies and programmes (WHO 2002a). Indeed, for a volume that seeks to shed light on the exceedingly complex challenge of appropriately translating international public health recommendations in multiple culturally diverse settings, the *Global Strategy* eloquently illustrates the adage 'Think globally, act locally'. This dimension is all the more evident given the idiosyncratic nature of nurturing and nourishing children based on the rules imposed by the group into which each of us is born. Perhaps the ultimate paradox in this connection is that there can be no universal approach to ensuring unhindered access to our species' *only* example of a universal food and feeding system – breast milk and breastfeeding – which are forever mediated by culture and clan.

Starting in early 2000, WHO and the United Nations Children's Fund (UNICEF) began jointly developing the *Global Strategy*, whose aim is to improve – through optimal feeding – the nutritional status, growth and development, and health, and thus the very survival of infants and young children. Its specific objectives are (WHO 2003a):

- To raise awareness of the main problems affecting feeding, identify approaches to their solution, and provide a framework of essential interventions
- To increase the commitment of governments, international organisations and other concerned parties for optimal feeding practices

- To create an environment that will enable mothers, families and other caregivers in all circumstances to make – and implement – informed choices about optimal feeding practices.

At the same time, the *Global Strategy* reaffirms the relevance and urgency of the four operational targets of the *Innocenti Declaration on the Protection, Promotion and Support of Breastfeeding* (UNICEF/WHO 1990):

- Appointing a national breastfeeding coordinator and establishing a multi-sectoral national breastfeeding committee
- Ensuring that every facility providing maternity services fully practises the *Ten steps to successful breastfeeding* (WHO 1989)
- Giving effect to the *International Code of Marketing of Breast-milk Substitutes* (WHO 1981a) and subsequent relevant World Health Assembly resolutions in their entirety
- Enacting legislation protecting the breastfeeding rights of working women and establishing means for its enforcement.

This chapter proposes a framework, in three interrelated parts, for visualising worldwide implementation of the *Global Strategy*.

- The *first* part describes the historical context and how the *Global Strategy* came to be formulated over time within a discrete and dynamic international organisation culture.
- The *second* part identifies important common features of the challenge of going to scale with the *Global Strategy* that are often ignored or seriously underplayed.
- The *third* part makes specific proposals for broadening the international public health nutrition policy agenda where:
  - Each proposal corresponds to a major challenge due to inadequate information or awareness, which can easily obstruct implementation of the *Global Strategy* **today**;
  - Each proposal corresponds to a key priority for driving a crucial cultural shift that, ideally, will facilitate implementation of the *Global Strategy* **tomorrow**.

The proposals are deceptively straightforward and brief. If taken seriously, however, all imply significant investment in changing awareness, attitudes and behaviour. Education, in the widest sense of the term, is obviously a key ingredient here, but it is only a means to achieving the desired end – a fully normalised society-wide transformation in how we ensure that all our children are appropriately nurtured and nourished.

The implications of extreme diversity will be explored less from the standpoint of the variations routinely encountered in sociocultural influences, which are the primary focus of the chapters that follow. Rather, they will be viewed mainly in terms of how fundamental economic and political assumptions – including attitudes towards breast milk and its routine replacement, and adherence to supposed free market principles governing the sale of breast-milk substitutes – mould governments' approach to determining and implementing their public health policies.

In this connection it is useful to recall WHO's status as an international intergovernmental organisation and the dual role of its individual members, first in terms of achieving consensus on global health policy, and then in actually giving effect to it within their own territory 'taking into account national circumstances' (WHO 2002a). From a narrow conflict of interest perspective, some might question the suitability of the same agents deciding on a strategy's content and then how, or even whether, to apply it. But such is the reality of national sovereignty, the undisputed first principle of today's multilateral organisations.

In the present context, 'going to scale' denotes the process of increasing the number of countries embracing the *Global Strategy*, the size of the populations targeted, and the proportion of people actually sharing the benefits of its adaptation and implementation. However, we should not lose sight of a key intrinsic element of interdependence in this regard. The highly complex – some might say plodding – international intergovernmental organisation model of producing consensus-based recommendations is anything but a top-down exercise. WHO's deliberate step-by-step participatory process more closely resembles a constant feedback loop whereby sovereign governments especially, and also numerous other non-state actors, exercise control over the inputs that finally coalesce into a more or less coherent set of international recommendations, which in turn serve as a basis for formulating national policies dealing with vital public health themes. As will become clear here and in subsequent chapters, the gradual evolution in international public health nutrition thinking and related policy formulation is thus as much a driver for change as it is the result of this change.

Beyond single references to the scientific literature to illustrate specific points, there will be no systematic effort to catalogue the benefits of appropriate infant and young child feeding. Readers wishing to update their knowledge of both science and recommended practice in this regard are invited to consult relevant resources, including those that WHO has prepared concerning breastfeeding healthy term (Pan American Health Organization (PAHO)/WHO 2004) and low birth weight infants (WHO 2006a), HIV and infant feeding (WHO 2007a), evidence of the long-term effects of breastfeeding (WHO 2007b), complementary feeding for breastfed (PAHO/WHO 2004) and non-breastfed (WHO 2005a) children, and feeding infants and young children during emergencies (WHO 2005b).

Where the risks of artificial feeding are concerned, the mass of evidence in the scientific literature continues to swell. Nevertheless, with only rare exceptions (for example Walker 1992, 1998, 2004) comprehensive accounts are lacking of the adverse health outcomes that result when infant formula routinely replaces breast milk. Indeed, it is not uncommon that even individual studies reporting poorer health among formula-fed children avoid naming formula feeding in their titles and abstracts (Smith *et al.* 2008). Such a candid accounting would, at a minimum, include:

- *For children*, increased risk of impaired postpartum cognitive and visual development (Michaelsen *et al.* 2003; Vohr *et al.* 2007; Kramer *et al.* 2008; Sussmann *et al.* 2009); child mortality (Chen & Rogan 2004; Department of International Development (DFID) 2006; Edmond *et al.* 2006); numerous serious diseases, including celiac disease (Chertok 2007), Crohn's disease (Klement *et al.* 2004), diabetes (Mayer-Davis 2008), diarrhoeal disease and respiratory ailments (Howie *et al.* 1990; Wilson *et al.* 1998; Quigley *et al.* 2007; Morteau *et al.* 2008; Newburg 2008; Wilson *et al.* 2008); asthma, ear infection, leukaemia and necrotising enterocolitis (Ip *et al.* 2007); pathogens in the gastrointestinal tract (Wilson *et al.* 2008); obesity (Von Kries *et al.* 2000; Plagemann & Harder 2005; American Institute for Cancer Research (AICR) 2008; American Psychological Association (APA) 2008; Apfelbacher 2008; August *et al.* 2008; Griffiths *et al.* 2008; Karaolis-Danckert *et al.* 2008; Kim & Peterson 2008; Maurage 2008; Hawkins *et al.* 2009; O'Tierney *et al.* 2009; Palou & Picó 2009; Simon *et al.* 2009); sepsis in very low birth weight infants (Hylander *et al.* 1998); SIDS (McVea *et al.* 2000; Ip *et al.* 2007; McKenna *et al.* 2007; Vennemann *et al.* 2009) and urinary tract disease (Pisacane *et al.* 1992; Levy *et al.* 2008); childhood behavioural or mental health problems (American Public Health Association (APHA) 2008); impaired arsenic metabolism in relevant environments (Fängström *et al.* 2008); and, in later life, increased risk of cardiovascular disease (Lawlor *et al.* 2005; Singhal 2006), higher blood pressure (Martin *et al.* 2004), higher blood cholesterol concentrations (Owen *et al.* 2008) and reduced lung function (Tennant *et al.* 2008; Ogbuanu *et al.* 2009)
- *For mothers*, increased risk of haemorrhaging (Sobhy & Mohame 2004) and inadequately spaced pregnancies (Bellagio Consensus 1988; Lawrence 2007); breast cancer (Collaborative Group on Hormonal Factors in Breastfeeding 2002; Martin *et al.* 2005; AICR 2008; Lord *et al.* 2008; Phipps *et al.* 2008; Sotgia *et al.* 2009; World Cancer Research Fund (WCRF) 2009), uterine cancer (Okamura *et al.* 2006) and ovarian cancer (Riman *et al.* 2004); diabetes (Stuebe *et al.* 2005; Ip *et al.* 2007); hip fractures and osteoporosis (Turck 2005); gallbladder disease (Liu *et al.* 2008); higher blood pressure (Jonas *et al.* 2008); myocardial infarction in middle to late adulthood (Stuebe *et al.* 2009); postpartum weight retention (Baker *et al.* 2008); rheumatoid arthritis (Karlson *et al.* 2004; Pikwer *et al.* 2009); postpartum relapses in women with multiple sclerosis (Langer-Gould *et al.* 2009); and maternally perpetrated child maltreatment, particularly child neglect (Strathearn *et al.* 2009).

Feeding infants and young children appropriately clearly depends on more than breast milk. Nevertheless, given breastfeeding's centrality to human health and development, and the short- and longer-term significance, in every environment, of getting things right in this regard, the current discussion bias leans consciously in this direction. In essence the premise is that if we can succeed here, so much else affecting the health and welfare of children and mothers will be that much more likely to fall into place. However, before going further with discussing the *Global Strategy* itself, a bit of history is in order to help us understand not only how we arrived at this particular public health policy crossroads, but also how we might move beyond it efficiently and effectively.

1.2 How it all began

In strict chronological terms, the *Global Strategy* was just over two years in the making. Viewed from a broader historical perspective, however, it was in fact the product of a gradual, and usually non-linear, progression in international public health nutrition thinking over more than three decades. This evolution was in large measure forcefully jumpstarted by the perfect storm in the mid-to-late 1970s (Akre 2006) of a unique set of socio-political forces – governmental, non-governmental and commercial – which resulted in the formulation and adoption of the *International Code of Marketing of Breast-milk Substitutes* (WHO 1981a).

Ensuring appropriate marketing and distribution of breast-milk substitutes is surely important; yet considerably more is required to secure the nutritional status of infants and young children while protecting the health of mothers. Awareness of human milk's unique species-specific properties and thus the inescapable implications for the health of all people throughout the life course, and the indispensable supportive policies and practices in the healthcare system and throughout the community, are but two examples of other necessary conditions. However, it is equally evident that this trade-related piece of the evolving international public health nutrition policy mosaic, which some observers narrowly cast in terms of the rich exploiting the poor, quickly captured worldwide media and political attention. One unfortunate – and doubtless unintended – result was to draw lopsided attention to the dangers associated with artificial feeding by populations in low-income countries rather than to the risks incurred in varying degrees by mothers and children *anywhere* if they do not breastfeed as they should.

Regrettably, the resulting skewed perception of marketing's relative significance and the absence of clarity in accompanying culture-based feeding beliefs and behaviours persist to this day. Part of the problem resides in emphasis on controlling the supply of breast-milk substitutes to the detriment of reducing demand for them, which can be achieved only by increasing demand for breast milk. This outcome in turn relies on mounting awareness of the significance of and society-wide support for the biological norm for feeding the young of our species (Akre 2006). As the World Health Assembly stressed in 1981, 'adoption of and adherence to the *International Code of Marketing of Breast-milk Substitutes* is a minimum requirement and only one of several important actions required in order to protect healthy practices in respect of infant and young child feeding' (WHO 1981b).

In addition, more than a quarter of a century after the adoption of the *International Code*, many people living in conditions of relative prosperity still naïvely conclude that, as far as *their* children are concerned, artificial feeding is adequate and safe because they have the means to make it so. Not surprisingly, this culturally conditioned response is both mirrored in and reinforced by public health policies mainly, but not exclusively, in high-income countries that have yet to embrace the notion that feeding a breast-milk substitute represents a deviation from the biological norm for the young of our species (WHO 1994) that carries with it serious consequences throughout the life course. This flawed perspective also shows how international public health nutrition policy needs to evolve to take breastfeeding to the next plateau of significantly changed awareness and behaviour (Akre 2006).

The ebb and flow of the focus of international child feeding policy recommendations can be compared to an indeterminate series of reclining hourglasses. Moving linearly over time, there continues to be a broader-to-narrower focus, and back again, on numerous interrelated and isolated variables. Article 2 of WHO's Constitution, which came into force in 1948, identifies promoting 'the improvement of nutrition' and 'maternal and child health and welfare' among its functions (WHO 2006b). However, nowhere is breastfeeding explicitly mentioned.

The first occasion for WHO's senior policy-making organ, the World Health Assembly, to speak of breastfeeding occurred only in 1974 when it 'noted the general decline in breastfeeding in many parts of the world, related to sociocultural and other factors, including the promotion of manufactured breast-milk substitutes'; the Health Assembly urged 'Member countries to review sales promotion activities on baby foods and to introduce appropriate remedial measures, including advertisement codes and legislation where necessary' (WHO 1974). The issue was taken up again in 1978 when the Health Assembly recommended that governments give priority to preventing malnutrition in infants and young children by supporting and promoting breastfeeding, taking legislative and social action to facilitate breastfeeding by working mothers, and 'regulating inappropriate sales promotion of infant foods that can be used to replace breast milk' (WHO 1978).

Meanwhile, with formula promotion in resource-poor settings picking up in the 1960s, so, too, did criticism of artificial feeding and marketing. This included: the evocative coinage 'commerciogenic malnutrition' advanced by the renowned expert in tropical paediatrics and nutrition Derrick Jelliffe in 1968 to describe what he saw as the result of unregulated marketing of infant formula among the poor (Jelliffe 1971); a feature article in the *New Internationalist* in 1973 calling for a campaign to stop formula promotion (Hendrikse & Morley 1973); and publication by the British non-governmental organisation War on Want in 1974 of a report on infant malnutrition and the promotion of artificial feeding in the 'third world' called *The Baby Killer* (Muller 1974). Then, in Washington DC, also in 1978, Senator Edward Kennedy presided over a hearing in the US Senate on 'marketing and promotion of infant formula in developing nations'. Acknowledging that 'it is always the children who suffer most' from poverty, malnutrition and disease, Senator Kennedy described (US Senate 1978) the hearing's purpose as focusing:

> 'on one small element of their problems . . . the use of a product intended to nourish life, to enable infants to thrive and grow, and see how it can have the unintended effects of fostering malnutrition and spreading disease. We will focus on the advertising, marketing, promotion and use of infant formula in developing nations . . .'

This hearing, which included prepared statements by two WHO representatives, contributed to the decision by WHO and UNICEF late the same year to organise their landmark joint meeting on infant and young child feeding to 'make the most effective use of [a] groundswell of opinion' (WHO 1981a) among governments, non-governmental organisations, professional associations, scientists, and manufacturers of infant foods. The meeting, which was convened in Geneva in October 1979, was attended by some 150 representatives of these same groups; discussions were organised on five themes (WHO 1979):

- Encouragement and support of breastfeeding
- Promotion and support of appropriate and timely complementary feeding
- Strengthening of education, training and information on infant and young child feeding
- Promotion of the health and social status of women in this connection
- Appropriate marketing and distribution of breast-milk substitutes.

While endorsing in its entirety the statement and recommendations that had been agreed by consensus at this joint WHO/UNICEF meeting on the five interrelated discussion themes, the World Health Assembly in May 1980 once more narrowed its policy focus. Making particular mention of the meeting's recommendation that 'there should be an international code of marketing of infant formula and other products used as breast-milk substitutes', the assembly requested WHO's Director-General to prepare such a code 'in close consultation with Member States and all other parties concerned' (WHO 1980).

Thus began a process of numerous and lengthy consultations both with governments, and groups and individuals represented at the October 1979 meeting. The debate on the form and content of four successive code drafts, accompanied by a flood of media coverage, culminated in May 1981 with the adoption of the *International Code of Marketing of Breast-milk Substitutes*, in the form of a recommendation, with only one country – the USA – voting against. Governments were called on to take action to give effect to the code 'as appropriate to their social and legislative framework, including the adoption of national legislation, regulations or other suitable measures', and to report annually on this basis to WHO (WHO 1981a). The Health Assembly, in turn, was to be informed of government action in biennial reports presented in even years (WHO 1981a). Responding to a request from a number of governments for an operational definition of a pivotal phrase in the *International Code* – 'infants who have to be fed on breast-milk substitutes' – in 1986 detailed guidelines were presented at the Health Assembly on the main health and socioeconomic circumstances where this is the case (WHO 1986a).

In 1989 WHO and UNICEF once again cast their policy net wider by issuing a joint statement, whose purpose was to increase awareness of the critical role that health services play in promoting breastfeeding, and to describe what should be done to provide mothers with appropriate information and support (WHO 1989). This statement served as the foundation for the Baby-friendly Hospital Initiative (WHO 1991a), which WHO and UNICEF formally launched in 1991 (this is discussed further in Chapter 2).

Between 1982 and 2000 the World Health Assembly adopted more than a dozen resolutions on infant and young child nutrition, appropriate feeding practices and related questions, and still others that drew attention to key policy instruments and initiatives. These included:

- Requesting WHO's Director-General to direct the attention of governments and other parties to two key observations regarding complementary feeding: that 'any food or drink given before complementary feeding is nutritionally required may interfere with the initiation or maintenance of breastfeeding and therefore should neither be promoted nor encouraged for use by infants during this period', and that 'the practice being introduced in some countries of providing infants with specially formulated milks (so called "follow-up milks") is not necessary' (WHO 1986b)
- Encouraging ratification and implementation of the Convention on the Rights of the Child (UN 1989) as a vehicle for family health development (WHO 1992a)
- Welcoming the *Innocenti Declaration on the Protection, Promotion and Support of Breastfeeding* (WHO 1991b)
- Endorsing the *World Declaration and Plan of Action for Nutrition adopted by the International Conference on Nutrition* (WHO 1993), which had been organised jointly by the Food and Agriculture Organization of the United Nations (FAO) and WHO.

Finally, we come full circle to adoption of the *Global Strategy* in 2002 as described above.

Although concluded a year after adoption of the *Global Strategy*, a brief word is nevertheless in order about the groundbreaking WHO coordinated research conducted between 1997 and 2003 among nearly 8500 breastfed children in Brazil, Ghana, India, Norway, Oman, and the USA. A serious flaw in the child growth reference which WHO had been recommending for universal use since the 1970s was that it was based on a single community sample of predominantly formula-fed infants, whose growth pattern was significantly different from that of their breastfed counterparts. The results of the WHO coordinated research have transformed understanding of child growth and development; they demonstrate for the first time that children born in different regions of the world and given the optimum start in life have the potential to grow and develop within the same range of height and weight for age (WHO 2006c). Moreover, the new growth curves prepared on this basis not only provide a single international standard that represents the best description of physiological growth for all children from birth to age 5; they also establish the breastfed baby as the *normative model* for growth and development (WHO 2006d).

1.3 Grasping the global challenge

In this section common features of the importance of going to scale with the *Global Strategy* are identified and discussed from the perspective of social determinants of health (Wilensky & Satcher 2009), including political, economic, geographical and nutritional aspects.

1.3.1 Starting with numbers

The *Global Strategy*'s freeze frame sketch of the challenge facing governments and the international community in 2002 began by recalling the role that malnutrition plays, directly or indirectly, in 60% of the 10.9 million deaths annually among children under 5. Well over two-thirds of these deaths, which are often associated with inappropriate feeding practices – lack of exclusive breastfeeding, complementary feeding that begins too early or too late, micronutrient deficiencies and consumption of nutritionally inadequate and unsafe foods – occur during the first year of life (WHO 2003a).

Research results presented in a series of interlocking papers at forums organised by the medical journal *The Lancet* in early 2008 (Global Health Network 2008) reconfirmed this grim picture. Indeed, the maternal and child undernutrition so highly prevalent in low- and middle-income countries was cited as responsible for fully 11% of the world's disease burden. Authors stressed that the high prevalence of malnutrition seriously undermines achievement of the Millennium Development Goals (UN 2008a). Noting that 80% of the world's undernourished children live in just 20 countries, authors stressed getting nutrition on the list of national priorities and keeping it there, and using resources to support actions that have been proven to have a direct effect on undernutrition in the most critical populations – mothers, and children under 24 months.

The final paper in the series is doubtless the most politically provocative insofar as the authors describe an international nutrition system – composed of international and donor organisations, academia, civil society and the private sector – which they consider fragmented, dysfunctional and desperately in need of reform. They argue that such a system should deliver in four functional areas: stewardship, mobilisation of financial resources, direct provision of nutrition services at times of natural disaster or conflict, and human and institutional resource strengthening. The authors conclude (Global Health Network 2008) that:

> 'The moment is ripe for these reforms. Their implementation would transform the political salience of undernutrition, and offer the chance of a better, more productive life to the 67 million children born each year [of an estimated 136 million births annually (WHO 2005c)] in the countries most severely afflicted by undernutrition.'

In the struggle to eradicate poverty, because breastfeeding is good for both mother and child, it can make a significant contribution to the family economy. If there is illness or infection it may be a life-saving gift. If there is poverty it may be the only gift (Lawrence 2007).

1.3.2   The escalating food crisis

Later in 2008 the dramatic convergence of a range of potent forces – including the impact of climate change, urbanisation, population growth, biofuel production, increased energy and transportation overhead, troubled financial markets combined with an international credit squeeze, and sharply higher commodity costs due, at least in part, to speculative purchases of agricultural commodities – all contributed in varying degrees to mounting world food prices and food shortages. The results not only served to confirm the stark conclusions of *The Lancet* series, they also appeared to compromise still further the ability of governments and the international community to respond to the nutritional needs of the most vulnerable population groups, including the mothers and children just described.

By the first quarter of 2008, as the price of basic foodstuffs soared, civil unrest had broken out in many countries including Cameroon, Côte d'Ivoire, Egypt, Ethiopia, Haiti, Indonesia, Italy, Mauritania, Philippines, Thailand, Uzbekistan and Yemen. At a moment when the spectre of food shortages, even famine, looms large for huge numbers of people, governments are finding themselves forced into artificially controlling the cost of, among other basic commodities, bread, maize, rice and dairy products (surely steep price increases for already expensive infant formula cannot be far behind). United Nations Secretary General Ban Ki-moon candidly qualified the situation this way (UN 2008b): 'The rapidly escalating crisis of food availability around the world has reached emergency proportions.' Indeed, at the close of 2008, another 40 million people – rising to a total of 963 million – had been pushed into hunger primarily due to higher food prices (FAO 2008).

The point here is not to detail the decidedly catastrophic consequences of the world food crisis for so many people (which are not the focus of this chapter) or to speculate on the relative merits of steps to avert or alleviate the crisis. It is rather to observe, in this light, how much more important still are the everyday means potentially at our collective disposal to prevent or at least to minimise the impact of a global food crisis on the most vulnerable populations in a resource-strapped world. In the present context, our immediate response is as familiar as it is elementary: doing everything we can to make sure that mothers and children everywhere breastfeed, exclusively for the first six months to optimally protect their health, including by promoting child spacing; and for as long as possible thereafter together with nutritionally adequate and safe complementary foods.

1.3.3   Health and climate change

Paradoxically, the escalating global food crisis offers governments and the international community compelling additional self-interest incentives at the crossroads of global food security and protecting health from climate change, which was the theme of World Health Day 2008. In their joint celebration of World Health Day, La Leche League International (LLLI) and the World Alliance for Breastfeeding Action (WABA) were inspired by WHO's key messages (in italics) to illustrate breastfeeding's vital contribution (Vickers 2008; WHO 2008a):

- *The health impacts of climate change will hit the poor the hardest.* Breastfeeding is the great equaliser; babies born to the poorest of the poor have the same starting point as those born to the richest of the rich.
- *Traditional public health tools are important components of effective response to climate change.* Breastfeeding is the ultimate 'traditional public health tool'.
- *Cross-sector, interdisciplinary partnerships are necessary to meet this global health threat.* Every time a mother puts her newborn to her breast, she symbolically links arm-in-arm with every other mother on the planet.
- *Action must begin now to protect health by applying both adaptation and mitigation . . .* Because breastfeeding provides such a powerful life start, a by-product of the support it deserves may well be global environmental protection.

And as the LLLI and WABA also noted, breastfeeding is inherently environmentally friendly, for example, no manufacturing plants, no intensive use of farmland and no packaging are required. Breastfeeding also helps counteract greenhouse gas emissions generated by the livestock sector, which is a major source of land and water degradation (FAO 2006).

1.3.4   Making sound economic sense

Ensuring the nutritional status of mothers is an ethical good in its own right. Furthermore, compared with the complex challenge of feeding infants artificially, breastfeeding is easy and inexpensive to do, thereby underwriting mothers' capacity to directly meet the nurturing and nutritional needs of their children. Also, because it is in their direct economic interest, all governments will want to invest in cost-effective actions to overcome the malnutrition in mothers and young children that was expected to claim 3.5 million lives in 2008 alone (Global Health Network 2008). For example, scaling up programmes dealing with deficiencies in iodine, vitamin A and iron, and adding folate and zinc supplements, to ensure provision for 80% of south Asians and sub-Saharan Africans is estimated to cost about US$347m per year; but it would yield a massive US$5bn from improved future earnings and reduced healthcare spending (Horton & Lomborg 2008).

1.3.4.1   The value of breast milk

Speaking of basic commodities, typically countries with large-scale commercial dairy production, for example among the 27 members of the European Union and in Canada, New Zealand, Switzerland and the USA, keep close tabs on virtually every drop of bovine milk produced. In contrast, tiny Norway (population 4.6 million) is the *only* country where human milk production – an estimated 10.3 million litres (nearly 10.9 million quarts) in 2004 alone (Norwegian Directorate for Health 2004) – is a routine feature of national food balance sheets (Oshaug & Botten 1994).

Some promising, if isolated, efforts have been made to place a monetary value on the actual and potential production of human milk elsewhere. For example, it was estimated that Australian women supplied 33 million kg of breast milk in 1992, compared with 16 million kg in 1972. Valued at AU$67 (the price of expressed human milk) the 1992 production level was worth AU$2.2bn or 6% of private spending on food (Smith 1999). In sub-Saharan Africa, where the production of human milk is considered to be about 50% of that of cow's milk, in 1997 the national annual median human milk production was estimated to be between 146 000 metric tonnes (Mali) and 1.3 million metric tonnes (Nigeria), and production per capita between 8 kg (Zimbabwe) and 15 kg (Mali) per year (Hatløy & Oshaug 1997).

It is difficult to place a precise economic value on breast milk. In addition to being so much more than a mere food, it is rarely traded in the marketplace. Hatløy and Oshaug included in their analysis of sub-Saharan African breast milk production a reference to the contemporaneous retail price of US$36–47 per litre in Norwegian hospitals. They then proceeded to assign a ridiculously low global price of US$1 per litre and, on this basis, to calculate the impact in just two countries had the value of human milk been included in calculating gross national product (GNP). For Mali, whose GNP per capita was US$270 in 1990, the estimated value of human milk would have added another US$15 per capita or an increase of more than 5%. For Senegal, with a GNP per capita of US$710, GNP would have increased by nearly 2% (Hatløy & Oshaug 1997). These excessively modest figures, which take no account whatsoever of the multiple costs of artificial feeding incurred by individuals and society as a whole over the life course, represent only a tiny fraction of human milk's total value. Nevertheless, extrapolated worldwide they promptly give the lie to the all too common – and frankly absurd, even offensive – assertion that breast milk is somehow free.

1.3.4.2   The value of breastfeeding

Breastfeeding itself has at least three price tags attached (Akre 2006):

- A *mother's time*, which far too many observers mistakenly, even disrespectfully, consider to be 'on the house'
- The *energy cost* of producing milk (though an incomparable value in terms of the benefits derived for both mother and child, the approximate daily additional 500 kcal still need to come from somewhere)
- The *opportunity cost* – the cost of a decision based on what must be given up – for example in the case of mothers who must choose between staying at home with their families and returning to paid employment outside the home to meet their financial needs.

Taken together these three price tags provide additional compelling evidence that breast milk is anything but free.

1.3.4.3   Nourishing the brain

Except for the marsupials, the human infant is the most immature of mammalian offspring (Lawrence 2007). At birth the infant's brain is the most undifferentiated organ in the body (Siegel 1999), and it doubles in size in the first year of life (Lawrence 2007). If genes and early experience shape the way neurones connect to one another, thereby forming the specialized circuits that give rise to mental processes, it is reasonable to conclude that whether this process is initially fired in a manner that is evolutionarily consistent with who we are as a species or relies on a food that is based on the milk of an *alien* species will make a significant difference in terms of developmental outcome. It is time for international public health nutrition policy to reflect this generic perspective as the only nutritional basis for ensuring the full genetic potential for every child's cognitive development.

In multivariable analyses of the early life determinants of childhood intelligence in a population-based birth cohort of individuals born in Brisbane, Australia, Lawlor *et al.* (2006) reported that the strongest and most robust predictors of intelligence were family income, parental education and breastfeeding, with these three variables explaining 7.5% of the variation in intelligence at age 14. What do we suppose would be the cumulative worth, over a lifetime, of the 1.6 and 9.8 additional IQ points that Daniels & Adair (2005) observed among Filipino children for the many millions of, respectively, normal and low birth weight children born every year if they were breastfed for 12–18 months? As paediatrician Nils Bergman puts it (Health Promotion Agency for Northern Ireland 2005):

> 'Breastfeeding is a behaviour which shapes and sculpts the brain and that brain shaping stays for life. Skin-to-skin contact is what the newborn requires in order for the brain to be shaped in the best possible way, and breastfeeding in the fullest sense is not about eating, but about brain growth, and the development of good relationships. Any other form of care is experienced by the newborn as separation, and prolonged separation causes permanent harm to babies' brains.'

1.3.4.4   The true cost of routine artificial feeding

As summarised above, even the most casual search for information concerning the multiple risks of routine artificial feeding turns up a mass of startling and persuasive information. Thus, it is time for international public health nutrition policy to reflect this reality by ceasing to emphasise the *benefits of breastfeeding*, which is normal feeding behaviour. Instead, we need to focus, directly and consistently, on the *short- and long-term risks* to mothers and children alike of *failing to breastfeed*, which constitutes a deviation from the biological norm (WHO 1994), with significant negative consequences over the entire life course.

Routine non-emergency artificial feeding engenders numerous direct and indirect costs for children and mothers, and thus society as a whole (see also Chapter 10). Three especially fertile areas of inquiry should be vigorously pursued in this connection (Akre 2006):

- The multiple, complex and lifelong economic implications of observing or disregarding the biological 'hominid blueprint' (Dettwyler 1995) for nourishing the young of our species (acknowledging that humans are primates, the hominid blueprint refers to what patterns in non-human primates suggest would be the natural age of weaning in modern humans if these behaviours were not modified by culture)

- The need for a unifying theory, integrating the short- and longer-term economic implications of the impact of more or less breastfeeding on the health and cognitive development of babies, on the health of children and adults, and on the health and wellbeing of mothers, families, and thus entire societies
- An analysis of the interdependence of early feeding patterns, and health maintenance and health expenditure throughout the life course for entire populations.

Among the most successful public health initiatives of the last 30–50 years, governments around the world have taken concerted action to curb tobacco use, and to improve passenger safety by promoting the use of seat belts, car seats for children and safety helmets. All these measures are based on the indisputable cost–benefit implications for both individuals and society as a whole in terms of, among other major variables, significantly reduced healthcare costs and premature mortality. Public health revolutions do not occur overnight. Yet, with everything that is already known about the health implications, across the entire life course, of failing to feed human babies human milk, the assumption is that relatively little additional work would be required to produce the convincing quantitative evidence needed as a further stimulus for increasing prevalence and duration of breastfeeding.

Running the numbers successfully and interpreting their significance accurately should serve as a tipping point – for achieving the critical mass required to reverse trends towards artificial feeding in some environments; for increasing breastfeeding prevalence and duration in others; and for restructuring the healthcare system, community and workplace in ways to ensure that, because these changes are understood to be in the best interest of society as a whole, they are welcomed by one and all. International public health nutrition policy needs to promote cost-effective decision making by ensuring that the science-based understanding of the health – and therefore the economic – implications of more or less breastfeeding are thoroughly assessed, convincingly presented and taken fully into account (Akre 2006).

1.3.4.5   Human milk banks

On this basis alone, it should be easy to imagine the day – and to begin taking serious steps to achieve it – when human milk banks for ill and preterm infants are as routine a component of the healthcare system as blood banks have become over the past 100 years (Bloodbook 2005). Human milk banking began early in the twentieth century, with the first such bank established in Vienna in 1909 followed by others in the USA and Germany (Jones 2003). The Human Milk Bureau opened in England in 1939, and by 1959 there were 100 milk banks in Germany alone (South African Breastmilk Reserve (SABR) 2006).

Over time, protocols were developed for sterilising, pasteurising, storing and freezing human milk. Thus, despite the marked initial decrease in their number in the 1980s with the advent of human immunodeficiency virus (HIV)/acquired immune deficiency syndrome (AIDS), evidence of safety and continuing research into the importance of human milk translates into the number of donor milk banks being once again on the rise around the world, including in Australia, Brazil, Bulgaria, Canada, the Czech Republic, Denmark, Finland, France, Germany, Greece, India, Japan, Norway, South Africa, Sweden, Switzerland, UK, Uruguay, USA and Venezuela.

Pasteurised donor milk is used for failure-to-thrive infants, infants with malabsorption and short-gut syndromes, renal failure, inborn errors of metabolism, paediatric burn patients, feeding intolerance, infectious diseases, necrotising enterocolitis and cardiac patients. At the King Edward Memorial Hospital in Perth (Australia), the recovery period of preterm infants who receive human milk has shortened by approximately two weeks. The estimated cost saving for *one* preterm infant who is given human milk versus an artificial substitute is AU$18 200 (US$17 000). In Queensland alone, 4300 preterm and 4000 term babies required donor milk during 2004 (Mothersmilkbank 2007).

1.3.5 When best is not good enough

In their 1989 foreword to the joint WHO/UNICEF statement on breastfeeding and maternity services (WHO 1989), the Director-General of WHO and the Executive Director of UNICEF observed that 'few today would openly contest the maxim "breast is best". Yet slogans, however accurate, are no substitute for action.' Slogans indeed. Two decades later, some observers advocate abandoning 'breast is best' altogether in favour of describing human mothers and babies who are breast-feeding as normal, routine and commonplace (Wiessinger 1996; Akre 2006; Berry & Gribble 2008). In addition to being consistent with how all 5000 or so other species of mammals regularly behave, by adopting this approach we effectively avoid implying that, somehow, artificial feeding is the norm and that breastfeeding is something better than the norm. On the contrary, the implication is rather that anything else should be regarded as a *deviation* from the norm.

Furthermore, this approach is wholly consistent with how public health recommendations generally are conceived, formulated, transmitted and understood. Certainly, few observers focus on the *benefits* of not smoking, ensuring that children are protected against the major childhood diseases, using a seat belt and placing children in sturdy car seats while driving, making sure that medicines and cleaning products are kept out of reach of young children, or always using requisite safety gear, for example helmets, gloves and eye protection, when engaging in potentially dangerous activities. Rather we emphasise the *risks* involved, to ourselves and others, if we fail to heed elementary health and safety precautions. And surely the competent national authorities responsible for promoting public health and safety are unlikely to agonise about the possibility of inflicting guilt on the citizenry by calling attention, bluntly and repeatedly, to the risks incurred when people act contrary to the warnings given. Why should it be any different for our messages about breast milk and breastfeeding? Clearly, it is time to stop referring to the benefits of acting consistently with who we are as a species and to zero in on the dangers – for mothers and children alike, and thus the entire population, throughout the life course – if we fail to do so.

1.3.6   Breastfeeding and breast cancer

After lung cancer, which is the most common cancer worldwide with 1.4 million deaths per year (WHO 2008b), there are just over one million cases of cancer of the breast annually (WHO 2003b) resulting in 548 000 deaths (WHO 2008b). The unequivocal results of a major study published in 2002 lend an important perspective to these mortality figures: the longer women breastfeed the more they are protected against breast cancer, and the short lifetime duration of breastfeeding typical of women in high-income countries makes a major contribution to the high incidence of breast cancer in these countries (Collaborative Group on Hormonal Factors in Breastfeeding 2002). The link being investigated between breastfeeding and a reduced risk of breast cancer is hardly new. What is newsworthy here, however, is how this study convincingly mines so large a quantity of robust data – concerning more than 50 000 women with invasive breast cancer and more than 95 000 controls from a total of 47 epidemiological studies in 30 countries – to reach its conclusions.

In 2008, an Expert Panel of the American Institute for Cancer Research went further in its comprehensive 517-page report, which was the result of a five-year process involving nine independent teams of scientists, hundreds of peer reviewers, and 21 international experts who reviewed and analysed over 7000 large scale studies on all aspects of cancer risk (AICR 2008). The Expert Panel reviewed data from 98 studies on lactation and breast cancer risk and concluded that the evidence linking lactation to lower risk for both pre- and postmenopausal breast cancer was convincing, meaning that the evidence met the panel's strictest criteria (evidence that lactation reduces risk of ovarian cancer was judged 'limited, but suggestive'). Moreover, according to the AICR report, breastfeeding a child probably reduces the chances of overweight for at least the early years of childhood. This is important, it noted, because excess body fat in childhood tends to carry over into adulthood, and excess body fat is a convincing cause of six common cancers: colon, kidney, pancreas, endometrium, adenocarcinoma of the oesophagus and postmenopausal breast cancer.

Although breast cancer continues to be most prominent in affluent countries, the risks of both breast cancer and death due to breast cancer are clearly increasing worldwide. Some 45% of the more than one million new cases of breast cancer diagnosed each year, and more than 55% of deaths related to breast cancer occur in low- and middle-income countries (Curado et al. 2008). As more countries modernise and more women adopt behavioural patterns such as delayed childbearing, lower parity and reduced breastfeeding, breast cancer rates will no doubt increase in lower- and middle-income countries as well (Porter 2008). And yet the link between artificial feeding and increased risk of breast cancer continues to rank as one of the best-kept secrets in terms of popular health knowledge as even a casual survey of the websites of cancer charities and associations makes clear (Akre 2006); related information is often unavailable, or when it is, it can be difficult to locate and outdated. In any case, as illustrated by the results of a survey commissioned by the World Cancer Research Fund six months after publication of the AICR report, this key information is not yet anchored in popular consciousness (AICR 2008). In a nationally representative sample of 1998 adults in the UK, only 19–25% of women and 13% of men thought breastfeeding reduced the mother's risk of cancer, while just 25–33% of women and 17% of men thought it reduced the child's risk of being overweight (WCRF 2008).

Ironically, this regrettable picture was reinforced with the publication in 2006 of the results of a substantial survey whose aim was to assess knowledge of breast cancer risk in a large sample of young people – over 19 000 male and female university students – from 23 countries in Africa, North and South America, Asia and Europe (Peacey *et al.* 2006). Curiously, data collected were limited to respondents' awareness of links with heredity, alcohol use, exercise, obesity, stress, smoking and diet. And yet, as the researchers themselves note, at least a fifth of breast cancer cases in Western countries are likely to be due to modifiable lifestyle factors, presumably including prevalence and duration of breastfeeding, which the survey ignored entirely.

1.3.7 Deconstructing infant formula

It is time to take infant formula down from its inappropriate nutritional pedestal and to transform its unjustified image among health professionals and the general public alike, as the 'obvious' substitute for breast milk. As WHO has made clear (WHO 1986a; WHO 2003a), in those few situations where infants cannot, or should not, be breastfed, the choice of the best alternative – expressed breast milk from an infant's own mother, breast milk from a healthy wet nurse or a human milk bank, or a breast-milk substitute – depends on individual circumstances.

Fortunately, in an emergency, infant formula prepared in accordance with applicable Codex Alimentarius standards (FAO/WHO 2007) can sustain infants who, for whatever reason, are denied access to human milk. However, when infant formula is pitched as somehow suitable for *routine non-emergency* use, this formerly life-sustaining crisis commodity is instantly transformed, indeed denatured, into a paediatric fast food. Moreover, the generalised use of an inert manufactured product that is typically based on the milk of an alien species carries with it significant and irreversible negative consequences, across the entire life course, for the health and wellbeing of children, mothers, and thus society as a whole. We need to remove infant formula, once and for all, from the kitchen pantry and permanently relegate it to the medicine cupboard, where it got its start as an emergency nutrition intervention. In the first decade of the third millennium, deconstructing infant formula – by transforming both popular and health professional perceptions of formula from the best nutritional alternative to breast milk to the *least-bad* alternative – may well be our single most important priority in this context (Akre 2006).

Concerning follow-up formula (FAO/WHO 1987) which, as noted earlier, the World Health Assembly described as 'not necessary' (WHO 1986b), WHO has made several relevant observations in the context of the *International Code* (WHO 1992b). While acknowledging that, strictly speaking, follow-up formula does not fall within the scope of the *International Code*, WHO nevertheless:

> '*has also made clear that, taking into account the intent and spirit of the Code, there would appear to be grounds for the competent authorities in countries to conclude otherwise in the light of the way follow-up formula is perceived and used in individual circumstances . . . the competent authorities may wish to take the position that follow-up formula should be considered a de facto breast-milk substitute. WHO recommends that infants be breastfed exclusively for the first six months of life and that, once complementary feeding has begun, breastfeeding should continue up to the age of two years or beyond. Seen in this context, it could be argued that breast milk is the most appropriate liquid part of a progressively diversified diet once complementary feeding has begun.*'

1.3.8   Infant formula as a crisis commodity

Meanwhile, for infants who have to be fed on a breast-milk substitute, nutritional science should continue to strive to render infant formula the least incomplete and the least inadequate breast-milk substitute possible. There are pressing unanswered – indeed, largely unasked – questions about infant formula that call for resolution multilaterally based on a thorough and disinterested reading of the latest scientific and epidemiological evidence or by undertaking new research. For example:

- The recommended period during which formula alone can be said to meet infants' nutritional needs, which is another way of saying when complementary feeding should begin for infants who are not breastfed
- The safety and efficacy of supplementing formula with DHA (docosahexaenoic acid) and ARA (arachidonic acid), respectively the omega-3 and omega-6 essential fatty acids which are said to be added to over 99% of US infant formulas and consumed by millions of infants in over 70 countries (Martek 2009).

1.3.8.1   *How long is long enough?*

Concerning the first point, while WHO undertook a systematic review of the nutrient adequacy of breast milk in 2000–2001 (WHO 2001c; WHO 2002b), no comparable inquiry has ever been conducted into the nutrient adequacy of infant formula as the sole source of nourishment. The norm of four to six months was established in the late 1970s (WHO 1979). Today, the relevant Codex Alimentarius standard calls for information to be included on the label that 'infants should receive complementary foods . . . from an age that is appropriate for their specific growth and development needs . . . and in any case from the age over six months'. However, the standard skirts age-specificity by defining formula somewhat circularly as a 'breast-milk substitute specially manufactured to satisfy, by itself, the nutritional requirements of infants *during the first months of life* up to the introduction of appropriate complementary feeding' [italics added] (FAO/WHO 2007). WHO's guiding principles for feeding non-breastfed children (WHO 2005a) provide some useful considerations in this connection, but they do not answer the question posed.

1.3.8.2   Essential fatty acids and food safety

DHA and ARA, which are naturally found in breast milk and other foods such as fish and eggs, are known to be important for infant eye and brain development. However, where including synthetic versions of these essential fatty acids in infant formula is concerned, recent reviews of research and expert recommendations are as varied as they are inconsistent, even contradictory. For example, infant food manu-facturers in the USA have produced and sold such formulas since 2002. And yet the US Food and Drug Administration's Center for Food Safety and Applied Nutrition advises consumers not only that 'there are no currently available published reports from clinical studies that address whether any long term beneficial effects exist' from including these fatty acids in infant formula, but also that 'systematic monitor-ing efforts are not in place to collect and analyze information' on any long-term benefits or adverse consequences of formulas containing them (US Food and Drug Administration (USFDA) 2006).

Meanwhile, participants in a one-day workshop in February 2008 sponsored by Martek Biosciences Corporation, which produces synthetic versions of DHA and ARA for use in infant formula, evaluated research exploring how these fatty acids affect infant brain and eye development. Participants concluded that both DHA and ARA should be added to infant formula in order to provide formula-fed infants these nutrients 'at a comparable rate to their breastfed counterparts' (Koletzko et al. 2008; NHS Tayside 2008).

In contrast, in January 2008 the Cornucopia Institute (2008a) described the DHA and ARA oils in question – extracted from laboratory-grown fermented algae and fungus and processed using a toxic chemical, hexane, a derivative of petroleum refining – as structurally different from those naturally found in human milk in addition to never before having been part of the human diet. Cornucopia also drew attention to the FDA's response to Martek Biosciences indicating that the FDA had not made any determination regarding the safety of these oils (USFDA 2001). In April 2008 Cornucopia filed a legal complaint with the US Department of Agriculture 'demanding that the agency enforce the organic regulations prohibiting toxic solvents [hexane] from being used in the production of organic food' (Cornucopia Institute 2008b). Cornucopia reports that it learned through a Freedom of Information request filed with the Food and Drug Administration that 'algal- and fungal-based DHA/ARA have been linked to serious side effects such as virulent diarrhoea and vomiting in infants consuming infant formula, many of whom required medical treat-ment and hospitalization' (Freedom of Information Act (FOIA) 2007; Cornucopia Institute 2008b). The complaint has not yet been adjudicated.

In the late 1990s, the world's best known source of rigorous systematic reviews of randomised controlled trials, the Cochrane Collaboration, began publishing reviews on the effect of feeding term and preterm infants with infant formula containing low levels of long-chain polyunsaturated fatty acids (LCPUFA). The most recent substantive updates, which are consistent with previous Cochrane reviews, 'found that feeding term infants with milk formula enriched with LCPUFA had no proven benefit regarding vision, cognition or physical growth' (Simmer *et al.* 2007a). In addition, 'the evidence does not support the claim that preterm infants have improved visual and intellectual development' or that LCPUFA supplementation significantly influences their long-term growth (Simmer *et al.* 2007b).

Certainly, nutritional science should continue to strive to make the crisis commodity that is infant formula the least incomplete and the least inadequate breast-milk substitute possible. But we should not be fooled by a 'bouillabaisse fallacy'. It is not just the number and types of ingredients found in formula based on our still primitive reading of their presence and significance in breast milk, it is also a matter of how they interact in an inert, indeed stagnant, replacement food, and how – or even if – a child's body absorbs and uses them.

1.4   Summary recommendations

Acceptance of the above analysis and the following resultant recommendations presupposes a reorientation of international public health nutrition priorities. This outcome, in turn, is contingent on a shift in thinking, a kind of multilateral cultural transformation. It also implies abandoning accepted wisdom and traditional unilateral behaviours in favour of focusing internationally on both the biological and cultural components – the biocultural dimension – to child feeding behaviour (Stuart-Macadam 1995). Neither transformation can be taken for granted. However, both are entirely justified based on the information and evidence already at our disposal.

The following specific proposals are presented in the interest of accelerating implementation of the *Global Strategy for Infant and Young Child Feeding* in ways that routinely take account of the biocultural dimension. The proposals are deceptively straightforward and brief; if taken seriously, however, all imply a significant investment in changing awareness, attitudes and behaviour throughout society. As noted in the introduction, they seek to broaden the international public health policy agenda where:

- Each proposal corresponds to a major challenge due to inadequate information or awareness, which can easily obstruct implementation of the *Global Strategy* **today.**
- Each proposal corresponds to a key priority for driving a crucial cultural shift that, ideally, will facilitate implementation of the *Global Strategy* **tomorrow.**

Before proceeding, a word is in order about the intended sense of the recurrent phrase 'the international public health nutrition community'. It very nearly means whatever readers want it to mean; as a generic collective term, the intention is to err on the side of completeness. Taking a lead from the *Global Strategy* itself, a pragmatic description of what is intended includes a variety of parties operating with or parallel to governments, for example international intergovernmental organisations, professional bodies, commercial enterprises, and nongovernmental organisations and associations, including community-based support networks and consumer groups.

1.4.1   Reframing routine artificial feeding

It is time for governments and the international public health nutrition community to acknowledge that routine non-emergency substitution of breast milk:

- Constitutes a significant deviation from the biological norm for the young of our species
- Has serious consequences, throughout the life course, for children, mothers and thus society as a whole
- Should be countered, firstly, by improving collective understanding of breast-feeding's significance for all humankind and, secondly, by restructuring the health services, community and workplace accordingly.

1.4.2   Replacing 'the benefits of breastfeeding' with 'the risks of not breastfeeding'

It is time for governments and the international public health nutrition community to cease emphasising the *benefits* of breastfeeding, which is normal feeding behaviour, and to focus instead on the *short- and long-term risks*, to mothers and children and thus to society as a whole, of *failing* to breastfeed.

1.4.3   Tracking the adverse health outcomes of artificial feeding

It is time for governments and the international public health nutrition community to track systematically, over the short and longer term, the adverse health outcomes for children and mothers due to routine non-emergency artificial feeding.

1.4.4   Focusing on breast milk's significance for cognitive and visual development

It is time for governments and the international public health nutrition community to adopt as their default perspective that human milk provides the *only* basis for human babies to achieve their full genetic potential in terms of cognitive and visual development.

1.4.5   Recognising artificial feeding's significance for increased risk of cancer

It is time for governments and the international public health nutrition community to recognise and act on: the link between artificial feeding and a significantly higher risk for mothers of both pre- and postmenopausal breast cancer, and uterine and ovarian cancer; and the impact of excess body fat due to artificial feeding in childhood, carried over into adulthood, as a risk factor for developing a variety of other cancers.

1.4.6   Calculating the amount and value of human milk produced and consumed worldwide

It is time for governments and the international public health nutrition community to routinely calculate the amount and value of human milk produced and consumed worldwide as a means of raising awareness of the global significance of this essential food resource.

1.4.7   Evaluating the global economic implications of child feeding mode

It is time for governments and the international public health nutrition community to evaluate the multiple, complex and lifelong economic implications, for individuals and society as a whole, of observing or disregarding the hominid blueprint for the natural age of weaning. Cost-effective decision making can be promoted by ensuring that the health – and therefore the economic – implications of more or less breastfeeding are thoroughly assessed, convincingly presented and taken fully into account.

1.4.8   Making human milk banks a routine component of healthcare infrastructure

It is time for governments and the international public health nutrition community to ensure that human milk banks are as routine a component of the healthcare system as blood banks have been for the past century.

1.4.9   Ensuring that the crisis commodity called 'infant formula' is the least nutritionally incomplete and inadequate possible

It is time for governments and the international public health nutrition community to ensure that the Codex Alimentarius infant formula standard consistently reflects the most up-to-date internationally agreed position on formula's age-related nutrient adequacy as a sole source of nourishment, and the safety and efficacy of adding omega-3 and omega-6 essential fatty acids.

1.4.10   Giving effect to the *International Code of Marketing of Breast-milk Substitutes* and relevant resolutions

It is time for governments and the international public health nutrition community to give effect, in their entirety, to the *International Code of Marketing of Breast-milk*

Substitutes and relevant World Health Assembly resolutions, as a key component of overall feeding policy and practice, a minimum requirement, and one of several important actions required in order to protect healthy practices in respect of infant and young child feeding.

1.5　Conclusion

Changing positively the perception and place of breastfeeding depends on how successful we are in transforming the way the community understands and relates to child feeding and development, and the implications for the health of children and mothers and thus society as a whole, throughout the life course. This starts with promoting an awareness of breastfeeding that is consistent with our common mammalian condition and, until recently in evolutionary terms, our common mammalian tradition. Replacing collective hubris with a dash of collective humility should also help as we struggle to unlock nature's secrets in this regard.

As we go to scale with a global feeding strategy, by all means, let us continue to expand our scientific knowledge and augment our epidemiological evidence of what it means in the modern world, nutritionally and developmentally, to be a newborn child and a mother of a newborn child. But as we do let us proceed respectfully, on the understanding that ours is, at base, a universally common set of nurturing and nutritional needs, and that, despite outward sociocultural diversity, these needs are precisely what our self-sameness imposes.

Nature does not readily submit to scrutiny via double-blind randomised trials, which in any case are unethical where our mothers and babies are concerned. On the other hand, 200 million years or so of mammalian evolution should be worth something in terms of our default position being intuitively weighted in favour of breastfeeding – an essential part of the human experience, and an unavoidable and indispensable feature of who we are as a species. Consistent with nature's plan, the ordinary miracle that is life itself, whether at the cellular level or in terms of begetting and giving birth to new life, is matched by our natural capacity to nurture, nourish and sustain life in our own unique species-specific way.

References

AICR (2008) Cancer experts: breastfeeding protects mothers, children. Press release, 14 January 2008 concerning *Food, Nutrition, Physical Activity, and the Prevention of Cancer: A Global Perspective*. At: http://www.aicr.org/site/News2?abbr=pr_&page=NewsArticle&id=13057 (accessed 7 February 2009).

Akre, J. (2006) *The Problem with Breastfeeding. A Personal Reflection*. Hale Publishing, Amarillo, Texas.

APA (2008) Chronic ear infections linked to taste damage, increased obesity risk in children and adults. Press release, 14 August 2008 concerning symposium presentations by Daly, K., Hayes, J. & Hoffman, H. At: http://www.apa.org/releases/earinfectionC08.html (accessed 7 February 2009).

Apfelbacher, C.J., Loerbroks, A., Cairns, J., Behrendt, H., Ring, J. & Kraemer, U. (2008) Predictors of overweight and obesity in five to seven-year-old children in Germany: results from cross-sectional studies. *BMC Public Health*, 8 (1): 171.

APHA (2008) Breastfeeding associated with decreased childhood behavioral problems. Press release, 29 October 2008 concerning research presented at the annual meeting of the APHA by Hobbs Knutson, K. & Arauz Boudreau, A. At: http://www.apha.org/about/news/pressreleases/2008/08_AM_research_breastfeeding.htm (accessed 7 February 2009).

August, G.P., Caprio, S., Fennoy, I., Freemark, M., Kaufman, F.R., Lustig, R.H., et al. (2008) Prevention and treatment of pediatric obesity: an endocrine society clinical practice guideline based on expert opinion. *Journal of Clinical Endocrinology & Metabolism*, 93 (12): 4576–4599.

Baker, J.L., Gamborg, M., Heitmann, B.I., Lissner, L., Sorensen, T.I.A. & Rasmussen, K.M. (2008) Breastfeeding reduces postpartum weight retention. *American Journal of Clinical Nutrition*, 88 (6): 1543–1551.

Bellagio Consensus (1988) Consensus statement: breastfeeding as a family planning method. *Lancet*, ii: 1204–1205.

Berry, N.J. & Gribble, K.D. (2008) Breast is no longer best: promoting normal infant feeding. *Maternal and Child Nutrition*, 4 (1): 74–79.

Bloodbook (2005) History of blood banks and the industry of blood banking worldwide, including blood types, blood storage, dates and a list of milestones in the history of blood banking. At: http://www.bloodbook.com/banking.html (accessed 7 February 2009).

Chen, A. & Rogan, W. (2004) Breastfeeding and the risk of postneonatal death in the United States. *Pediatrics*, 113: 435–439.

Chertok, I.R. (2007) The importance of exclusive breastfeeding in infants at risk of celiac disease. *American Journal of Maternal Child Nursing*, 32 (1): 50–54.

Collaborative Group on Hormonal Factors in Breastfeeding (2002) Breast cancer and breastfeeding: collaborative reanalysis of individual data from 47 epidemiological studies in 30 countries, including 50 302 women with breast cancer and 96 973 women without the disease. *Lancet*, 360 (9328): 203–210.

Cornucopia Institute (2008a) *Replacing Mother – Imitating Human Breast Milk in the Laboratory. Novel Oils in Infant Formula and Organic Foods: Safe and Valuable Functional Food or Risky Marketing Gimmick?* Cornucopia, Wisconsin. At: http://cornucopia.org/index.php/replacing-mother-infant-formula-report/ (accessed 7 February 2009).

Cornucopia Institute (2008b) Organic infant formula ingredients processed with toxic chemical. Press release. At: http://cornucopia.org/index.php/organic-infant-formula-ingredients-processed-with-toxic-chemical/ (accessed 7 February 2009).

Curado, M.P., Curado, B., Edwards, B., Shin, H.R., Storm, H., Ferlay, J., et al. (eds) (2008) *Cancer Incidence in Five Continents*. Vol. IX. IARC Scientific Publications No. 160. IARC, Lyon.

Daniels, M.C. & Adair, L.S. (2005) Breast-feeding influences cognitive development in Filipino children. *Journal of Nutrition*, 135: 2589–2595.

DFID (2006) Breastfeeding in the first hour of life could save almost one million babies' lives each year. Press release. At: http://www.dfid.gov.uk/News/files/pressreleases/breastfeeding.asp (accessed 7 February 2009).

Dettwyler, K.A. (1995) A time to wean: the hominid blueprint for the natural age of weaning in modern human populations. In: Stuart-Macadam, P. & Dettwyler, K.A. (eds) *Breastfeeding. Biocultural Perspectives*. Aldine de Gruyter, New York, pp. 39–73.

Edmond, K.M., Zandoh, C., Quigley, M.A., Amenga-Etego, S., Owusu-Agyei, S. & Kirkwood, B.R. (2006) Delayed breastfeeding initiation increases risk of neonatal mortality. *Pediatrics*, 117 (3): e380–e386.

Fängström, B., Hamadani, J., Nermell, B., Grandér, M., Palm, B. & Vahter, M. (2008) Impaired arsenic metabolism in children during weaning. *Toxicology and Applied Pharmacology*, 6 January 2009 [Epub ahead of print].

FAO (2006) *Livestock a Major Threat to Environment: Remedies Urgently Needed*. Food and Agriculture Organization of the United Nations, Rome. At: http://www.fao.org/newsroom/en/news/2006/1000448/index.html (accessed 7 February 2009).

FAO (2008) Number of hungry people rises to 963 million. FAO Newsroom, Rome. At: http://www.fao.org/news/story/en/item/8836/icode/ (accessed 7 February 2009).

FAO/WHO (1987) *Codex Standard for Follow-Up Formula*, CODEX STAN 156–1987, amended 1989. At: http://www.codexalimentarius.net/web/index_en.jsp (accessed 7 February 2009).

FAO/WHO (2007) *Standard for Infant Formula and Formulas for Special Medical Purposes Intended for Infants*, CODEX STAN 72–1981, Revision 2007. At: http://www.codexalimentarius. net/web/index_en.jsp (accessed 7 February 2009).

FOIA (2007) CAERS reports allegedly related to DHA & ARA. Freedom of Information Act request #07–7305 by The Cornucopia Institute. CAERS Report #07–7305A. United States Food and Drug Administration, Center for Food Safety and Applied Nutrition, CFSAN Adverse Events Reporting System (CAERS).

Global Health Network (2008) Launch of *The Lancet's* Series on Maternal and Child Undernutrition. Woodrow Wilson International Center for Scholars, Washington, DC, and the Science and Media Centre, London. At: http://www.thelancet.com/online/focus/undernutrition and http://www.wilsoncenter.org/index.cfm?fuseaction=events.event_summary&event_id= 305075 (accessed 7 February 2009).

Griffiths, I.J., Smeeth, L., Hawkins, S.S., Cole, T.J. & Dezateux, C. (2008) Effects of infant feeding practice on weight gain from birth to 3 years. *Archives of Disease in Childhood*, 19 November 2008 [Epub ahead of print].

Hatløy, A. & Oshaug, A. (1997) *Human Milk. An Invisible Food Resource*. Food consumption and nutrition division discussion, p. 33. International Food Policy Research Institute, Washington, D.C. At: http://www.ifpri.org/divs/fcnd/dp/papers/dp33.pdf (accessed 7 February 2009).

Hawkins, S.S., Cole, T.J., Law, C. & the Millennium Cohort Study Child Health Group (2009) An ecological systems approach to examining risk factors for early childhood overweight: findings from the UK Millennium Cohort Study. *Journal of Epidemiology and Community Health*, 63: 147–155.

Health Promotion Agency for Northern Ireland (2005) *All-island breastfeeding conference highlights significant health impact of breastfeeding*. Press release. At: http://www.healthpromotionagency. org.uk/Work/Publicrelations/PressReleases/breastfeedingconference05.htm (accessed 7 February 2009).

Hendrikse, R.G. & Morley, D. (1973) The baby food tragedy. *New Internationalist*, p. 12.

Horton, S. & Lomborg, B. (2008) The hungry billion. *The Guardian, commentisfree*, 7 April. At: http://commentisfree.guardian.co.uk/sue_horton_and_bjrn_lomborg/2008/04/the_hungry_ billion.html (accessed 7 February 2009).

Howie, P.W., Forsyth, J.S., Ogston, S.A., Clark, A. & Florey, C.D. (1990) Protective effect of breast feeding against infection. *British Medical Journal*, 300 (6716): 11–16.

Hylander, M.A., Strobino, D.M. & Dhanireddy, R. (1998) Human milk feedings and infection among very low birth weight infants. *Pediatrics*, 102 (3): E38.

Ip, S., Chung, M., Raman, G., Chew, P., Magula, N., DeVine, D., *et al*. (2007) Breastfeeding and maternal and infant health outcomes in developed countries. *Evidence Report/Technology Assessment*, 153: 1–186.

Jelliffe, D. (1971) Commerciogenic malnutrition? Time for a dialogue. *Food Technology*, pp. 55–56.

Jonas, W., Nissen, E., Ransjo-Arvidson, I.W., Henriksson, P. & Uvnas-Moberg, K. (2008) Short- and long-term decrease of blood pressure in women during breastfeeding. *Breastfeeding Medicine*, 3 (2): 103–109.

Jones, F. (2003) *The History of Milk Banking*. Human Milk Banking Association of North America. At: http://www.hmbana.org/index.php?mode=history (accessed 7 February 2009).

Karaolis-Danckert, N., Buyken, A.E., Kulig, M., Kroke, A., Forster, J., Kamin, W., *et al*. (2008) How pre- and postnatal risk factors modify the effect of rapid weight gain in infancy and early childhood on subsequent fat mass development: results from the Multicenter Allergy Study 90. *American Journal of Clinical Nutrition*, 87 (5): 1356–1364.

Karlson, E.W., Mandl, L.A., Hankinson, S.E. & Grodstein, F. (2004) Do breast-feeding and other reproductive factors influence future risk of rheumatoid arthritis? Results from the Nurses' Health Study. *Arthritis and Rheumatism*, 50 (11): 3458–3467.

Kim, J. & Peterson, K.E. (2008) Association of infant child care with infant feeding practices and weight gain among US infants. *Archives of Pediatrics and Adolescent Medicine*, 162 (7): 627–633.

Klement, E., Cohen, R.V., Boxman, J., Joseph, A. & Reif, S. (2004) Breastfeeding and risk of inflammatory bowel disease: a systematic review with meta-analysis. *American Journal of Clinical Nutrition*, 80 (5): 1342–1352.

Koletzko, B., Lien, E., Agostoni, C., Böhles, H., Campoy, C., Cetin, I., *et al.* (2008) The roles of long-chain polyunsaturated fatty acids in pregnancy, lactation and infancy: review of current knowledge and consensus recommendations. *Journal of Perinatal Medicine*, 36 (2): 1–23.

Kramer, M.S., Aboud, F., Mironova, E., Vanilovich, I., Platt, R.W., Matush, L., *et al.* (2008) Breastfeeding and child cognitive development. New evidence from a large randomized trial. *Archives of General Psychiatry*, 65 (5): 578–584.

Langer-Gould, A., Huang, S.M., Stanford, C.A., Leimpeter, A.D., Albers, K.B., Van Den Eeden, S.K., *et al.* (2009) Exclusive breastfeeding and the risk of postpartum relapses in women with multiple sclerosis. Study presented at the American Academy of Neurology's 61st Annual Meeting, 25 April–2 May 2009, Seattle, WA, USA. At: http://www.abstracts2view.com/aan2009seattle/view.php?nu=AAN09L_S01.006 (accessed 5 March 2009).

Lawlor, D.A., Najman, J.M., Batty, G.D., O'Callaghan, M.J., Williams, G.M. & Bor, W. (2005) Infant feeding and components of the metabolic syndrome: findings from the European Youth Heart Study. *Archives of Disease in Childhood*, 90 (6): 582–588.

Lawlor, D.A., Najman, J.M., Batty, G.D., O'Callaghan, M.J., Williams, G.M. & Bor, W. (2006) Early life predictors of childhood intelligence: findings from the Mater-University study of pregnancy and its outcomes. *Paediatric and Perinatal Epidemiology*, 20 (2): 148–162.

Lawrence, R.A. (2007) The eradication of poverty one child at a time through breastfeeding: a contribution to the global theme issue on poverty and human development, October 22, 2007. *Breastfeeding Medicine*, 2 (4): 193–194. At: http://www.liebertonline.com/doi/pdfplus/10.1089/bfm.2007.9982 (accessed 7 February 2009).

Levy, I., Comarsca, J., Davidovits, M., Klinger, G., Sirota, L. & Linder, N. (2008) Urinary tract infection in preterm infants: the protective role of breastfeeding. *International Journal of Pediatric Nephrology*, 24 (3): 527–531.

Liu, B., Beral, V. & Balkwill, A. (2008) On behalf of the million women study collaborators: child-bearing, breastfeeding, other reproductive factors and the subsequent risk of hospitalization for gallbladder disease. *International Journal of Epidemiology*, 38 (1): 312–318.

Lord, S.J., Bernstein, L., Johnson, K.A., Malone, K.E., McDonald, J.A., Marchbanks, P.A., *et al.* (2008) Breast cancer risk and hormone receptor status in older women by parity, age of first birth, and breastfeeding: a case-control study. *Cancer Epidemiology Biomarkers and Prevention*, 17: 1723–1730.

Martek Biosciences Corporation (2009) New study: higher DHA levels improve neurodevelopmental outcomes in premature girls. PR/Newswire-FirstCall, 26 January 2009. At: http://news.prnewswire.com/DisplayReleaseContent.aspx?ACCT=104&STORY=/www/story/01–26–2009/0004960211&EDATE= (accessed 7 February 2009).

Martin, R.M., Ness, A.R., Gunnell, D., Emmett, P., Davey Smith, G. & ALSPAC Study Team (2004) Does breast-feeding in infancy lower blood pressure in childhood? The Avon Longitudinal Study of Parents and Children (ALSPAC). *Circulation*, 109 (10): 1259–1266.

Martin, R.M., Middleton, N., Gunnell, D., Owen, C.G. & Davey Smith, G. (2005) Breast-feeding and cancer: The Boyd Orr Cohort and a systematic review with meta-analysis. *Journal of the National Cancer Institute*, 97 (19): 1446–1457.

Maurage, C. (2008) Children's nutrition and health in adulthood. *Appetite*, 51 (1): 22–24.

Mayer-Davis, E.J., Dabelea, D., Lamichhane, A.P., D'Agostino, R.B. Jr., Liese, A.D., Thomas, J., *et al.* (2008) Breast-feeding and type 2 diabetes in the youth of three ethnic groups: the SEARCH for diabetes in youth case-control study. *Diabetes Care*, 31 (3): 470–475.

McKenna, J.J., Ball, H.L. & Gettler, L.T. (2007) Mother-infant cosleeping, breastfeeding and sudden infant death syndrome: what biological anthropology has discovered about normal infant sleep and pediatric sleep medicine. *American Journal of Physical Anthropology*, 45 Suppl: 133–161.

McVea, K.L., Turner, P.D. & Peppler, D.K. (2000) The role of breastfeeding in sudden infant death syndrome. *Journal of Human Lactation*, 16: 13–20.

Michaelsen, K.F., Lauritzen, L., Horby Jorgensen, M. & Lykke Mortensen, E. (2003) Breast-feeding and brain development. *Scandinavian Journal of Nutrition*, 47 (3): 147–151.

Morteau, O., Gerard, C., Lu, B., Ghiran, S., Rits, M., Fujiwara, Y., *et al.* (2008) An indispensable role for the chemokine receptor CCR10 in IgA antibody-secreting cell accumulation. *Journal of Immunology*, 181: 6309–6315.

Mothersmilkbank (2007) *Mothersmilkbank progress report: 2007.* Banora Point, NSW Australia 2486. At: http://www.mothersmilkbank.com.au/news.htm (accessed 7 February 2009).

Muller, M. (1974) *The Baby Killer. A War on Want Investigation into the Promotion and Sale of Powdered Baby Milks in the Third World.* War on Want, London.

Newburg, D.S. (2008) Neonatal protection by an innate immune system of human milk consisting of oligosaccharides and glycans. *Journal of Animal Science,* 21 November 2008 [Epub ahead of print].

NHS Tayside (2008) Breast is best, but infant formula must contain DHA omega-3 and AA omega-6, say experts. Press release. At: http://www.nhstayside.scot.nhs.uk/news/200802/27–02–08%20Breast%20is%20best,but%20infant%20formulamust%20contain%20DHA%20omega-3%20and%20AA%20omega-6,say%20experts.pdf (accessed 7 February 2009).

Norwegian Directorate for Health (2004) *Utviklingen I Norsk Kosthold.* Matforsyningsstatistikk og Forbruksundersøkelser, Sosial-og helsedirektoratet. Directorate for Health and Social Affairs, Department of Nutrition, IS-1218. [In Norwegian.]

Ogbuanu, I.U., Karmaus, W., Hasan Arshad, S., Kurukulaaratchy, R.J. & Ewart, S. (2009) The effect of breastfeeding duration on lung function at age 10 years: a prospective birth cohort study. *Thorax,* 64 (1): 62–66.

Okamura, C., Tsubono, Y., Ito, K., Niikura, H., Takano, T., Nagase, S., *et al.* (2006) Lactation and risk of endometrial cancer in Japan: a case-control study. *Tohoku Journal of Experimental Medicine,* 208 (2): 109–115.

Oshaug, A. & Botten, G. (1994) Human milk in food supply statistics. *Food Policy,* 19 (5): 479–482.

O'Tierney, P.F., Barker, D.J., Osmond, C., Kajantie, E. & Eriksson, J.G. (2009) Duration of breast-feeding and adiposity in adult life. *Journal of Nutrition,* 139 (2): 422S–425S.

Owen, C.G., Whincup, P.H., Kaye, S.J., Martin R.M., Davey Smith, G., Cook, D.G., *et al.* (2008) Does initial breastfeeding lead to lower blood cholesterol in adult life? A quantitative review of the evidence. *American Journal of Clinical Nutrition,* 88 (2): 305–314.

PAHO/WHO (2004) *Guiding Principles for Complementary Feeding of the Breastfed Child.* Pan American Health Organization/World Health Organization, Division of Health Promotion and Protection/Food and Nutrition Program, Washington, DC. English and Spanish. At: http://www.who.int/nutrition/publications/infantfeeding/en/index.html (accessed 7 February 2009).

Palou, A. & Picó, C. (2009) Leptin intake during lactation prevents obesity and affects food intake and food preferences in later life. *Appetite,* 52 (1): 249–252.

Peacey, V., Steptoe, A., Davídsdóttir, S., Baban, A. & Wardle, J. (2006) Low levels of breast cancer risk awareness in young women: an international survey. *European Journal of Cancer,* 42 (15): 2585–2589.

Phipps, A.I., Malone, K.E., Porter, P.L., Daling, J.R. & Li, C.I. (2008) Reproductive and hormonal factors for postmenopausal luminal, HER-2 overexpressing, and triple-negative breast cancer. *Cancer,* 113 (7): 1521–1526.

Pikwer, M., Bergström, U., Nilsson, J.A., Jacobsson, L., Berglund, G. & Turesson, C. (2009) Breast feeding, but not oral contraceptives, is associated with a reduced risk of rheumatoid arthritis. *Annals of the Rheumatic Diseases,* 68 (4): 526–530.

Pisacane, A., Graziano, L., Mazzarella, G., Scarpellino, B. & Zona, G. (1992) Breast-feeding and urinary tract infection. *Journal of Pediatrics,* 120 (1): 87–89.

Plagemann, A. & Harder, T. (2005) Breast feeding and the risk of obesity and related metabolic diseases in the child. *Metabolic Syndrome and Related Disorders,* 3 (3): 222–232.

Porter, P. (2008) 'Westernizing' women's risks? Breast cancer in lower-income countries. *New England Journal of Medicine,* 358 (3): 213–216.

Quigley, M.A., Kelly, Y.J. & Sacker, A. (2007) Breastfeeding and hospitalization for diarrheal and respiratory infection in the United Kingdom Millennium Cohort Study. *Pediatrics,* 120 (2): e837–e842.

Riman, T., Nilsson, S. & Persson, I. (2004) Review of epidemiological evidence for reproductive and hormonal factors in relation to the risk of epithelial ovarian malignancies. *Acta Obstetricia et Gynecologica Scandinavica,* 83 (9): 783–795.

SABR (2006) *History of Human Milk Banks.* South African Breastmilk Reserve, Johannesburg. At: http://www.sabr.org.za/about/ (accessed 7 February 2009).

Siegel, D.J. (1999) *The Developing Mind. How Relationships and the Brain Interact to Shape Who We Are*. Guilford Press, New York.

Simmer, K., Patole, S.K. & Rao, S.C. (2007a) Longchain polyunsaturated fatty acid supplementation in infants born at term. *Cochrane Database of Systematic Reviews* (4): CD000376. At: http://www.cochrane.org/reviews/en/ab000376.html (accessed 7 February 2009).

Simmer, K., Schulzke, S.M. & Patole, S. (2007b) Longchain polyunsaturated fatty acid supplementation in preterm infants. *Cochrane Database of Systematic Reviews*, (1): CD000375. At: http://www.cochrane.org/reviews/en/ab000375.html (accessed 7 February 2009).

Simon, V.G., de Souza, J.M. & de Souza, S.B. (2009) Breastfeeding, complementary feeding, overweight and obesity in pre-school children. *Revista de Saúde Pública*, 43 (1): 60–69.

Singhal, A. (2006) Early nutrition and long-term cardiovascular health. *Nutrition Reviews*, 64 (5 Pt 2): 544–549.

Smith, J.P. (1999) Human milk supply in Australia. *Food Policy*, 24 (1): 71–91.

Smith, J.P., Dunstone, M.D. & Elliott-Rudder, M.E. (2008) 'Voldemort' and health professional knowledge of breastfeeding – do journal titles and abstracts accurately convey findings on differential health outcomes for formula fed infants? Australian Centre for Economic Research on Health, ACERH Working Paper Number 4, December 2008. At: http://www.acerh.edu.au/publications/ACERH_WP4.pdf (accessed 9 March 2009).

Sobhy, S.I. & Mohame, N.A. (2004) The effect of early initiation of breast feeding on the amount of vaginal blood loss during the fourth stage of labor. *Journal of the Egyptian Public Health Association*, 79 (1–2): 1–12.

Sotgia, F., Casimiro, M.C., Bonuccelli, G., Liu, M., Whitaker-Menezes, D., Er, O., *et al.* (2009) Loss of caveolin-3 induces a lactogenic microenvironment that is protective against mammary tumor formation. *American Journal of Pathology*, 174 (2): 613–629.

Strathearn, L., Mamun, A.A., Najman, J.M. & O'Callaghan, M.J. (2009) Does breastfeeding protect against substantiated child abuse and neglect? A 15-year cohort study. *Pediatrics*, 123 (2): 483–493.

Stuart-Macadam, P. (1995) Biocultural perspectives on breastfeeding. In: Stuart-Macadam, P. & Dettwyler, K.A. (eds) *Breastfeeding. Biocultural Perspectives*, pp. 1–37. Aldine de Gruyter, New York.

Stuebe, A.M., Rich-Edwards, J.W., Willett, W.C., Manson, J.E. & Michels, K.B. (2005) Duration of lactation and incidence of type 2 diabetes. *Journal of the American Medical Association*, 294: 2601–2610.

Stuebe, A.M., Michels, K.B., Willett, W.C., Manson, J.E., Rexrode, K., & Rich-Edwards, J.W. (2009) Duration of lactation and incidence of myocardial infarction in middle to late adulthood. *American Journal of Obstetrics and Gynecology*, 200: 138.e1–138.e8.

Sussmann, J.E., McIntosh, A.M., Lawrie, S.M., & Johnstone, E.C. (2009) Obstetric complications and mild to modern intellectual disability. *British Journal of Psychiatry*, 194: 224–228.

Tennant, P.W.G., Gibson, J.G. & Pearce, M.S. (2008) Lifecourse predictors of adult respiratory function: results from the Newcastle Thousand Families Study. *Thorax*, 63: 823–830.

Turck, D. (2005) Article in French. Breastfeeding: health benefits for child and mother. *Archives de Pédiatrie*, 12 S3: S145–S165.

UN (1989) *Convention of the Rights of the Child*. Adopted and opened for signature, ratification and accession by General Assembly resolution 44/25 of 20 November 1989; entry into force 2 September 1990, in accordance with article 49. At: http://www.unhchr.ch/html/menu3/b/k2crc.htm (accessed 7 February 2009).

UN (2008a) *UN Millennium Development Goals*. Department of Public Information, United Nations, New York. At: http://www.un.org/millenniumgoals/ (accessed 7 February 2009).

UN (2008b) United Nations Secretary-General. Emergency and long-term steps needed to address escalating world food crisis, says Secretary-General to special Economic and Social Council meeting. SG/SM/11511, ECOSOC/6329, 14 April 2008. At: http://wwww.reliefweb.int/rw/rwb.nsf/db900sid/YSAR-7DPSM2?OpenDocument (accessed 7 February 2009).

UNICEF/WHO (1990) *Innocenti Declaration on the Protection, Promotion and Support of Breastfeeding*. UNICEF/WHO, Florence. At: http://www.unicef.org/programme/breastfeeding/innocenti.htm (accessed 7 February 2009).

USFDA (2001) GRAS notice 000041, May 17, 2001. US Food and Drug Administration, Washington. At: http://www.cfsan.fda.gov/~rdb/opa-g041.html (accessed 7 February 2009).

USFDA (2006) Infant formula: frequently asked questions. US Food and Drug Administration, Center for Food Safety and Applied Nutrition. At: http://www.cfsan.fda.gov/~dms/inf-faq.html (accessed 7 February 2009).

US Senate (1978) *Examination on the Advertising, Marketing, Promotion, and Use of Infant Formula in Developing Nations*, p. 1. Hearing before the subcommittee on Health and Scientific Research of the Committee on Human Resources. Fifty-fifth Congress, May 23, 1978. US Government Printing Office, Washington, D.C.

Vennemann, M.M., Bajanowski, T., Brinkmann, B., Jorch, G., Yücesan, K., Sauerland, C., *et al.* (2009) Does breastfeeding reduce the risk of sudden infant death syndrome? *Pediatrics*, **123**: e406–e410.

Vickers, M.C. (2008) *Breastfeeding as a Shield Against the Health Effects of Climate Change*. For La Leche League International and the World Alliance for Breastfeeding Action. At: http://www.waba.org.my/pdf/World%20Health%20Day%202008.pdf (accessed 7 February 2009).

Vohr, B.R., Poindexter, B.B., Dusick, A.M., McKinley, L.T., Higgins, R.D., Langer, J.C., *et al.* (2007) Persistent beneficial effects of breast milk ingested in the neonatal intensive care unit on outcomes of extremely low birth weight infants at 30 months of age. *Pediatrics*, **120** (4): e953–e959.

Von Kries, R., Koletzko, B., Sauerwald, T. & Von Mutius, E. (2000) Does breast-feeding protect against childhood obesity? In: Koletzko, B. (ed.) *Short and Long Term Effects of Breast Feeding on Child Health*, pp. 29–39. Kluwer Academic/Plenum Publishers, London.

Walker, M. (1992) *Summary of Hazards of Infant Formula, Part 1* (for health workers). International Lactation Consultant Association, Raleigh, NC, USA.

Walker, M. (1998) *Summary of Hazards of Infant Formula, Part 2* (for health workers and mothers). International Lactation Consultant Association, Raleigh, NC, USA.

Walker, M. (2004) *Summary of Hazards of Infant Formula, Part 3* (focusing on contamination). International Lactation Consultant Association, Raleigh, NC, USA.

WCRF (2008) Most women unaware breastfeeding can prevent cancer. Press release, WCRF (UK). At: http://www.wcrf-uk.org/press_media/releases/28042008.lasso (accessed 7 February 2009).

WCRF (2009) Landmark report: many cancers could be prevented across the globe. Press release, WCRF (UK) At: http://www.wcrf-uk.org/audience/media/press_releases.htm (accessed 5 March 2009).

WHO (1974) Twenty-seventh World Health Assembly, resolution WHA27.43. WHO, Geneva.

WHO (1978) Thirty-first World Health Assembly, resolution WHA31.47. WHO, Geneva.

WHO (1979) Joint WHO/UNICEF meeting on infant and young child feeding, Geneva, 9–12 October 1979 (statement, recommendations, list of participants). WHO, Geneva.

WHO (1980) Thirty-third World Health Assembly, resolution WHA33.32. WHO, Geneva.

WHO (1981a) *International Code of Marketing of Breast-Milk Substitutes*. WHO, Geneva. At: http://www.who.int/nutrition/publications/code_english.pdf (accessed 7 February 2009).

WHO (1981b) Thirty-fourth World Health Assembly, resolution WHA34.22. WHO, Geneva.

WHO (1986a) *Guidelines Concerning the Main Health and Socioeconomic Circumstances in which Infants have to be Fed on Breast-Milk Substitutes*. Thirty-ninth World Health Assembly, document WHA39/1986/REC/1, Annex 6, Part 2. WHO, Geneva.

WHO (1986b) Thirty-ninth World Health Assembly, resolution WHA39.28. WHO, Geneva.

WHO (1989) *Protecting, Promoting and Supporting Breastfeeding: the Special Role of Maternity Services*. A joint WHO/UNICEF Statement. WHO, Geneva.

WHO (1991a) *Baby-Friendly Hospital Initiative*. At: http://www.who.int/nutrition/topics/bfhi/en/index.html (accessed 7 February 2009).

WHO (1991b) Forty-fourth World Health Assembly, resolution WHA44.33. WHO, Geneva.

WHO (1992a) Forty-fifth World Health Assembly, resolution WHA45.34. *Infant and Young Child Nutrition*. WHO, Geneva.

WHO (1992b) Forty-fifth World Health Assembly, document WHA45/1991/REC/1, Annex 9, paragraphs 45–51. WHO, Geneva. Summary at: http://www.who.int/nutrition/follow-up_formula_eng.pdf (accessed 7 February 2009).

WHO (1993) Forty-sixth World Health Assembly, resolution WHA46.7. WHO, Geneva.

WHO (1994) *Infant and Young Child Nutrition (Progress and Evaluation Report; and Status of Implementation of the International Code of Marketing of Breast-milk Substitutes)*. Forty-seventh World Health Assembly, Report by the Director-General, document WHA47/1994/REC/1, Annex 1, paragraph 138. WHO, Geneva.

WHO (2001a) *The Optimal Duration of Exclusive Breastfeeding, Report of an Expert Consultation*. WHO, Geneva. At: http://www.who.int/nutrition/publications/optimal_duration_of_exc_bfeeding_report_eng.pdf (accessed 7 February 2009).

WHO (2001b) *WHO Technical Consultation on Behalf of the UNFPA/UNICEF/WHO/UNAIDS Interagency Team on Mother-to-child Transmission of HIV*, October 2001, document WHO/RHR/01.28. WHO, Geneva.

WHO (2001c) *The optimal Duration of Exclusive Breastfeeding: A Systematic Review*. WHO, Geneva. At: http://www.who.int/nutrition/publications/optimal_duration_of_exc_bfeeding_review_eng.pdf (accessed 7 February 2009).

WHO (2002a) Fifty-fifth World Health Assembly, resolution WHA55.25. *Infant and Young Child Feeding*. WHO, Geneva.

WHO (2002b) *Nutrient Adequacy of Exclusive Breastfeeding for the Term Infant during the First Six Months of Life*. WHO, Geneva. At: http://www.who.int/nutrition/publications/nut_adequacy_of_exc_bfeeding_eng.pdf (accessed 7 February 2009).

WHO (2003a) *Global Strategy for Infant and Young Child Feeding*. Fifty-fifth World Health Assembly. WHO, Geneva. At: http://www.who.int/nutrition/publications/gs_infant_feeding_text_eng.pdf (accessed 7 February 2009).

WHO (2003b) Global cancer rates could increase by 50% to 15 million by 2020. WHO, Geneva. Press release, 3 April 2003. At: http://www.mindfully.org/Health/2003/Cancer-Rates-15M3apr03.htm (accessed 7 February 2009).

WHO (2005a) *Guiding Principles on Feeding Non-breastfed Children 6–24 Months of Age*. English and French. WHO, Geneva. At: http://www.who.int/nutrition/publications/guidingprin_nonbreastfed_child.pdf (accessed 7 February 2009).

WHO (2005b) *Guiding Principles for Feeding Infants and Young Children during Emergencies*. WHO, Geneva. At: http://www.who.int/nutrition/publications/guiding_principles_feedchidren_emergencies.pdf (accessed 7 February 2009).

WHO (2005c) Chapter 4. Attending to 136 million births, every year. In: *World Health Report 2005*. WHO, Geneva.

WHO (2006a) In: Edmond, K. & Bahl, R. *Optimal Feeding of Low-birth-weight Infants*. WHO, Geneva. At: http://whqlibdoc.who.int/publications/2006/9789241595094_eng.pdf (accessed 7 February 2009).

WHO (2006b) Constitution of the World Health Organization, article 2. *Basic documents, Forty-fifth edition, Supplement*. WHO, Geneva. At: http://www.who.int/governance/eb/who_constitution_en.pdf (accessed 7 February 2009).

WHO (2006c) *WHO Child Growth Standards*. Backgrounder 1. WHO, Geneva. At: http://www.who.int/nutrition/media_page/backgrounders_1_en.pdf (accessed 7 February 2009).

WHO (2006d) World Health Organization releases new child growth standards (press release). WHO, Geneva. At: http://www.who.int/mediacentre/news/releases/2006/pr21/en/index.html (accessed 7 February 2009).

WHO (2007a) *WHO HIV and Infant Feeding Technical Consultation – Consensus Statement*. English, French, Portuguese and Spanish. WHO, Geneva. At: http://www.who.int/child_adolescent_health/documents/if_consensus/en/index.html (accessed 7 February 2009).

WHO (2007b) In: Horta, B., Bahl, R., Martines, J. & Victora, C. *Evidence on the Long-term Effects of Breastfeeding*. WHO, Geneva. At: http://www.who.int/child_adolescent_health/documents/9241595230/en/index.html (accessed 7 February 2009).

WHO (2008a) *Protecting Health from Climate Change*. WHO, Geneva. At: http://www.who.int/world-health-day/en/ (accessed 7 February 2009).

WHO (2008b) Cancer. Fact sheet no. 297. WHO, Geneva. At: http://www.who.int/mediacentre/factsheets/fs297/en/index.html (accessed 7 February 2009).

WHO & UNICEF (2006) *Infant and Young Child Feeding Counselling. An Integrated Course*. Session 2: Why breastfeeding is important. WHO, Geneva. At: http://whqlibdoc.who.int/publications/2006/9789241594752_eng.pdf (accessed 7 February 2009).

Wiessinger, D. (1996) Watch your language! *Journal of Human Lactation*, **12** (1): 1–4.

Wilensky, G.R. & Satcher, D. (2009) Don't forget about the social determinants of health. *Health Affairs*, **28** (2): w194–w198.

Wilson, A.C., Forsyth, J.S., Greene, S.A., Irvine, L., Hau, C. & Howie, P.W. (1998) Relation of infant diet to childhood health: seven year follow up of cohort of children in Dundee infant feeding study. *British Medical Journal*, **316** (7124): 21–25.

Wilson, N.L., Robinson, L.J., Donnet, A., Bovetto, L., Packer, N.H. & Karlsson, N.G. (2008) Glycoproteomics of milk: differences in sugar epitopes on human and bovine milk fat globule membranes. *Journal of Proteome Research*, **7**: 3687–3696.

2 A Biocultural Basis for Protecting, Promoting and Supporting Breastfeeding

Andy Bilson and Fiona Dykes

2.1 Introduction

The relationship between a mother and her baby is both beautiful and complex. We can marvel at the mother's production of food that is nutritious and promotes her health and the child's resistance to disease, and we can see the growing evidence from neuroscience that the interaction between parents and their children shapes the development of the child's brain in profound ways. These abilities and complex relationships are the result of a process of adaptation and change that has spanned thousands of years and one we are far from understanding. However, within our Western scientific culture we have progressively introduced modern technologies that interfere with this complex interaction, examples being infant formula feeding, caesarean births and separation of mother and baby by use of cots and incubators.

In this chapter we focus upon the Baby-Friendly Hospital Initiative (BFHI). The BFHI is one of the key strategies that the *Global Strategy for Infant and Young Child Feeding* recommends is implemented in every maternity service, globally. We argue for an approach to implementing the BFHI based on an understanding of our lives as embodied beings. An understanding based on biology, and the ways in which it interfaces with culture, provides us with a different starting point for our thinking about what is beneficial for babies and their mothers. This understanding also supports us in reconceptualising the ways in which we endeavour to change the practices of health professionals in this field (the key focus of our chapter). We suggest that adopting a biocultural perspective supports an approach to change in organisations and practices that moves beyond traditional rational mechanisms of command and control to ones which value emotional engagement. Implementation of the BFHI may be seen as a case study in which to consider this approach.

2.2 WHO/UNICEF Baby-Friendly Hospital Initiative

The superiority of breastfeeding for the growth and development of infants and for the health of the mother has led to a clear recognition at global, national and local levels of the need to promote practices that value the natural processes of breastfeeding and infant care by parents. In light of this knowledge, the protection, promotion and support of breastfeeding has become a major international public health goal that is given high priority by the World Health Organization (WHO) and

United Nations Children's Fund (UNICEF) as illustrated by a series of initiatives outlined below.

In 1989 WHO and UNICEF published a joint statement *Protecting, Promoting and Supporting Breastfeeding* (WHO/UNICEF 1989). This statement included ten best practice standards for maternity units, named the 'Ten Steps to Successful Breast Feeding', hereafter abbreviated to 'Ten Steps'. The 'Ten Steps' were constructed by the WHO/UNICEF to reflect what the two organisations felt were the key actions to promote breastfeeding in maternity hospitals (WHO 1998).

In 1990, WHO/UNICEF issued the *Innocenti Declaration on the Protection, Promotion and Support of Breastfeeding* (WHO 1990). This internationally endorsed declaration contained a comprehensive set of social policy targets to be reached by governments to assist a change of culture and facilitate increased breastfeeding initiation and duration rates. The declaration also contained a commitment to ensure that all maternity facilities meet the 'Ten Steps'.

In 1991 WHO/UNICEF launched the BFHI. The purpose of this initiative was to support the development of an infrastructure by maternity care facilities that enabled maternity services to implement the 'Ten Steps' (WHO/UNICEF 1989). WHO and UNICEF then set up national teams in participating countries to coordinate and monitor implementation in hospitals. BFHI accreditation is issued to those deemed to have reached a minimum externally auditable standard in relation to the 'Ten Steps'.

In 2003, the *Global Strategy for Infant and Young Child Feeding* was launched (WHO 2003). This was developed through a highly participatory global consultation process lasting two years. It is grounded on epidemiological and scientific evidence, while recognising the complex political and sociocultural influences on infant feeding practices. It was envisaged that the strategy would act as a catalyst for revitalising international attention towards the impact of feeding practices on the wellbeing of infants and young children. To achieve optimal infant and young child feeding practices the strategy calls for a renewed commitment to the *WHO International Code of Marketing of Breast-milk Substitutes* (WHO 1981), the *Innocenti Declaration on Protection, Promotion and Support of Breastfeeding* (WHO 1990) and the BFHI (WHO/UNICEF 1989).

The *Global Strategy* calls on governments to develop, implement and evaluate a comprehensive national policy on infant and young child feeding and thereby to enable full operationalisation of its aims. This requires social, political and economic changes and concomitant public investment to be made to remove the constraints on women in achieving and maintaining optimum infant and young child feeding practices. However, the extent to which the *Global Strategy* is implemented across the globe will, as with the WHO Code, relate to government commitment, prioritisation and competing political agendas.

As stated, the comprehensive BFHI is a cornerstone of the *Global Strategy*. It aims to remove or reduce many of the hospital-based constraints that disadvantage breastfeeding women, to include the banning of advertising of breast-milk substitutes in maternity hospitals and ending the separation of babies from their mothers in hospital nurseries. Implementation of the BFHI has been associated with significant increases in breastfeeding rates (Prasad & Costello 1995; Cattaneo & Buzzetti

2001; Kramer *et al.* 2001; Philipp *et al.* 2001, 2003; Alam *et al.* 2002; Caldeira & Goncalves 2007).

It is important to distinguish between the aims of the BFHI – to optimise breast-feeding practices – and the process by which this is to be achieved. The initiative is challenging to implement in that it advocates the making of relatively uniform changes across the globe in enormously diverse cultural settings. Implementation in a country in the former Soviet Union, which operates in a command and control culture of governance within health facilities, would be unlikely to be directly trans-ferable to a hospital in the UK or Africa. Even within one country the mechanism by which change is managed and sustained will inevitably be influenced by the organ-isational culture of the maternity hospital within which the initiative is implemented.

The style of BFHI implementation will inevitably reflect the local institutional culture and the ways in which change is managed. It may therefore be implemented in a 'top-down' or 'bottom-up' way or perhaps a combination of both. Walker and Gilson (2004) summarise these two key ways in which policy is implemented: 'Top-down' implementation involves central planners pre-planning and organising rational implementation of a list of standards or conditions. 'Bottom-up' sees policy change as much more dynamic and iterative. It places emphasis on understanding the local culture and implementing change in a creative, systemic and culturally sensitive way.

The top-down approach to changing health and social care practice has also been called a scientific-bureaucratic approach by Harrison (1999), who argues that it:

'centres on the assumption that valid and reliable knowledge is mainly to be obtained from the accumulation of research conducted by experts according to strict scientific criteria. . . . It further assumes that working clinicians are likely to be both too busy and insufficiently skilled to interpret and apply such knowledge for themselves, and therefore holds that professional practice should be influenced through the systematic aggregation by academic experts of research findings on a particular topic, and the distillation of such findings into protocols and guidelines which may then be communicated to practitioners with the expectation that practice will be improved. . . . The logic, though not always the overt form, of guidelines is essentially algorithmic . . .'

Harrison (1999, p. 3)

Frequently, attempts to change healthcare practice within institutions involve a top-down, rationalist strategy. At the same time the ability to change organisational culture is frequently taken for granted (Ormorod 2003) and its capacity to shape what can be thought, said, or done is underestimated by those managing change (Davies *et al.* 2000; Bilson & White 2004; Lawler & Bilson 2005). Yet, research into teams and professions in health and social care (Bloor 1976; Pithouse 1987; Hall 1997; White 1998; Latimer 2000) shows how cultures are locally accom-plished and reproduced and can sustain the practices of professions, occupations, organisations and teams and therefore invoke serious resistance to attempts to make interventions into culture.

Bilson and Thorpe (2007) argue that there are major difficulties in the way many countries manage policy implementation in health services. They assert that one of the reasons for the failure of initiatives is due to a lack of understanding of organisational problems that stem from complex interrelationships within the organisation and with its environment and that are not susceptible to the rational planning approaches commonly applied (see also Chapman 2004). Within the framework of rational planning attempted solutions to problems are based on redesign of organisations in top-down ways by setting targets and performance indicators, increasing external control structures and other attempts to drive through changes. Indeed, research on staff into the impact of the top-down approach to managing change, in practice settings, has demonstrated the dissatisfaction and dissonance created by it (Harrison & Lim 2000; Harrison 2002; Attree 2005).

One of the key issues when implementing change is sustainability, which, of course, reflects how effectively change is managed. Although these data are available in some countries, for example the UK, in others they are difficult to access, and from personal experience in other countries the second author (FD) is aware that some maternity units were awarded the BFHI in the 1990s and are still calling themselves 'Baby-Friendly' and displaying the Global Baby-Friendly accreditation certificate on their walls. However, they have never been reassessed as the country in question has not put in place a clear reassessment strategy.

Research that focuses on implementation of the BFHI gives us more of a global picture of management of change issues. For example, Moore *et al.* (2007) identified a number of barriers in implementing a BFHI policy and associated education in five New Zealand hospitals. These barriers included: hospitals being in varying stages of BFHI policy development; hospital policy not necessarily based on government policy; hospital policies communicated in differing ways and dependent on resources; factors outside hospital control impacting on capacity to improve breastfeeding rates: and complex organisational matters posing a barrier to educating personnel involved in the birthing process. Furber and Thomson (2006), in England, reported midwives 'breaking the rules' and they 'knowingly concealed' their actions. Rules were broken if they were felt to contravene a woman-centred approach and/or informed decision making by women despite what the 'evidence' said. Rule breaking also occurred when the rules contravened midwives' own beliefs and some of the deeply entrenched cultural norms within the institution. Merewood and Phillipp (2001) discussed the implementation of the BFHI in the USA at the hospital level and acknowledged that this was a major undertaking that required strategic planning, implementing and maintaining change throughout the whole institution, staff education at all levels, and expense. In addition it requires committed leadership, the involvement of many departments, and the support of senior hospital staff members. Hofvander (2005) in Sweden identified the need for strong support from the government and medical profession as well as an organised central lead group. Clearly, substantially more in-depth research is needed in this area and in the next section we suggest that a biocultural understanding of institutional practices and organisational change will support not only implementation of initiatives but also sustainability.

2.3   A biocultural approach to institutional change

In this section we suggest embracing an understanding of issues in infant feeding that includes a different perspective on how to promote change in organisational practices. This is based on biological ideas mainly developed in the field of systems theory (Maturana & Bunnell 1998; Bilson & Ross 1999; Bilson 2004, 2006a,b; Chapman 2004; Lawler & Bilson 2005; Bilson & Thorpe 2007). We suggest that an approach to organisational and cultural change based on biological understandings may lead to a new set of reflections on how to promote breastfeeding and support for breastfeeding mothers. We introduce the writing of Humberto Maturana, a Chilean biologist, whose work draws on research into perception, systems theory and other aspects of biology to provide a view of humans as embodied, emotional, reasoning beings. Maturana describes his biology of cognition, which addresses some of the key problems that are more usually the subject of philosophical and moral reasoning. This biology of cognition provides an explanation of how our human worlds are constructed through the intertwining of emotional and rational processes. It has had wide impact in fields as diverse as sociology (Luhman 1989, 1990, 1993), management science (Mingers 1995, 2002), computing (Cordoba & Midgley 2000), family therapy (Dell 1982, 1985; Leyland 1988), psychology (Ruiz 1996), the law (Teubner 1987), complexity theory (Capra 2003) and many more.

The biology of cognition leads to a way of thinking about human systems (organisations, teams, families etc.) in which we consider them as 'networks of conversations' (Maturana 1988; Bilson 1997). In using the term conversation, we are not simply referring to speech but to a much more encompassing and interlocking network of behaviours: an embodied 'dance' between participants that involves the use of language interlocking patterns of behaviour and it is braided in emotion. This latter is an important point because in the Western cultural tradition the role of emotions is played down in an attempt to maintain 'rationality'. This biological view is rather that emotions both determine and are determined by interactions in the conversation. In particular we move between conversations emotionally and attention to emotions is an essential part of working with organisations.

One implication of the above is that a change in a system is brought about by a change in the network of conversations that the members of the system generate. However, the normal interactions of a member of a system are from within the network of conversations that constitute it, and are therefore confirmatory of the system. In other words, human systems tend to be conservative. From this viewpoint the culture of a particular human system, be it a team, an organization, or nation, is a manner of living that brings forth a particular world. Cultures have developed through the history of the closed network of conversations that constitute them and are learned (actually lived) by new participants in these conversations. Culture shapes all of our experiences as Maturana (2007, p. 113) states:

'Experiences are distinctions that we make of what happens in us or to us as languaging beings . . . and since a culture is a closed network of conversations,

we necessarily live the consequences of these experiences in our living according to the culture in which we live . . .'

Thus culture develops over the history of the system and not only shapes what can be done but also how things are experienced. It is passed on and maintained in the ongoing conversations through a range of emotional, verbal and non-verbal interactions that shape the behaviour and world view of participants. These cultures are based on assumptions that are mostly unexamined and taken for granted. They create the work environment and shape what is possible to do or to see. In work they constitute the 'way we do things here' that is learned by new entrants to an organisation or team. Because of this people are resistant to cultural change as Beer (1975, p. 11) argues: 'individuals are highly resistant to changing the picture of the world that their culture projects to them.'

A key aspect of Western capitalist culture is concerned with effectiveness, efficiency, production and so on, which restricts choice, attempts to control outcomes, often removing human judgement, and, as such, essentially limits the humanness of our participation in the world of work (Lipsky 1980; Ritzer 1992; Dykes 2002, 2005a,b, 2006). This is at the root of proceduralised approaches such as the scientific-bureaucratic one described above. Ritzer (1992) asserts that this leaves us in what the sociologist Max Weber called an 'iron cage of rationality'. Similarly Maturana and Bunnell (1998) note that such systems restrict the possibilities for acting out of awareness and that they demand that we behave like robots. The alternative approach suggested here is to let go of the desire to control and instead aim to increase responsibility and vision through inspiration and promoting critical reflection.

An organisation can be seen to have multiple networks of conversations and cultures that will shape local responses to attempts to change practices such as promoting breastfeeding. Likewise mothers themselves will participate in a range of cultures and subcultures. From such a standpoint there can be no single method for promoting change applicable to all organisations and all situations within an organisation. Instead biologically informed systems theorists such as Maturana, Beer and Bateson suggest that we need to open a space for reflection and release the restrictions on individual judgement. As Maturana and Bunnell (1998, p. 143) state:

'As we release these restrictions, as we let humans be humans, without this demand of robotizations, then creativity, cooperation, . . . and co-inspiration appear. If we have the same inspiration we don't need control, we have freedom, and we have responsibility. In a way all these reflections lead us to discover that we can do all we wish to do together as a co-inspiration when we let human beings appear.'

A fundamental underpinning of 'top-down' approaches is an assumption about causation; this we challenge arguing that human systems do not operate on linear causation but on circular or more complex chains of causation. By this we mean that simple formulations of the form 'A causes B' do not accurately describe what happens. In circular models of causation A has an effect on B; B has an effect on C; and so on around the circuit until eventually Z has an effect on A and the effects then continue to reverberate throughout the system. In such a system there is no simple cause and effect. It is possible to punctuate this sequence to suggest that A has caused B, or, if a different starting point is chosen, it can be said that B caused the chain of events that caused A. One implication of this is that changes in any part of a system will affect all other parts and a second is that an input into a system can reverberate around the system continuing to make a difference long after the initial stimulus. This is referred to as circular causation (see Bilson 2004 for a fuller discussion).

Bilson (2004) argues that a key issue raised by the concept of circular causation is the need for a re-conceptualisation of power and control. From this viewpoint a person cannot control a system such as an organisation or team. They can make an intervention and 'perturb' the system, but how it responds will depend on its own state and how it perceives the intervention. This applies to interventions such as target setting and performance indicators. These are unlikely to achieve their desired ends for a number of reasons; for example control through rigidly set targets will upset the delicate balances that maintain the stability of the organisation. Gregory Bateson warns against fixing any one particular variable in a dynamic system 'because fixing the value of any variable will in the end disrupt the homeostatic process' (Bateson & Bateson 1988, p. 119).

Watzlawich *et al.* (1974) suggest that a linear view of causation often leads to what they call a 'more of the same loop' in which the failure of successive attempted solutions lead to an escalation of the attempted solutions rather than a re-evaluation of them. In time the solutions themselves become the problem. Such an escalation is well illustrated in responses to 'whole system' problems in health and social care in England (see Bilson & Thorpe 2007). Here, repeated government attempts to deal with lack of coordination between social care and health services have led to escalating attempts to apply 'top-down' control. Within the space of a few years attempted solutions have progressively included: advice; permissive powers for joint planning; the power to share budgets between health and social work; new joint services; punishing local authorities through charges for delayed discharges of older people from hospitals; setting up rating schemes for social care and health organisations and taking over the management of failing organisations; establishing a multidisciplinary 'single assessment process' so that staff in all agencies use the same forms and work to the same strict timescales; the co-location of staff; joint teams and finally major reorganisations combining services from multiple organisations. Thus, in England, we have seen attempts to resolve the problem of the lack of coordination between agencies which have escalated dramatically. However, not only does the original problem remain unsolved but also new problems arise because of the disruption the attempted solutions have created.

2.4   Conclusion

The key purpose of the BFHI is to intervene in the culture of hospitals to protect, promote and support breastfeeding. Although the 'Ten Steps' framework is, of its very nature, proceduralising, we argue that it can be implemented and, when successful, probably is implemented, in a flexible, reflexive emotionally engaging manner. The biological concepts outlined here suggest that if we are to intervene in culture, we have a responsibility for the manner in which we intervene. This is particularly important for the BFHI since it aims to repair the damage caused by an over-medicalised response to maternity care and infant feeding. There is thus a distinct danger if we act again within a top-down medical framework of reducing individual responsibility and reinforcing rather than challenging the over-medicalisation we seek to change and this is one possible pitfall for achieving the aims of the BFHI in a sustainable way.

If we intervene in the ways that seem logical in our Western culture, ways that Maturana and Bunnell (1998) have summed up as using 'demand, force, threats, and power, or through more subtle ways of restricting vision, such as competition and ambition' then we will create a culture that restricts our ability to see others, to cooperate, to reflect and to act responsibly. Authority, command and power restrict responsibility and reduce our ability to be fully human, but the cultural lenses through which we see our world often hide this from us. This may then lead to compliance on the one hand, and resistance on the other, as described by Furber and Thomson (2006).

Thus we are left with an apparent paradox of desiring change but, if we take the lessons of a biocultural understanding seriously, having to reject responses based on control. We need to see people, not rules and to promote a culture of cooperation in which reflexivity plays a key role. This has implications for implementing and sustaining any intervention into culture. We need to change hearts and minds and this requires an understanding of the complex biocultural underpinnings of human behaviour and of the ways in which organisational change may be achieved with this knowledge in mind.

So what are the implications for the BFHI? It is crucial that we promote practices and hospital environments that support breastfeeding, such as early experience of feeding, skin-to-skin contact between mothers and babies, and prevent the promotion of bottle feeding. This imperative is reinforced by the *Global Strategy for Infant and Young Child Feeding*, which, as stated, recommends implementation of the BFHI in all maternity units, globally.

The style of implementation of this initiative is equally crucial. Those taking a lead on implementation of the BFHI may have high levels of passion and indeed personal emotional engagement; although this can provide energy and drive it may also promote a culture in which challenge and critical reflection are discouraged in a desire to drive the initiative forwards. At the same time those promoting the BFHI, whether internationally, nationally or locally, will have the difficult task of stepping out of a dominant Western medical culture that often promotes the 'robotisation' of staff. This suggests that attempts to implement BFHI will need to promote responsibility and vision of staff and parents rather than compliance with rigid procedures and practices applied to varied cultural settings. This may mean a change from, for example, measuring targets for how many staff have been trained in a policy, to finding ways to assess how a hospital engages its staff and parents in reflexively undertaking local problem solving.

There is still need for research into what are the best processes by which such a flexible approach can be achieved and we suggest that the focus needs to shift from the dominant medical research paradigm, which is objective, detached and rational, to one that emotionally engages research participants, encourages reflexivity and values diversity (see Bilson 1997 for further discussion of these issues). The paradox of promoting a non-medicalised medical response provides a challenge to policy makers, practitioners and researchers alike. We are not providing answers, rather posing questions, but we believe that a biocultural understanding provides a framework for contemplating alternative ways of implementing and indeed sustaining change within health and social care organisations.

References

Alam, M.U.M., Rahman, M. & Rahman, F. (2002) Effectiveness of baby friendly hospital initiative on the promotion of exclusive breast feeding among the Dhaka city dwellers in Bangladesh. *Mymensingh Medical Journal: MMJ*, 11 (2): 94–99.

Attree, M. (2005) Nursing agency and governance: registered nurses' perceptions. *Journal of Nursing Management*, 13: 387–396.

Bateson, G. & Bateson, M.C. (1988) *Angels Fear: An Investigation into the Nature and the Meaning of the Sacred*. Rider, London.

Beer, S. (1975) *Designing Freedom*. John Wiley, London.

Bilson, A. (1997) Guidelines for a constructivist approach: steps towards the adaptation of ideas from family therapy for use in organizations. *Systems Practice*, 10: 153–178.

Bilson, A. (2004) Escaping from intrinsically unstable and untrustful relations: implications of a constitutive ontology for responding to issues of power. *Journal of Cybernetics and Human Knowing*, 11: 21–35.

Bilson, A. (2006a) Promoting compassionate concern in social work: reflections on ethics, biology and love. *British Journal of Social Work*, 37: 1371–1386. doi:10.1093/bjsw/bcl060.

Bilson, A. (2006b) Rationality, reflection and research. In: White, S., Fook, J. & Gardener, F. *Critical reflection and professional development: state of the art*. Oxford University Press, Maidenhead.

Bilson, A. & Ross, S. (1999) *Social Work Management and Practice: Systems Principles*, 2nd edn. Jessica Kingsley, London.

Bilson, A. & Thorpe, D. (2007) Towards aesthetic seduction using emotional engagement and stories. *Kybernetics*, 36 (7/8): 936–945.

Bilson, A. & White, S. (2004) The limits of governance: interrogating the tacit dimension. In: Gray, A. & Harrison, S. (eds) *Governing Medicine*. Oxford University Press, Maidenhead.

Bloor, M. (1976) Bishop Berkeley and the adeno-tonsillectomy enigma: an exploration of variation in the social construction of medical disposal. *Sociology*, 10: 43–61.

Caldeira, A.P. & Goncalves, E. (2007) Assessment of the impact of implementing the baby-friendly hospital initiative. *Jornal de Pediatria*, 83 (2): 127–132.

Capra, F. (2003) *The Hidden Connections: A Science for Sustainable Living*. Doubleday, New York.

Cattaneo, A. & Buzzetti, R. (2001) Effect on rates of breast feeding of training for the Baby-Friendly Hospital Initiative. *British Medical Journal*, 323: 1358–1362.

Chapman, J. (2004) *System Failure*, 2nd edn. Demos, London.

Cordoba, J.R. & Midgley, G. (2000) Rethinking stakeholder involvement: an application of the theory of autopoiesis and boundary critique to information systems planning. In: Clarke, S. & Lehaney, B. (eds) *Human Centered Methods in Information Systems: Current Research and Practice*. Idea Group, Hershey.

Davies, H.T.O., Nutley, S.M. & Mannion, R. (2000) Organisational culture and quality of health care. *Quality in Health Care*, 9: 111–119.

Dell, P.F. (1982) Family theory and the epistemology of Humberto Maturana. In: Kaslow, F.W. (ed.) *The International Book of Family Therapy*. Brunner/Mazel, New York.

Dell, P.F. (1985) Understanding Bateson and Maturana: toward a biological foundation for the social sciences. *Journal of Marital and Family Therapy*, 11 (1): 1–20.

Dykes, F. (2002) Western medicine and marketing – construction of an insufficient milk syndrome. *Health Care for Women International*, 23: 492–502.

Dykes, F. (2005a) A critical ethnographic study of encounters between midwives and breastfeeding women on postnatal wards. *Midwifery*, 21: 241–252.

Dykes, F. (2005b) 'Supply' and 'demand': breastfeeding as labour. *Social Science and Medicine*, 60: 2283–2293.

Dykes, F. (2006) *Breastfeeding in Hospital: Midwives, Mothers and the Production Line*. Routledge, London.

Furber, C.M. & Thomson, A.M. (2006) 'Breaking the rules' in baby-feeding practice in the UK: deviance and good practice? *Midwifery*, 22: 365–376.

Hall, C. (1997) Social work as narrative: storytelling and persuasion in professional texts. Ashgate, Aldershot.

Harrison, S. (1999) New labour, modernisation and health care governance. Paper presented at the political studies association/social policy association conference. New Labour, New Health, London, September 1999.

Harrison, S. (2002) New labour, modernisation and the medical labour process. *Journal of Social Policy*, 31: 465–485.

Harrison, S. & Lim, J. (2000) Clinical governance and primary care in the english national health service: some issues of organization and rules. *Critical Public Health*, 10: 321–329.

Hofvander, Y. (2005) Breastfeeding and the Baby-Friendly Hospital Initiative (BFHI): organisation, response and outcome in Sweden and other countries. *Acta Paediatrica*, 94 (1): 105–123.

Kramer, M.S., Chalmers, B., Hodnett, E.D., Sevkovskaya, Z. & Dzikovich, I. (2001) Promotion Of Breastfeeding Intervention Trial (PROBIT): a randomised trial in the Republic of Belarus. *Journal of the American Medical Association*, 285: 413–420.

Lawler, J. & Bilson, A. (2005) Towards a more reflexive research aware practice: the influence and potential of professional and team culture. In: Bilson, A. *Evidence Based Practice in Social Work*. Whiting and Birch, London, 2005.

Leyland, M.L. (1988) An introduction to some of the ideas of Humberto Maturana. *Journal of Family Therapy*, 1: 357–374.

Lipsky, M. (1980) *Street-level Bureaucracy. Dilemmas of the Individual in Public Services*. Russell Sage Foundation, New York.

Luhmann, N. (1989) *Ecological Communication*. Polity Press, Cambridge.

Luhmann, N. (1990) The cognitive program of constructivism and a reality that remains unknown. In: Krohn, W., Küppers, G. & Nowotny, H. (eds) *Selforganization: Portrait of a Scientific Revolution*. Kluwer Academic Publishers, Dordecht.

Luhmann, N. (1993) Ecological communication: coping with the unknown. *Systems Practice*, 6: 527–539.

Maturana, H.R. (1988) Reality: the search for objectivity or the quest for a compelling argument. *Irish Journal of Psychology*, 9: 25–82.

Maturana, H.R. (2007) The biological foundations of virtual realities and their implications for human existence. *Constructivist Foundations*, 3 (2). 109–111.

Maturana, H.R. & Bunnell, P. (1998) Biosphere, homosphere, and robosphere: what has that to do with business? At: http://www.solonline.org/res/wp/maturana/index.html (accessed 8 July 2008).

Merewood, A. & Phillipp, B.L. (2001) Implementing change: becoming baby-friendly in an inner city hospital. *Birth*, 28: 36–40.

Mingers, J. (1995) *Self-Producing Systems: Implications and Applications of Autopoiesis*. Plenum Publishing, New York.

Mingers, J. (2002) Can Social Systems be autopoietic? Assessing Luhmann's social theory. *Sociological Review*, 50 (2): 278–299.

Moore, T.R., Gauld, R. & Williams, S. (2007) Implementing baby friendly hospital initiative policy: the case of New Zealand public hospitals. *International Breastfeeding Journal*, 2: 8.

Ormorod, S. (2003) Organisational culture in health service policy and research: 'third-way' political fad or policy development? *Policy and Politics*, 31 (2): 227–237.

Pithouse, A. (1987) *Social Work: the Social Organisation of an Invisible Trade*. Avebury Gower, Aldershot.

Phillip, B.L., Merewood, A., Miller, L.W., Chawla, N., Murphy-Smith, M.M., Gomes, J.S. *et al.* (2001) Baby-Friendly Hospital Initiative improves breastfeeding initiation rates in a US hospital setting. *Pediatrics*, 108: 677–681.

Philipp, B.L., Malone, K.L., Cimo, S. & Merewood, A. (2003) Sustained breastfeeding rates at a US baby-friendly hospital. *Pediatrics*, 112: e234–e236.

Prasad, B. & Costello, A.M. (1995) Impact and sustainability of a 'baby friendly' health education intervention at a district hospital in Bihar, India. *British Medical Journal*, 310: 621–623.

Ritzer, G. (1992) *The McDonaldization of society*. Pine Forge Press, Thousand Oaks.

Ruiz, A. (1996) The contributions of Humberto Maturana to the sciences of complexity and psychology. *Journal of Constructivist Psychology*, 9 (4): 283–302.

Teubner, G. (ed.) (1987) *Autopoiesis and Law*. De Gruytner, Berlin.

Walker, L. & Gilson, L. (2004) We are bitter but are satisfied: nurses as street-level bureaucrats in South Africa. *Social Science and Medicine*, 59: 1251–1261.

Watzlawick, P., Weakland, J.H. and Fisch, R. (1974) *Change: Principles of Problem Formation and Resolution*. Norton, New York.

White, S. (1998) Examining the artfulness of risk talk. In: Jokinen, A., Juhila, K. & Poso, T. (eds) *Constructing Social Work Practices*. Ashgate, Aldershot.

WHO (1981) *International Code of Marketing of Breast-milk Substitutes*. WHO, Geneva.

WHO (1990) *Innocenti Declaration on the Protection, Promotion and Support of Breastfeeding*. WHO, Florence.

WHO (1998) *Evidence for the Ten Steps to Successful Breastfeeding*. WHO, Geneva.

WHO (2003) *Global Strategy for Infant and Young Child Feeding*. WHO & UNICEF, Geneva.

WHO/UNICEF (1989) *Protecting, Promoting and Supporting Breastfeeding: the Special Role of Maternity Services*. WHO & UNICEF, Geneva.

3 Feeding Preterm Infants in Sweden: Challenges to Implementing the *Global Strategy* in a Pro-Breastfeeding Culture

Renée Flacking

3.1 Introduction

Breastfeeding of preterm babies (born before the 37th gestational week) is highlighted as particularly important in the *Global Strategy for Infant and Young Child Feeding* (World Health Organization (WHO) 2003) due to the increased risk of infection, morbidity and mortality in this vulnerable group. The recommendation in the *Global Strategy* that babies 'should be exclusively breastfed for the first six months of life' (WHO 2003, p. 8) presents challenges in breastfeeding of preterm babies. In pro-breastfeeding countries such as Sweden there may be excessive emphasis on meeting the *Global Strategy* recommendations with insufficient regard to the challenges of breastfeeding a preterm baby and the building of relationships between the parents and infant. A professional discourse that focuses on breast milk as nutrition tends to underemphasise the relational aspects of breastfeeding. Emphasis on nutritional aspects of breastfeeding tends to be stronger in neonatal units as preterm babies are particularly vulnerable. In addition, the contextual setting of a neonatal unit presents challenges for experiencing breastfeeding as a mutual pleasure in which the fulfilment of the baby's behavioural and emotional needs, as well as the mother's physiological and emotional needs, are valued.

This chapter will illuminate the challenges experienced by breastfeeding mothers of preterm babies in a pro-breastfeeding culture, with a focus on relationality between the mother and baby and the process of becoming a mother. In doing so it will address issues on the spatial and cultural context, the enactment of care routines related to feeding, and attitudes of neonatal unit staff. Furthermore, the consequences of the experiences within a neonatal unit, for the process of breastfeeding and relationality at home, are discussed. Finally, some conclusive remarks are presented on the need for a change of paradigm in neonatal care and breastfeeding in mothers of preterm infants.

3.2 Breastfeeding preterm babies in Sweden

Breastfeeding of preterm babies is of great interest from several perspectives. Even though preterm babies constitute a fairly small percentage of all babies, they comprise a very vulnerable group with regard to neonatal morbidity and mortality. Infants born preterm may have reduced cognitive function and behavioural problems during infancy and later childhood (see for example: Holmgren & Hogberg 2001; Marlow *et al.* 2005; Delobel-Ayoub *et al.* 2006). As research on breastfeeding in preterm babies has shown that breast milk has potentially more positive effects in preterm babies compared with babies born at term, with regard to nutritional, immunological and cognitive outcomes (Lucas *et al.* 1998; Anderson *et al.* 1999; Schanler *et al.* 1999; Edmond & Bahl 2007), the breastfeeding duration in preterm babies has become highly significant from a medical perspective and recognised as a particularly important in the *Global Strategy for Infant and Young Child Feeding*. Compared with studies of mothers of term babies, little research has sought to describe the emotional experiences of mothers of preterm babies' with regard to breastfeeding and mothering. Rather, most research in the area of breastfeeding in preterm babies has focused on nutritional aspects of breastfeeding or on explanatory factors for non-initiation or early cessation of breastfeeding.

Sweden has been regarded as a pro-breastfeeding culture for decades. With a breastfeeding frequency of 98% at one week of age and where 70% are still breastfed at six months of age (The National Board of Health and Welfare 2007), one can clearly state that breastfeeding is the most common way to feed the baby in the first months of life. From a political and societal perspective, breastfeeding is valued, facilitated and sanctioned by the Swedish legislation, in which the Swedish parental leave constitutes the most job-protected paid leave among the Organisation for Economic Co-operation and Development (OECD) countries, which is regarded as highly beneficial for a long period of breastfeeding (Galtry 2003; WHO 2003; Swedish Social Insurance Agency 2005).

In 1998, a prospective study was undertaken to investigate the breastfeeding rate at discharge and up to eight months of postnatal age in 70 mothers with low birth weight babies (<2500 g) admitted to a neonatal intensive care unit (NICU) (Flacking *et al.* 2003). Findings showed that 93% of the babies were breastfed at discharge (74% exclusively). The ones who were not breastfed had mothers who received treatment by chemotherapy or had a previous breast surgery. Findings from a large follow-up population-based register study of about 37 000 babies born in 1993–2001, in which about 2000 babies were born preterm (Flacking *et al.* 2007b), concerning the mothers' breastfeeding duration, are shown in Figure 3.1. Despite the low rate of breastfeeding in very preterm babies (<32 gestational weeks) at six months (45%), it was comparable with and in some cases higher than the rates in term babies reported in other countries, for example in Australia (46%), Canada (41%), USA (32.5%) and Italy (19%) (Callen & Pinelli 2004; Scott *et al.* 2006).

Thus it appears that, in Sweden, even though breastfeeding rates are lower in mothers of preterm babies than in mothers of babies born at term, the norm to

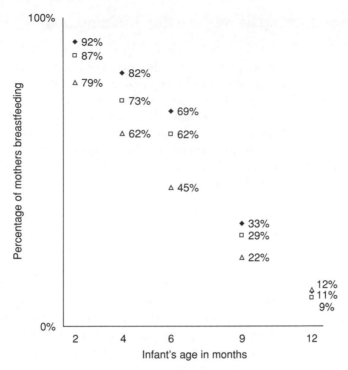

Figure 3.1   Breastfeeding frequencies at postnatal ages of 2, 4, 6, 9 and 12 months. Symbols: ◆ mothers of infants born at >36 weeks (n = 35.250); □ mothers of infants born at 32–36 weeks (n = 1866); △ mothers of infants born at <32 weeks (n = 225).

breastfeed prevails, with 60% of all preterm babies being breastfed at six months of age. High rates of breastfeeding might be seen as synonymous with 'successful breastfeeding' and assumed to be mediated by the provision of good care. Thus with targets set within neonatal units, mothers could possibly be coerced to initiate and sustain breastfeeding by the staff and the means to negotiate breastfeeding, from the mothers' perspective, could be reduced. This prompted a qualitative exploration of how mothers of preterm babies in Sweden experienced the process of becoming a mother and breastfeeding (Flacking *et al.* 2006; Flacking *et al.* 2007a). In-depth interviews were conducted with 25 mothers of 26 babies born at a gestational age of 24–31 weeks. The mothers were recruited from seven neonatal units in Sweden, three at university hospitals and four at county hospitals; each selected with the purpose of having access to mothers who had different experiences of physical environments and care routines after the birth of their babies. In the two following sections, findings from this study, as well as findings from other research, will illuminate the challenges that the *Global Strategy for Infant and Young Child Feeding* presents, with regard to its imperative for mothers to breastfeed and the apparent lack of emphasis on breastfeeding in terms of relationality between the mother and baby.

3.3   Breastfeeding as relationship building in the early phase

Most neonatal units in Sweden support the early initiation of breastfeeding as evidence shows that breastfeeding can be initiated as soon as the baby is physiologically stable, regardless of gestational age or weight, and that babies' early sucking behaviour is the result of learning, enhanced by contingent stimuli (Nyqvist *et al.* 1999; Nyqvist 2008). In addition, most neonatal unit staff emphasise to parents the benefits of breast milk and its importance for a baby's growth and immune system (Petersen *et al.* 2004). Thus, mothers are encouraged at an early stage to express breast milk, which almost all mothers continue to do up until hospital discharge (Flacking *et al.* 2003).

In the early phase, most often occurring during intensive care, when the preterm babies are able to lay on their mothers' breast but still medically dependent and immature, breastfeeding has been described by mothers as not primarily about the intake of breast milk but as a way to be together (Flacking *et al.* 2006, 2007a). Hence, breastfeeding is not considered as nutritive, as the baby's sucking behaviour is still too immature, but is regarded as highly relational. Mothers describe the initial physical closeness of skin-to-skin contact and breastfeeding as something that supports the mother–baby relationship from three aspects: as a sign of the baby's vitality and strength; as a step towards normality; and as an experience of being an important person to her baby.

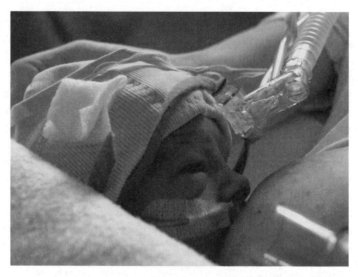

Figure 3.2   Vincent, born after 30 weeks of gestation, 4 days of age, weighing 1400 g and lying at his mother Sofia's breast. Photograph taken by Vincent's father Anders Östman. Printed with permission of the family.

Lena, a primiparous mother, described the first time she held her 5-day-old daughter Anna, who was born in the 25th gestational week:

'It (breastfeeding) felt so right. So, both kangaroo-holding itself and just to lay her at my breast becomes something that's approaching the normal. I don't think that she got any breast milk the first time, but the second time she did. From then on we always breastfed when we had her kangaroo.'

During this phase, breastfeeding was described by mothers as something that occurred naturally, in that sense that breastfeeding was not 'technified' but where the mother's and baby's physiological, maturational and emotional state and needs were regarded. Describing her experiences of breastfeeding support, Karin said:

'They didn't make a big affair like: "Oh, now he has to get it right and you have to be aware not to pump before." It was mostly "Well, let's try this and if it works it's great but it can take time." I didn't feel any pressure but I felt support[ed].'

Breastfeeding is a form of interplay where both the mother and the baby are active. Mothers reflected on their babies as active as the babies licked, opened their mouths and sucked a few times. They described their baby's behaviour as strong and competent – because their baby 'understood how to do it' or 'found my nipple with his mouth even though I was so clumsy'. Seeing the baby as highly competent in combination with early encouragement and initiation of breastfeeding may indicate to the mother that breastfeeding is possible, despite an early gestational age at birth or a potential neonatal disorder. The early initiation might be one reason why it is found that neither gestational age nor neonatal disorders had an effect on the breastfeeding initiation and duration in a cohort of mothers of very preterm babies in Sweden (Flacking *et al.* 2007c).

Bruschweiler Stern (1998) emphasises the importance of providing a safe holding environment from experienced, warm and accepting staff who develop a therapeutic alliance with the mother by validating her in the new role and do so without criticism and disqualification. Mothers in our study experienced not only to be 'held' by the staff but by their babies. During this early phase, mothers were comforted by their babies and, by being in close connection to each other, the mothers could 'mentally survive' and they experienced skin-to-skin care and breastfeeding as something that was 'healing'. When staff emphasise that the main purpose of breastfeeding is a mutual pleasure, comfort and attachment, without any demands of 'succeeding' and as a fulfilment of the emotional needs of the infants and mothers, breastfeeding and skin-to-skin contact become activities that are relationally strengthening. Maternal emotions with regard to feeding preterm babies have been largely superseded by the predominant focus on breastfeeding as mere nutrition; regarding breastfeeding as an activity which can or should be introduced at a certain gestational week and where the baby's sucking behaviour and intake should be supervised, assessed and evaluated (Morton 2002; Isaacson 2006; Sweet

2006, 2008). An experience of breastfeeding as mutually pleasurable enhances the mother's feelings of competence and trust in her baby, which strengthen the 'emotional tie' between mother and baby (Widstrom *et al.* 1990; Klaus 1998). Even though breastfeeding is triggered through biological mechanisms, the perception of breastfeeding varies according to cultural values of motherhood (Small 1998; Schmied & Barclay 1999; Hauck & Irurita 2002; Scott & Mostyn 2003) and the way in which a mother may negotiate the experience of breastfeeding (Murphy 1999; Marshall *et al.* 2007). It could be assumed that when breastfeeding initiation follows early skin-to-skin holding, it progresses in a natural way in which the process does not become disturbed by technified interventions or 'hands-on' (Weimers *et al.* 2006; Law *et al.* 2007; Hannula *et al.* 2008). This gives the sense of breastfeeding as a reciprocal interplay that may be facilitated and fortified. In term babies, research has shown the importance of skin-to-skin contact or close proximity for breastfeeding initiation, when other factors are held constant (Righard & Alade 1990; Ball *et al.* 2006). Hence, when breastfeeding follows skin-to-skin care or when the mother and her baby remain in close proximity, the experience of breast-feeding may embrace more relational aspects and can be negotiated from a personal perspective rather than an institutionalised requirement of succeeding. However, mothers may experience such a requirement of succeeding and a change in the breast-feeding dynamic – from breastfeeding as a relational interplay to becoming just mere nutrition, when the baby's medical condition improves or when the baby is transferred from the intensive-care room/unit to a low-dependency care room/unit, as a greater focus may be placed on growth. This change of discourse will be discussed in the following section.

3.4   Breastfeeding at the 'training camp'

Some mothers describe the change in discourses and staff practices around breast-feeding, from regarding breastfeeding as a relational interplay to just mere nutrition, as entering a 'training camp'. The 'training camp' usually takes place in the low-dependency care rooms/units, which in Sweden often are called 'growth-rooms'. At the 'training camp' the policy of providing a place in relation to what is expected to be 'produced' becomes quite burdensome, especially as this takes place in a highly public environment with few means of privacy. Aspects of the 'training camp' will now be discussed.

3.4.1   The institutional setting

Due to the initial and prolonged separation that occurs in most neonatal units throughout the world, mothers have few opportunities to be with their babies day and night in hospital or to be with their babies in privacy. Recommendations relating to feeding in exceptionally difficult circumstances in the *Global Strategy for Infant and Young Child Feeding* state that 'Wherever possible, mothers and babies should remain together and be provided the support they need to exercise the most appropriate feeding option under the circumstances' (p. 10). Although breast-feeding is indeed the most appropriate option for preterm babies in neonatal units worldwide, mothers and babies are commonly separated because of lack of spatial possibilities. This reflects a prevailing discourse that disregards the preterm baby as a person with physiological and emotional needs, dismisses the emotional needs of the parents, and does not acknowledge the family (parents and their baby) as an inseparable entity. As the initial and prolonged separation between mother and baby is perceived as 'formally sanctioned', it can make the mother feel unimportant, reducing her status to that of a visitor. In practice, mothers may only be offered a room when they breastfeed both day and night or when the baby is close to discharge, in order to learn about her infant's behaviour patterns and to experience 24-hour caregiving (Nye 2008). Again this emphasises nutritional need rather than comfort and closeness. In addition, the provision of a room 24–48 hours prior to discharge only (Nye 2008), might be seen as a surveillance exercise directed towards the mother and her ability to take care of her baby. This combined with the public environ-ment and lack of privacy resonates with both Goffman (1961) and Foucault's (1977) notion of the institution in which there is a supervision of conduct and activities of each individual in order to assess, judge and evaluate performance. Thus, the institutionalised environment in a neonatal unit comprises a space and a place for the assessment of 'organised' activities in the 'training camp'.

3.4.2   The enactment of care routines

As breastfeeding is the cultural norm in Sweden generally and within neonatal units, bottle feeding constitutes a deviation from the norm (Kliethermes *et al.* 1999). In addition, the non-use of bottles in neonatal units is in compliance to the ninth step in the *Ten Steps to Successful Breastfeeding*: 'Give no artificial teats or pacifiers to breastfeeding infants' (WHO 1998). Mothers used the term 'unwritten law' when describing the non-bottle feeding culture. This was exemplified when the staff lowered their voices when mentioning the use of bottles and their reluctance to suggest the use of a bottle unless the mother had mentioned it first herself. This was illustrated by Elin, a first-time mother:

'Nobody mentioned the bottle for the first eight weeks. It was like a disaster just to mention it. And I didn't know, so I thought, well, I have to stay here until he's one year old. It would have been a relief to know that if it doesn't work there's an alternative but it didn't seem to be one for him. To mention "the bottle" is worse than swearing in church.'

In Sweden the transition from gavage feeding to breastfeeding does not 'normally' include the use of bottle feeding, which may be in contrast to other countries (Flacking *et al.* 2003; Sweet 2006; Nye 2008). According to Sweet (2006), the use of bottle feeds in Australian neonatal units enable 'an objective assessment of infant intake' (p. 9). In Swedish neonatal units the transition from gavage feeding to breastfeeding is regulated and objectively assessed, not with bottles, but by the use of specific care routines, for example scheduling of gavage feeding. This conditions mothers to see breastfeeding as a routinised activity. Scheduled feeding is antithetical to the eighth step in the *Ten Steps to Successful Breastfeeding*: 'Encourage breastfeeding on demand' (WHO 1998). In preterm babies it has been shown that frequent positive learning experiences and a supportive context, in which the behavioural cues are acknowledged, enhance the baby's ability to breastfeed at an earlier age (Nyqvist *et al.* 1996, 1999). Unfortunately, 'frequent learning experiences' may not be supported by the care routine of scheduled feeding. By encouraging mothers to attempt breastfeeding at every scheduled feeding, it suggests that there is not only a set time for initiating breastfeeding, but also a limited time for breastfeeding attempts. In addition, the preterm baby's behavioural cues in terms of sleep-wakefulness stages are not acknowledged, nor is the baby acknowledged as an individual with individual needs (Als & Gilkerson 1997). As an example of her desire to maintain some flexibility, Sara described how she, while being at the neonatal unit, sometimes held her daughter in her arms wrapped in a blanket and just cuddled her as she slept when it was time to breastfeed:

'And then they [the staff] would say: "You have to try more often!" "Let her breastfeed as much as you can!" This gave me the impression that she would breastfeed much sooner if I only tried. It resulted in a feeling of failure, very early on – that breastfeeding was progressing too slowly. And I felt guilty for becoming disappointed in her. Breastfeeding was just a task, nothing pleasurable.'

Another care routine, test weighing, that is weighing the baby before and after breastfeeding to assess breast milk intake, is advocated in some Swedish neonatal units, as well as in neonatal units in other parts of the world (Nye 2008). In other Swedish neonatal units, babies are weighed less frequently, perhaps once a day or every other day, to assess weight increase in relation to how much has been supplemented by gavage feeding the preceding day.

Some mothers may experience the scheduled feeding and the weighing as necessary, as they constitute a structure in the experienced uncertainty of providing the infants with breast milk and assessing the intake. However, most mothers feel that having to disregard their baby's signals and needs and their own needs for closeness and interaction due to these rigid care routines are highly negative aspects. Such a disregard for breastfeeding as something pleasurable and relation strengthening implies a concept of breastfeeding being a task and breast milk a product. Petra, a first-time mother whose son Alfred was born in the 25th gestational week, illustrated her experiences of breastfeeding after the transfer to the 'growth unit':

'Breastfeeding became the worst part of the whole hospital stay! It's like falling at the winning post. It's like a marathon – all you can do is run! And then consider that I had a son that weighed 600 grams and was born in the 25th week. I got into a circle where my only relation with my son was bad breastfeeding attempts. To be weighed back and fore, that becomes a really weird relation. I kept on weighing him for a month when he took 5 ml. There is nothing natural about that

[weighing]. It's all about food. It's like having anorexia or bulimia, outside your-self. It felt like I was part of a sick experiment. The staff wanted me to breastfeed more than I did. Even though he was asleep the staff said, "You should always offer" [cheerful voice]. I had such an anxiety about the breastfeeding attempts so I thought "to hell with it". And then I had plenty of breast milk! I was mad and frustrated. It was all about mums and breast and babies and breastfeeding – they had some kind of a fixation. They lose focus on what it's all about. I think it would have been better if we could have had some peace and quiet and a pleasurable time.'

As this narrative illustrates, when reducing breastfeeding to merely a nutritional, one-directional activity and when the emotional needs are dismissed, breastfeeding may be experienced negatively (Sweet 2006). Care routines, such as scheduled feeding and weighing the baby before and after breastfeeding, reflect medical discourses indicating that such 'objective' and 'vital' assessments are superior to more vague measurements in terms of a baby's behaviour or maternal experiences. The challenge lies within the need to balance the insurance of optimal breast milk intake and yet not disregard the relational aspects. This challenge becomes manifest as there is a lack of knowledge on how to support the mother–baby dyad in the transition from gavage feeding to breastfeeding with regard to both intake and relationality (Flacking 2007). Hence, more research is required to ensure that health workers have the 'specific knowledge' needed to support the breastfeeding process in mothers and babies during difficult circumstances. However, the 'specific knowledge' does not only encompass the technified interventions provided but the support given by staff, as the staff behaviour also plays a part in the routinisation of breastfeeding, which will now be discussed.

3.4.3   The staff

Some staff tend to reinforce care routines regardless of the needs of the mother. This is exemplified by Birgitta:

'It felt like he was allowed to breastfeed but the clock ruled so much. I had to put him to the breast a quarter of an hour before feeding time. I had a quarter of an hour to hurry him and try to get him to feed. It's for the staff's sake; it's easier to keep track on even times. And then someone [staff] would stand in the doorway, stamp the floor, wanting to fetch milk for all of the babies at the same time. There wasn't any tranquillity. And then they [staff] thought it was odd that he only took 15 ml. It was hard doing it against time.'

Other staff are supportive and aware of the mothers' and infants' needs and wishes and act without judging, encourage without pressure, supply relevant knowledge, and treat the mother and baby as individuals. Pia, a fourth-time mother, whose son Harry was born in the 24th gestational week, believed very strongly in the emotional and physiological benefits of breastfeeding. Pia had previously breastfed two of her children for a year each and one for two years. As Harry was very ill and had undergone six surgeries within the first months of life, breastfeeding was not really initiated until he was about 40 weeks of postmenstrual age. She described how the staff adjusted to her needs and provided her with a double bed in a room of her own when she asked for this, so that she could breastfeed lying down, as she had been used to with her previous children. The double bed was a necessity, as Harry required oxygen and needed to be constantly monitored, and thus she needed the space to have the oxygen-tube and monitor devices in the bed. Pia said that she was helped to breastfeed in a way that she personally chose:

> 'I mean he lay next to me and I had my breast as when you put a dummy in the mouth. I persisted putting my breast in his mouth whenever he looked as if he wanted to suck. It wasn't feeding but more of a way for him to learn how to do it. I lay there in my bed and he got accustomed to just lying there and sucking and feeling my heartbeats. I believe that's good and calming and everything.'

Other mothers felt that the culture was too pro-breastfeeding and indeed oppressive and not respectful of individual needs. Hence, many mothers felt that a natural process got lost because of the staff being so 'breastfeeding-hysterical', as one mother put it:

> 'I think it would have been better if there hadn't been such a fixation around it. If it had come more naturally, slowly, 'cause you have such a long time ahead of you. I believe that something that is as natural as this and just is shouldn't be made into such a big thing 'cause then it won't be natural.'

The transition, in focus, from the relational and mutually pleasurable aspects of breastfeeding to a more task-oriented perspective might indicate that staff are more relationship-focused in the early phase and acknowledge the importance of bonding and attachment (Bowlby 1969; Klaus et al. 1996; Kennell & Klaus 1998), whereas with time they become more task-oriented (Fenwick et al. 1999). This task orientation resonates with the work of Dykes with regard to term babies (Dykes 2005, 2006). She argues that with a professional discourse that disregards the relational interplay, breastfeeding may be perceived as a labour and a productive project. Thus, when there is a disregard for breastfeeding as a relational interplay and something that is and should be negotiable from the perspective of the individual, breastfeeding may become reduced to a task and not a mutually pleasurable activity.

3.5 Breastfeeding at home – trying to experience a balance in needs

When coming home after the baby's hospitalisation many mothers experience not only relief but also emotional exhaustion. It has been suggested that psychological distress in mothers of preterm babies may be associated with social isolation, post-traumatic symptoms and feelings of guilt and shame persisting years after the birth (Singer *et al.* 1999; Eriksson & Pehrsson 2002; Garel *et al.* 2007). This, of course, affects the experience of becoming a mother as well as the experience of breastfeeding. The mothers need to adjust to a new situation, in which they are the primary caregivers rather than the neonatal unit staff. In the current situation mothers may role model the care giving style that they observed the neonatal unit (Jackson *et al.* 2003). Therefore mothers may adhere to care routines that reflect a lack of individualisation, objectification of the baby and a belief that breastfeeding can always be assessed and evaluated in terms of breast milk intake. This may lead to dissonance with regard to adaptation to motherhood.

In our study, some mothers saw breastfeeding as a profound symbol of motherhood, as also argued by Sweet (2008). Marianne, a first-time mother, whose daughter Agnes was born in the 29th gestational week, commented 17 months after birth:

'That was the only thing I could do that was right. Everything else I had done was wrong. Everything was my fault, that she was born preterm and everything. And the only thing that was left, where I could prove that I actually was a real mum, was to breastfeed. That was the only thing that could make her dependent on me.'

Mothers also highlighted aspects of healing, compensation and a natural way to be together as part of the mutuality and pleasure of breastfeeding. This resonates with the findings of Kavanaugh *et al.* (1997) with regard to mothers of preterm babies in the USA, who also experienced the closeness and enjoyment of breastfeeding in the post-discharge period. In our study, Pia described how she experienced breastfeeding Harry:

'I really enjoy breastfeeding. I feel it's so cosy so there's nothing more pleasant. You know, at night when he sleeps next to me, it's a bit like going back to the natural way. I lived in Africa when I was young and I never heard any babies cry, the mothers had their babies on their backs. Maybe our way of living is not adjusted to that but maybe one should reflect upon it. The breast milk has such a healing effect but also, I think it's some kind of compensation for being born so very preterm, being ill and having to grow up in an intensive care unit, as he has had to. This calmness, it's such a sense of pleasure to lie and breastfeed and having him inside my robe and he's skin-to-skin – it's a compensation to him for having such a tough start. We're having it very peaceful at home, apart from all hospital visits, and he needs all that as he had such a chaotic start. I can sense that he feels well by that and then I feel well. That's why it's so important for me to breastfeed.'

However, other mothers continued to experience breastfeeding as a task and a one-directional activity. They demonstrated difficulties in understanding and responding to their baby's signals and needs along with their own emotional needs. Anna, a single first-time mother, described her situation at home after discharge:

'I thought it was really hard as I didn't know how much milk he got when he breastfed. At the neonatal unit he got much more milk at night so that he

wouldn't wake up before it was time for the next feed, as the staff had to make it work with all the infants. But at home, he needed to breastfeed more often and that became too tough!'

The consequence of not having been enabled to learn and respond to the baby's signals and own needs or empowered to cope with 'unpredictability' (Sachs 2005) during the neonatal unit stay, may hence result in a perceived insufficient milk supply and a subsequent early cessation of breastfeeding (Hill *et al.* 1994; Kavanaugh *et al.* 1995; Hill *et al.* 2007). Although some mothers in our study ceased breastfeeding as a result of breastfeeding becoming a task and not pleasurable, other mothers continued to breastfeed, despite not wanting to, out of a sense of obligation to fulfil the role of being a 'good mother'. Hence, when mothers sustain breastfeeding to accomplish 'good mothering', regardless of their own inclinations, breastfeeding may have a negative influence on the mother–baby relationship. This was illustrated by Petra, nine months after discharge:

'It's obvious that when you get such a feeding start, you'll take it home with you. Breastfeeding is just feeding and that's because of the hospital stay. I had a duty and a responsibility when I got home and that was to make him grow and survive. Breastfeeding was actually a bit like when I was working as a home help. I wanted to do a good job! You are so anxious that you won't be a good mum. If ordinary mothers feel that they want to breastfeed for six months, then we should breastfeed for eight months. We always have to be a little bit better – because I'm a preemie-mum. I've had a baby that's preterm, in danger and sensitive to infections and I feel that it's my duty to give him the best and that's breast milk. I feel that freedom came and I think my relationship with him improved when I weaned from breastfeeding. And yet I struggled for nine months.'

It may be hypothesised that the relationship between continuation of breastfeeding and a woman's sense of identity as a good mother are likely to be stronger in very pro-breastfeeding cultures seen in the Scandinavian countries. The strength of this discourse contributed to embarrassment towards bottle feeding in public as articulated by Sara: 'When I went to town for coffee or lunch with my friends, then I breastfed even though I had weaned, because I felt ashamed about using the bottle.' Another dominant discourse that strongly encourages women to persevere with breastfeeding stems from the *Global Strategy*'s emphasis upon exclusive breastfeeding for six months. Thus 'successful breastfeeding' is related to continuation of breastfeeding and, furthermore, breastfeeding in its purest form, i.e. no other fluids or foods given during this 'window' of time. The *Global Strategy* also advocates breastfeeding for up to two years or beyond along with appropriate complementary foods. In concordance with the *Global Strategy*, the health and welfare institutions in Sweden present strong discourses that normalise breastfeeding for all, as illustrated by Katarina: 'How do you know what's best for a baby? I imagine it's the National Board of Health and Welfare that provides the norms for what is to be said at the child health centres.' It could be argued that the *Global Strategy for Infant and Young Child Feeding* reduces the means to negotiate breastfeeding as it is stated: 'The vast majority of mothers can and should breastfeed' (WHO 2003, p. 10), in order to 'achieve optimal growth, development and health' in their babies (p. 8). With such a top-down directive, the conflict arises, in the staff and in the mothers, when breastfeeding becomes non-negotiable and assumed. As breastfeeding is such an intimate interplay, breastfeeding cannot be something that 'should' be executed and as Winnicott (1990) states, 'The mother's pleasure has to be there or else the whole procedure is dead, useless, and mechanical' (p. 27). I now argue for a balance between these discourses that consider the nutritional aspects and yet do not disregard the relational aspect of motherhood and breastfeeding.

3.6 Paradigm shift

A paradigm shift with regard to breastfeeding is required, especially in the area of breastfeeding in mothers of preterm infants. As breastfeeding is an intimate interaction, the professional discourses with focus on breast milk as nutrition and disregard for the relational interplay should be amended. Steps should hence be taken to increase the means of experiencing breastfeeding as a mutual pleasure in which fulfilment of the baby's behavioural and emotional needs, as well as the mother's physiological and emotional needs, are regarded. There is a persisting challenge to assist mothers and their preterm babies in the transition to breastfeeding with regard to these relational aspects. More research is required that focuses on care routines applied in the transitional phase from gavage feeding to breastfeeding, where not only weight gain or 'successful' breastfeeding rates are considered as outcome measures but where the relational aspects are also regarded. It is unacceptable that aspects of relationality are disregarded in breastfeeding of preterm babies, as these mothers and babies constitute a vulnerable population that is need of a relation-strengthening physical and emotional environment (Bruschweiler Stern 1998). In addition, the *Global Strategy*'s imperative that mothers should breastfeed ought to be discussed and reflected on in concordance with this, so that all mothers feel enabled and supported to breastfeed but still experience it as negotiable from the perspective of the individual. Its achievement requires an environmentally facilitative culture that supports the mother's belief in herself as a mother and enables her to feel free to act in accordance with her wishes (Winnicott 1990).

3.7 Conclusion

The examples from the Swedish setting indicate that an early initiation of skin-to-skin care followed by breastfeeding is perceived as relation-strengthening. Thus, of outmost importance is to eliminate the institutionalised separation between mothers and their babies, which occurs in most neonatal units. When the spatial environment facilitates the mother and baby to remain together and when the mother has the means to room-in with her baby 24 hours a day throughout the hospital stay, as recommended by the WHO (1998), this will become supportive for the mother-baby relation and for experiencing a mutually pleasurable breastfeeding. Such spatial environments will also enable mothers of preterm babies to initiate and sustain kangaroo mother care to include continuous skin-to-skin contact day and night throughout the stay, frequent and exclusive or nearly exclusive breastfeeding, and early discharge from hospital. This form of care is reported to be a successful way to empower mothers to become familiar with their babies and strengthen their own mothering at their own pace (Feldman *et al.* 2002; Conde-Agudelo *et al.* 2003). Even though skin-to-skin care or remaining in close proximity to each other may not be achievable in periods of highly intensive care, a majority of preterm babies can safely remain near their mothers during a hospital stay (De Carvalho Guerra Abecasis & Gomes 2006). A change of paradigm in neonatal care is required in which the institutional forces are limited and the role of the neonatal unit staff is altered from 'doing' and supervising to become a resource and a facilitator thus empowering mothers to become more self-sufficient. In addition, such a shift of paradigm will enhance mothers' means to experience breastfeeding as relational and not merely nutritional.

References

Als, H. & Gilkerson, L. (1997) The role of relationship-based developmentally supportive newborn intensive care in strengthening outcome of preterm infants. *Seminars in Perinatology*, **21**: 178–189.

Anderson, J.W., Johnstone, B.M. & Remley, D.T. (1999) Breast-feeding and cognitive development: a meta-analysis. *American Journal of Clinical Nutrition*, **70**: 525–535.

Ball, H.L., Ward-Platt, M.P., Heslop, E., Leech, S.J. & Brown, K.A. (2006) Randomised trial of infant sleep location on the postnatal ward. *Archives of Disease in Childhood*, **91**: 1005–1010.

Bowlby, J. (1969) *Attachment and Loss, Vol. 1 Attachment*. Random House, London.

Bruschweiler Stern, N. (1998) Early emotional care for mothers and infants. *Pediatrics*, **102**: 1278–1281.

Callen, J. & Pinelli, J. (2004) Incidence and duration of breastfeeding for term infants in Canada, United States, Europe, and Australia: a literature review. *Birth*, **31**: 285–292.

Conde-Agudelo, A., Diaz-Rossello, J.L. & Belizan, J.M. (2003) Kangaroo mother care to reduce morbidity and mortality in low birthweight infants. *Cochrane Database of Systematic Reviews*, (**2**): CD002771.

De Carvalho Guerra Abecasis, F. & Gomes, A. (2006) Rooming-in for preterm infants: how far should we go? Five-year experience at a tertiary hospital. *Acta Paediatrica*, **95**: 1567–1570.

Delobel-Ayoub, M., Kaminski, M., Marret, S., Burguet, A., Marchand, L., N'Guyen, S. *et al.* (2006) Behavioral outcome at 3 years of age in very preterm infants: the EPIPAGE study. *Pediatrics*, **117**: 1996–2005.

Dykes, F. (2005) 'Supply' and 'demand': breastfeeding as labour. *Social Science and Medicine*, **60**: 2283–2293.

Dykes, F. (2006) *Breastfeeding in Hospital: Mothers, Midwives, and the Production Line*. Routledge, London.

Edmond, K. & Bahl, R. (2007) *Optimal Feeding of Low-Birth-Weight Infants: Technical Review*. WHO, Geneva.

Eriksson, B.S. & Pehrsson, G. (2002) Evaluation of psycho-social support to parents with an infant born preterm. *Journal of Child Health Care*, **6**: 19–33.

Feldman, R., Eidelman, A.I., Sirota, L. & Weller, A. (2002) Comparison of skin-to-skin (kangaroo) and traditional care: parenting outcomes and preterm infant development. *Pediatrics*, **110**: 16–26.

Fenwick, J., Barclay, L. & Schmied, V. (1999) Activities and interactions in level II nurseries: a report of an ethnographic study. *Journal of Perinatal and Neonatal Nursing*, **13**: 53–65.

Flacking, R. (2007) Breastfeeding and becoming a mother – influences and experiences of mothers of preterm infants. Thesis, Department of Women's and Children's Health, Uppsala University.

Flacking, R., Nyqvist, K.H., Ewald, U. & Wallin, L. (2003) Long-term duration of breastfeeding in Swedish low birth weight infants. *Journal of Human Lactation*, **19**: 157–165.

Flacking, R., Ewald, U., Nyqvist, K.H. & Starrin, B. (2006) Trustful bonds: a key to 'becoming a mother' and to reciprocal breastfeeding. Stories of mothers of very preterm infants at a neonatal unit. *Social Science and Medicine*, **62**: 70–80.

Flacking, R., Ewald, U. & Starrin, B. (2007a) 'I wanted to do a good job': experiences of 'becoming a mother' and breastfeeding in mothers of very preterm infants after discharge from a neonatal unit. *Social Science and Medicine*, **64**: 2405–2416.

Flacking, R., Nyqvist, K.H. & Ewald, U. (2007b) Effects of socioeconomic status on breastfeeding duration in mothers of preterm and term infants. *European Journal of Public Health*, **17**: 579–584.

Flacking, R., Wallin, L. & Ewald, U. (2007c) Perinatal and socioeconomic determinants of breastfeeding duration in very preterm infants. *Acta Paediatrica*, **96**: 1126–1130.

Foucault, M. (1977) *Discipline and Punish: The Birth of the Prison*. Penguin Books, Harmodsworth.

Galtry, J. (2003) The impact on breastfeeding of labour market policy and practice in Ireland, Sweden, and the USA. *Social Science and Medicine*, **57**: 167–177.

Garel, M., Dardennes, M. & Blondel, B. (2007) Mothers' psychological distress 1 year after very preterm childbirth. Results of the EPIPAGE qualitative study. *Child: Care, Health and Development*, **33**: 137–143.

Goffman, E. (1961) *Asylums: Essays on the Social Situation of Mental Patients and Other Inmates*. Anchor Books, New York.

Hannula, L., Kaunonen, M. & Tarkka, M.T. (2008) A systematic review of professional support interventions for breastfeeding. *Journal of Clinical Nursing*, **17**: 1132–1143.

Hauck, Y.L. & Irurita, V.F. (2002) Constructing compatibility: managing breast-feeding and weaning from the mother's perspective. *Qualitative Health Research*, **12**: 897–914.

Hill, P.D., Hanson, K.S. & Mefford, A.L. (1994) Mothers of low birthweight infants: breastfeeding patterns and problems. *Journal of Human Lactation*, **10**: 169–176.

Hill, P.D., Aldag, J.C., Zinaman, M. & Chatterton, R.T. (2007) Predictors of preterm infant feeding methods and perceived insufficient milk supply at week 12 postpartum. *Journal of Human Lactation*, **23**: 32–38, quiz 39–43.

Holmgren, P.A. & Hogberg, U. (2001) The very preterm infant – a population-based study. *Acta Obstetricia et Gynecologica Scandinavica*, **80**: 525–531.

Isaacson, L.J. (2006) Steps to successfully breastfeed the premature infant. *Neonatal Network*, **25**: 77–86.

Jackson, K., Ternestedt, B.M. & Schollin, J. (2003) From alienation to familiarity: experiences of mothers and fathers of preterm infants. *Journal of Advanced Nursing*, **43**: 120–129.

Kavanaugh, K., Mead, L., Meier, P. & Mangurten, H.H. (1995) Getting enough: mothers' concerns about breastfeeding a preterm infant after discharge. *Journal of Obstetric, Gynecologic and Neonatal Nursing*, **24**: 23–32.

Kavanaugh, K., Meier, P., Zimmermann, B. & Mead, L. (1997) The rewards outweigh the efforts: breastfeeding outcomes for mothers of preterm infants. *Journal of Human Lactation*, **13**: 15–21.

Kennell, J.H. & Klaus, M.H. (1998) Bonding: recent observations that alter perinatal care. *Pediatrics in Review*, **19**: 4–12.

Klaus, M. (1998) Mother and infant: early emotional ties. *Pediatrics*, **102**: 1244–1246.

Klaus, M.H., Kennell, J.H. & Klaus, P.H. (1996) *Bonding: building the foundations of secure attachment and independence*. Addison Wesley, Reading.

Kliethermes, P.A., Cross, M.L., Lanese, M.G., Johnson, K.M. & Simon, S.D. (1999) Transitioning preterm infants with nasogastric tube supplementation: increased likelihood of breastfeeding. *Journal of Obstetric, Gynecologic and Neonatal Nursing*, **28**: 264–273.

Law, S.M., Dunn, O.M., Wallace, L.M. & Inch, S.A. (2007) Breastfeeding best start study: training midwives in a 'hands off' positioning and attachment intervention. *Maternal and Child Nutrition*, **3**: 194–205.

Lucas, A., Morley, R. & Cole, T.J. (1998) Randomised trial of early diet in preterm babies and later intelligence quotient. *British Medical Journal*, **317**: 1481–1487.

Marlow, N., Wolke, D., Bracewell, M.A. & Samara, M. (2005) Neurologic and developmental disability at six years of age after extremely preterm birth. *New England Journal of Medicine*, **352**: 9–19.

Marshall, J.L., Godfrey, M. & Renfrew, M.J. (2007) Being a 'good mother': managing breastfeeding and merging identities. *Social Science and Medicine*, **65**: 2147–2159.

Morton, J.A. (2002) Strategies to support extended breastfeeding of the premature infant. *Advances in Neonatal Care*, **2**: 267–282.

Murphy, E. (1999) 'Breast is best': infant feeding decisions and maternal deviance. *Sociology of Health and Illness*, **21**: 187–208.

Nye, C. (2008) Transitioning premature infants from gavage to breast. *Neonatal Network*, **27**: 7–13.

Nyqvist, K.H. (2008) Early attainment of breastfeeding competence in very preterm infants. *Acta Paediatrica*, **97**: 776–781.

Nyqvist, K.H., Ewald, U. & Sjoden, P.O. (1996) Supporting a preterm infant's behaviour during breastfeeding: a case report. *Journal of Human Lactation*, **12**: 221–228.

Nyqvist, K.H., Sjoden, P.O. & Ewald, U. (1999) The development of preterm infants' breastfeeding behavior. *Early Human Development*, **55**: 247–264.

Petersen, K., Petersen, M. & Flacking, R. (2004) Sensitive to what the mother wants – a qualitative study regarding staffs' experience of supporting mothers and infants in the transition from gavage-feeding to breastfeeding in the neonatal unit. Department of Health and Society, Dalarna University.

Righard, L. & Alade, M.O. (1990) Effect of delivery room routines on success of first breast-feed. *Lancet*, **336**: 1105–1107.

Sachs, M. (2005) Following the line: an ethnographic study of the influence of routine baby weighing on breastfeeding women in a town in the Northwest of England. Unpublished thesis, Maternal & Infant Nutrition & Nurture Unit, University of Central Lancashire, UK.

Schanler, R.J., Shulman, R.J. & Lau, C. (1999) Feeding strategies for premature infants: beneficial outcomes of feeding fortified human milk versus preterm formula. *Pediatrics*, **103**: 1150–1157.

Schmied, V. & Barclay, L. (1999) Connection and pleasure, disruption and distress: women's experience of breastfeeding. *Journal of Human Lactation*, **15**: 325–334.

Scott, J.A. & Mostyn, T. (2003) Women's experiences of breastfeeding in a bottle-feeding culture. *Journal of Human Lactation*, **19**: 270–277.

Scott, J.A., Binns, C.W., Oddy, W.H. & Graham, K.I. (2006) Predictors of breastfeeding duration: evidence from a cohort study. *Pediatrics*, **117**: e646–655.

Singer, L.T., Salvator, A., Guo, S., Collin, M., Lilien, L. & Baley, J. (1999) Maternal psychological distress and parenting stress after the birth of a very low-birth-weight infant. *Journal of the American Medical Association*, **281**: 799–805.

Small, M. (1998) *Our Babies, Ourselves: How Biology and Culture Shape the Way We Parent*. Anchor Books, New York.

Swedish Social Insurance Agency (2005) *Social Insurance in Sweden 2005*. Swedish Social Insurance Agency, Stockholm. [In Swedish].

Sweet, L. (2006) Breastfeeding a preterm infant and the objectification of breastmilk. *Breastfeeding Review*, **14**: 5–13.

Sweet, L. (2008) Birth of a very low birth weight preterm infant and the intention to breastfeed 'naturally'. *Women Birth*, **21**: 13–20.

The National Board of Health and Welfare (2007) Breast-feeding, children born 2005. *Statistics – Health and Diseases* 2007: **12**. Centre for Epidemiology, Stockholm.

Weimers, L., Svensson, K., Dumas, L., Naver, L. & Wahlberg, V. (2006) Hands-on approach during breastfeeding support in a neonatal intensive care unit: a qualitative study of Swedish mothers' experiences. *International Breastfeeding Journal*, **1**: 20.

WHO (1998) *Evidence for the Ten Steps to Successful Breastfeeding*. WHO, Geneva.

WHO (2003) *Global Strategy for Infant and Young Child Feeding*. WHO, Geneva.

Widstrom, A.M., Wahlberg, V., Matthiesen, A.S., Eneroth, P., Uvnas-Moberg, K., Werner, S. *et al.* (1990) Short-term effects of early suckling and touch of the nipple on maternal behaviour. *Early Human Development*, **21**: 153–163.

Winnicott, D.W. (1990) *The Child, the Family, and the Outside World*. Addison-Wesley, Reading.

4 From 'to Learn' to 'to Know': Women's Embodied Knowledge of Breastfeeding in Japan

Naoko Hashimoto and Christine McCourt

4.1 Introduction

This chapter focuses on biocultural influences on infant feeding in the context of Japanese society. Centred on women's experiences and relationship with their babies, it illuminates the different influences at play in women's experiences and practices, including those of Japanese traditional culture, society and philosophy, and recent social changes in response to the US-led post-war administration, globalisation and greater openness to 'Western' cultural influences. The chapter illustrates that, although Japanese society retains a primarily 'breastfeeding culture', supported by various features of Japanese traditional culture, aspects of recent social and technological change, including modernisation of the maternity services under Western influence, have undermined women's exclusive breastfeeding, and the practice of mixed feeding has increased considerably. Japanese women continue to see breastfeeding as the norm, and are commonly committed to breastfeeding for long durations. However, the influence of health professionals and services, media and commercial influences, which have tended to undermine women's confidence in and practise of exclusive breastfeeding, interacting with the philosophical acceptance of bodily limitation within Japanese culture, have led to currently high rates of mixed feeding, despite these positive norms.

The steep decline of exclusive breastfeeding and increased rates of partial breast-feeding[i] been a political concern in Japan since the 1970s. Historically, infant feeding and weaning practice[ii] guidelines in Japan have fallen short of the World Health Organization's *Global Strategy for Infant and Young Child Feeding* (WHO 2003), having recommended introduction of weaning foods earlier than six months and cessation of breastfeeding before two years. However more recent government recommendations are more in alignment with the *Global Strategy* recommendations (Japan Ministry of Health, Labour and Welfare 2000, 2007). Furthermore

---

[i] The term used in the Japanese context translates as 'mixed feeding'.
[ii] In Japanese, 'introducing food to children' is called '*ri-nyuu*', which is translated into 'weaning'. Since the Japanese original guideline used the term '*ri-nyuu*', we use the English term 'weaning' in this chapter, rather than the term 'complementary feeding', as used in the WHO Global Strategy.

there is an emphasis in the new guidelines on supporting infant feeding with regard to developing a healthy relationship between mothers and their babies (Japan Ministry of Health, Labour and Welfare 2007). The 2007 guidelines recommend introduction of complementary food between five and six months and the cessation of breastfeeding is recommended between 12 and 18 months. Also, the previous guidelines followed a hierarchical style, giving 'instructions' to mothers with a rigid time schedule, whereas the new guidelines provide more flexibility recognising parental choice. An interesting observation from reading the discussion records (Japan Ministry of Health, Labour and Welfare 2006), is that the focus of the discussion centred on keeping the balance between the existing and the revised guidelines, a pragmatic or mediatory approach intended to avoid creating pressure about exclusive breastfeeding, to avoid confusion in weaning practice, and also to create a relaxed social environment for all mothers, regardless of their method of feeding. This reflects the Japanese cultural value system, which negates a clear division between the inside and outside of cultural values and thereby encourages syncretism.

The study we draw upon here arose out of Hashimoto's concerns relating to the public use of the 1995 infant feeding and weaning guidelines. As a Japanese mid-wife, she viewed Japanese mixed feeding as 'a cultural production', which emerged from the result of negotiation between the traditional Japanese breastfeeding and the modern social and cultural changes. From her observation in the community, Japanese women experienced difficulties in sustaining exclusive breastfeeding: they had a strong wish to breastfeed their babies, but somehow it did not work for many of them. To investigate these concerns, Hashimoto undertook a study of Japanese women's experience of breastfeeding in the community in Tokyo where she works as a community midwife. Using a narrative ethnographic approach, the study aimed to describe breastfeeding from women's point of view, to learn from women and their babies, in order to fill the gap between the medical and cultural discourse 'breast is best' and the women's actual experience of it. In the current Japanese social context, 99% of childbirth takes place in hospitals; women stay for five or six days after birth and are expected to learn 'proper' breastfeeding. Breastfeeding policy and practice varies in each institution but 'mother and baby in separation', 'regular feeding', and 'usage of bottles' are still found as a common medical discourse, even though some of the institutions are working towards the WHO/UNICEF Baby-Friendly Hospital Initiative[iii] and various lay and non-governmental organisation (NGO) groups are actively working to support breastfeeding.

In Japanese public discourse, breastfeeding is talked about as a strong cultural expectation for a mother. All health practitioners talk with a mother about infant feeding, thus any problem in breastfeeding is viewed as an individual difficulty. The accumulation of individual difficulty in breastfeeding is found in the national survey, which showed a decline of numbers in exclusive breastfeeding and the

[iii] The number of Baby-Friendly accredited hospitals reached 56 by October 2008 (Japan Breast Feeding Association 2008).

substantial number of women mixed feeding[iv] since the 1960s. The question was, therefore, how could we study the gap that exists between 'an individual problem' and 'a social phenomenon'. Using Western anthropological concepts, this study defined it as 'researching' between 'micro' and 'macro' perspectives of human life. Using an ethnographic approach, each individual life was studied as an example representing the cultural features of the phenomenon. Small-scale and local practices, experiences and perspectives were studied embedded within their larger social and cultural context (Eriksen & Nielsen 2001). The study showed that Japanese women's pragmatic approach of 'negotiation' enables them to maintain higher rates of breastfeeding (exclusive and partial breastfeeding) with a baby-centred approach in the face of significant social change, compared with many technologically developed societies.

The chapter begins by briefly describing the methodology. Before discussing some of the key themes, we look at the social and historical background of infant feeding and care in Japan, since these are important to an understanding of the complexity of feeding practices today. To understand the experience in a cross-cultural frame, we also refer to two anthropological concepts: the concept of 'bodily experience', in which the human's bodily parts are engaged with the event; and the concept of 'habitus', which argues that people's ordinary actions are unconsciously learnt through seeing other people 'doing' and through embodied practices in interaction with the social and physical environment (Bourdieu 1987). The action may be universal, but the meaning is variable as it is constructed through social and cultural elements. We conclude by putting forward some implications for the promotion of breastfeeding across different and complex cultural contexts, and try to make a bridge between the Western notions and Japanese notions of breastfeeding. Finally, the implications for the WHO *Global Strategy* to support breastfeeding and healthy infant feeding practices are drawn out.

4.2   The study

The study was designed to investigate the initial question of why some of the women did and some did not breastfeed their babies. Although there may be differences in hospital care settings, still there are issues that the professional or authoritative knowledge is failing to look at, so the study attempted to illuminate this 'missing part' of the knowledge. Therefore, the study used an ethnographic/narrative approach, through which the researcher can see and talk to women at the same time, and everyday life experience in the field can support understanding of the cultural aspects of breastfeeding. The main part of the study involved six women's narratives at approximately one-month intervals until their baby's first birthday, and a closing interview undertaken at between 14 and 18 months following the birth, to cover the time around cessation of breastfeeding.

[iv] By mixed-feeding, we refer to the introduction of formula milk feeds to complement breastfeeding. By exclusive breastfeeding we refer to breastfeeding without the introduction of formula feeds, or complementary foods, within the first six months of a baby's life.

4.3   Social and historical background

This section looks first at aspects of Japanese culture that have influenced the continuing Japanese cultural preference for breastfeeding, and then turns to socio-historical influences on more recent development of 'mixed feeding' as a cultural practice. Figure 4.1 shows the shift of infant feeding pattern in Japan, as collected in a retrospective survey, every five years, from 1960 to 2000 (Mother's and Children's Health and Welfare Association 2004). Table 4.1 compares the Japanese figures with UK rates (based on Hamlyn *et al.* 2000).

4.3.1   Japanese people's traditional attitudes towards breastfeeding

Looking historically, a number of cultural traditions and rituals supported the strong breastfeeding culture in Japan. The British social anthropologist Macfarlane (1997) argued that women in Japanese society traditionally had the longest duration of breastfeeding among the Asian countries. In Japan, dairy farming was not

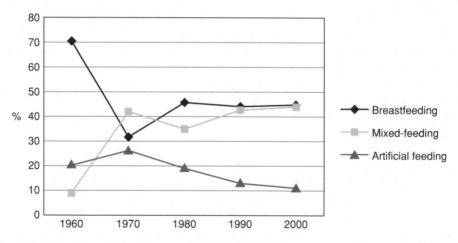

Figure 4.1   Feeding of infants by age 1960–2000. Based on surveys on the growth of infants and preschool children, 1960, 1970, 1980, 1990 and 2000 (Mother's and Children's Health and Welfare Association 2004).

Table 4.1   The percentage of breastfeeding (exclusive and partial breastfeeding) rate in 2000 in the UK (based on Hamlyn *et al.* 2000) and in Japan (based on Mother's and Children's Health and Welfare Association 2004)

UK (%)	Birth: 69	1 week: 55	6 weeks: 43	4 months: 28	6 months: 21
Japan (%)	N/A		1 month and over, under 2 months: 88.8	3 months and over, under 4 months: 69.9	4 months and over, under 5 months: 60.4

traditionally practised, so that use of animal milk was not an established substitute for breastfeeding, and use of wet-nursing was rare and confined to royalty and aristocracy. As a result, Japanese culture took a unique and relatively recent form of shift in breastfeeding from 'own mother' to 'bottles of formula' (Yamamoto 1983), whereas most cultures experienced a shift from 'own mother' to 'animal's milk', 'wet-nurse' and then 'bottles of formula' (Battersby 2006). Although current-day Japanese mothers could be considered as the second generation of mixed feeding culture, most Western societies have already reached the third or fourth generation that departed from the idea of 'breastfeeding one's own baby' as the norm.

Until the 1960s, when mass production of powder milk was established, the mother having enough breast milk was seen as central to her baby's survival (Yamamoto 1983). Therefore each locality has its own rituals and wisdom for the women to have enough breast milk. For example, childbirth and infant feeding was supported by female relatives cooking foods rich in fluid and carbohydrates such as miso soup and fish, rice and noodles, and also herbs and vegetables such as 'renkon' (lotus roots), 'hakobe' (chickweed) and 'gobou' (burdock roots) (Nishikawa 1992). Women and their own mothers also commonly go to the Shinto temple to pray. Natural objects such as 'ichou' (a maidenhair tree or ginkgo) or a mountain and objects that look like a woman's breast are also a focus for praying (Sawada 1983).

Practical care such as breast massage was common. For example, a childcare book written in 1703 advised that women's breasts should be massaged every day or should be suckled by a girl aged under 4 years to help breast milk flow and prevent engorgement (Sawada 1983). In the modern context, a Japanese obstetrician referred to 'breast massage' as a medical skill and launched it as a part of midwifery education in the 1930s (Oketani 1983). In the 1980s, a Japanese midwife developed breast massage skills further, under the name of 'oketani' massage (Oketani 1983), and 'self-care massage technique' was introduced by an obstetrician in the 1990s (Nezu 1992). Hospitals today commonly have an outpatient section of 'breast care' or 'breast massage', for women with mastitis, insufficient breast milk, and also for care related to completing breastfeeding. This hospital-based support programme is also recommended in the current infant feeding guidelines (Japan Ministry of Health, Labour and Welfare 2007).

The Japanese breastfeeding culture was supported by people's child-centred attitudes, and the physical closeness between a mother and her baby, which was an important way of protecting children's health. Although farming was the main family business, a baby's own mother or other family members such as a grandmother and other siblings carried them on their back ('onbu') while they worked, which made it easy for the baby to be breastfed whenever and wherever he or she wished. Mothers and children commonly slept together ('soine') and children were always carried by somebody's back or arms. This Japanese tradition was described as the heaven of children ('kodomo-tengoku' in Japanese) in Western travel diaries in the early twentieth century (Kiriyama 2004).

Breastfeeding was traditionally used in a social ritual, a way of bonding community members, called 'chichi-tsuke' ('chichi' means 'breasts', 'tsuke' means 'attaching'). Several women in the community breastfed the new baby as part of this ritual, and then they took a role of community parents, supporting the new parents. It was a people's wisdom in which the community as a whole took care of the new parents and their babies. Similar social rituals of breastfeeding, such as 'milk-kinship' have been described by anthropologists in other cultures (Maher 1992; Parkes 2005). In the modern Japanese context, physical closeness is described as the importance of 'skin-ship[v]', which is seen as 'enhancing children's state of health' (Japan Ministry of Health, Labour and Welfare 2007).

One of the modern shifts in Japanese breastfeeding culture may be related to people's attitudes towards women's upper body. In Japan, women's breasts were not traditionally seen as a source of embarrassment, since people adopted a Japanese manner (*'mite-minufuri'*) of pretending not to see. This is considered a learnt behaviour; although people were living in traditional Japanese housing, sharing rooms with other family members, private space was created by people's tacit manner. Breastfeeding in public was commonly seen up to the 1960s. However, Westernised views of women's bodies transformed people's perceptions; thus breastfeeding in public is not found in current cultural practice.

4.3.2   The post-war administration and the shift in breastfeeding

Before the 1960s, Japanese childbirth mainly took place at home or in a small community hut, in which the women came to stay for childbirth and female relatives came to look after the new mother and the baby. The first term for professional 'midwife' (*san-ba*: *'san'* means birth, *'ba'* means older women) was recorded in the early sixteenth century, and midwives were considered an equal and invited to family rituals following the childbirth. The certification system for medical professionals was launched in 1874, and the first rules of midwife registration were issued in 1875. The Japanese midwives supported childbirth at home as well as helping women with breastfeeding and overall care of the baby.

The traditional way of childbirth and mutual aid by the community members, and the role of formally trained midwives, was reformed under the supervision of the American General Head Quarters (GHQ) during the post-war reconstruction (Oobayashi 1985). Births started to shift into hospital settings, and since the 1980s, 99% of births take place in hospital, where regular feeding is taught by the clock, baby and mother in separation, and supplementary bottle feeds are commonly practised as hospital protocol. The Japanese hospital protocol was developed in the 1960s using North American hospital practices as a model. This model advocated restricted timing of feeds, separation of mother and baby, with mothers only being permitted to view their baby through a nursery window and being summoned to a feeding room every four hours. They were required to put on a gown and paper cap and wash their hands before entering the feeding room. The baby's weight was checked before handing to the mothers, and the mother's nipples were wiped by a

---

[v] This is a Japanese-English word, presumably created by combining the English terms 'skin-to-skin contact' and 'relationship'.

medicated swab before and after feeding, and the baby was latched onto the mother's breast for a limited time (Pearse 1990). Although Japanese medical professionals were working with these protocols, the American hospitals then abolished them due to the negative impacts on breastfeeding and mother–baby relationships, and started 'rooming-in' practices (Fukuda 1996). The WHO/UNICEF Baby-Friendly Initiative has been recommended in Japanese health policy since the 1990s, and the hospitals started to change their policies. However, hospital practices typically still do not meet the initiative's standards. Papers discussing the way of introducing 'a rooming-in system' in hospital practice, i.e. baby being next to the mother in a cot still recommended some traditional practices, for example a period of 24 hours of careful observation of the newborn baby in an infant room before rooming-in commenced, mothers cleaning their nipples with wipes before and after feeds, instructing the mothers when and how they need to add formula milk or glucose water after breastfeeding and test weighing to determine if supplementation was required (Senoo et al. 1995; Hachiya 1998; Sueshige et al. 1998; Takei 1998).

The traditional Japanese breastfeeding practice, having the longest duration of breastfeeding internationally, was also changed when an American childcare book was translated into Japanese in 1966, and widely read as a guide to modern child-care (Yamamoto 1983). As a result, breastfeeding came to be practised in a very restricted manner. Such 'Western' cultural practices around childcare have been exported as authoritative knowledge to a number of cultures, later leaving a legacy of mother and infant 'unfriendly' practices, as Western hospitals begin to question and then abandon them as 'not evidence based' (Jordan 2003).

The dramatic decline of exclusive breastfeeding between 1960 and 1970 may also have been influenced by the rapid change in people's lifestyle in the 1960s. Young couples moved into cities, living as a nuclear family, and housing, furniture and product design also changed accordingly. When a young couple has a baby, the new mother needs support but the husband is often too busy at work. Thus the woman usually goes back to her own parents' home, from 36 weeks in pregnancy until one month after birth, and her own mother looks after the new mother and new baby. This system, called 'sato-gaeri' in Japanese ('sato' means 'an old nest' and 'gaeri' means 'returning'), appeared as a modern cultural practice in the 1970s, in response to such changes. A Japanese traditional custom is also practised, in which the woman stays in bed for the first two weeks. Washing, cleaning, and cooking are all prohibited, since this is thought to block the path of blood that would affect breastfeeding, delay physical recovery from birth and, in the later stage of life, cause a severe menopause. The woman is encouraged to breastfeed her baby as often as possible. This family support could be considered as positive practice, which draws on older traditions of family support following childbirth. However, since the previous generation of mothers – today's grandmothers – were encouraged to introduce bottled and formula milk, and many did not exclusively breastfeed, this is not necessarily effective for supporting breastfeeding, as will be explained in the next section. Grandmother's experiences, influenced by modern 'expert' discourses of infant feeding under Western (especially US) influence from the 1960s, has made it more difficult for them to support the traditional norms of breastfeeding.

The rapid shift into 'mixed feeding', which ensued in this period, was explicitly promoted by medical discourses. In the 1950s, a group of paediatricians announced a recommendation of 'optimal breastfeeding' in which babies should be breastfed, but 5–10% of total feeding should be by another supplement such as thin water squeezed from steamed rice (Takahashi 1996). Once powdered milk became available at reasonable cost and quality, it was advocated as 5–10% of baby's total intake. Women were instructed in this feeding method as it was considered to constitute 'safer breastfeeding' by the public health services (Takahashi 1996). Although this was later found to be suboptimal practice, and exclusive breastfeeding was advocated as the 'best breastfeeding' from the 1970s, current grandmothers are likely to have mixed-fed their babies, having been taught this as authoritative knowledge. In the 'sato-gaeri' settings, new mothers experienced a conflict with their own mothers, while the grandmother became a person who told her daughter to add powder milk.

In the Japanese medical and public discourses, it is common to hear the phrase 'Just in case your baby has not got enough'. This discourse also shows the lack of confidence of medical professionals to be able to reassure new mothers about the sufficiency of their feeding. Yamamoto (1983) argues that more theoretical writings about breastfeeding meant the loss of common sense or embodied knowledge of breastfeeding as expert books were produced for both professional and popular reading. This is indicative of different forms of knowledge impacting on practice and privileging particular forms of learning: less theoretical or more embodied forms are progressively devalued and a problematic space is opened up between theory and practice – as in our case, between the authoritative practice and the everyday experience of infant feeding.

4.4   Breastfeeding as bodily experience: findings from Japanese women's narratives

In this section we discuss key themes from the women's narratives to provide insight into Japanese women's embodied knowledge of breastfeeding in the modern Japanese social and cultural context. The key theme to emerge was breastfeeding as bodily experience, which has been described by Ericksen and Nielsen (2001) as people's physical parts, such as hands, mouth, fingers, being engaged with their experiences. The key concept of 'bodily experience' as described in our study is explored in three dimensions; 'bodily reflection', 'bodily communication' and 'bodily limitations', which are used to illuminate the shift in the women's experience of breastfeeding from 'to learn' to ' to know'.

4.4.1   Bodily reflection

The six women involved in the study gave birth at different hospitals, and their first breastfeeding was initiated with instruction from the hospital nurses or midwives.

In the closing interview, Hashimoto asked about their feelings about the hospital stay, which they did not talk about during the preceding interviews. One woman (who had continued to breastfeed) related this as follows;

> *'Staying in hospital . . . five days' stay was enough to know about breastfeeding. Breastfeeding was different from something like . . . I do once or twice a day . . . At least, I did five or six times, and I felt hospital stay was long enough to know about it . . .'*
>
> Mrs M, interviewed at 18 months post partum

Another woman said:

> *'Hospital stay . . . it was not enough to learn breastfeeding . . .'*
>
> Mrs H, interviewed at 13 months post partum

These two excerpts illuminated the contrast in the bodily experience of exclusive breastfeeding and mixed feeding. The women's experience is revealed by the key terms 'to learn' and 'to know'. Mrs M, the first woman, stopped using bottles on the third day in hospital. She decided not to use bottles following her feeling of her breasts becoming full, and seeing that her night gown was wetted by breast milk. By the time of the first interview, breastfeeding seemed to have become part of everyday life. Following her narratives, the message of 'the woman and her baby in tune' appeared after baby's fourth month. For the first few months, her baby cried frequently during the night and was diagnosed as having eczema at four months. Thus Mrs M chose to go with a restricted diet, avoiding eggs and flour products in order to continue breastfeeding. Breastfeeding was practised in baby's accord, which came to 14 times a day maximum. However, she did not have any doubt that 'her baby had enough' with her husband supporting this perception. Her own mother, who lived near her home and visited them almost every day, did not say anything to her about her breastfeeding, but told her to follow her intuition, rather than reading the childcare books. In her narrative, her husband and her mother took the role of 'supporting her in silence', which is called '*mi-mamoru*' in Japanese ('*mi*' means 'seeing' and '*mamoru*' means 'protecting').

The shift from 'to learn' to 'to know' seems to be hindered by other people's interactions about breastfeeding:

> *'I have not enough breast milk . . . because my baby starts to cry one hour after breastfeeding, so I used formula milk. At night, I use formula milk, and then next time I breastfeed . . . When the hospital midwife said I did not have enough breast milk, I was so disappointed. My mother always tells "breast milk is best" . . . she seemed to have a lot of breast milk . . . cannot understand why I cannot have breast milk . . . I would like to breastfeed as much as I could . . . so I feel a bit stressed . . .'*
>
> Mrs H, interviewed at one month post partum

Mrs H's mother gave practical help, which supported her child caring, but her narratives were characterised by the sense of 'nagging'. Mrs H continued breastfeeding while also using formula milk:

'I continue to breastfeed, but I feel she does not get enough. She does not cry, but I just feel she does not get enough. So I add formula milk twice a day after breastfeeding. I started to think to add some food . . . maybe rice gruel? . . . but is it still too early? . . .'

Mrs H, interviewed at four months post partum

This excerpt illuminates a shift, since this was the first time she used the words 'I feel', rather than 'I think'. As a result of breastfeeding, even though it was practised as a form of partial breastfeeding, the shift from 'to learn' to 'to know' appeared after five months in her narratives.

In the narratives of Mrs N, who was a second-time mother and experienced mixed feeding for the first child, mixed feeding appeared as her embodied knowledge of breastfeeding:

'I breastfeed seven . . . eight times a day. If he does not get enough, I use milk . . . once or twice a day. I just breastfeed, when he cries . . . when I feel my breast is empty, after dealing with a lot of housework, I just go straight to milk [here this means bottle feeding] . . . From the experience of eldest, I know I could not get enough breast milk . . . I made a lot of efforts for the first baby . . . ate more, and slept more, but it did not work and I felt so miserable and depressed . . . From the experience of eldest, I know breastfeeding [here this means mixed feeding] helps my baby to grow healthy . . .'

Mrs N, interviewed at one month post partum

The women's breastfeeding practice, whether exclusive or partial breastfeeding, was performed in an embedded manner. The previous experience of infant feeding was used to enhance the process of shift from 'to learn' to 'to know', and physical closeness in breastfeeding is a key to enabling this shift to take place.

Using the concept of bodily experience, breastfeeding could be defined as a bodily performance in which a woman and her baby's bodily parts are engaged in inter-actions and reflect each other's bodily responses. For example, the women could feel the rhythms in their baby's suckling and also how their breasts responded, which we refer to as 'bodily reflection'. The process of shifting from 'to learn' to 'to know' seems to relate to each woman's as well as baby's level of bodily reflection.

The women also learnt breastfeeding by seeing other women breastfeeding, which also enhances their bodily reflection. Referring to the Japanese cultural ways of leaning, 'silence' is considered as a key element of stimulating 'inner reflections'. In traditional physical performances, such as the 'Japanese tea ceremony', silence is used to reflect one's own self. The process of teaching is started by observing the teacher or other senior students' performance. The students are expected to have 'good eyes' to know the key elements of a practice. The new students are directly engaged in the performance and are expected to repeat it until they come to know it. This cultural way of learning was also found in the women's breastfeeding. They used the theoretical knowledge later, in the advanced stage of the 'learning process.'

4.4.2 Bodily communication

It became clear through the observations of interactions between women and babies during the study that other people's attitudes influenced the process of bodily reflection. A woman and her baby needed a quiet and relaxed environment to sense each other's bodily reflections. Too much talk from others, even from hospital staff teaching how to breastfeed, may hinder the onset of bodily reflection because the baby and the woman, as a unique couple, need a time and space on their own to be able to immerse themselves in breastfeeding. After several months, once women latched their baby on, they said things such as 'it will not take long', or after some time 'he will go to sleep very soon', while touching baby's hands and feet and sensing they were getting warmer. They did not have this skill, which can be described as 'bodily communication', from the beginning; rather it developed over time.

Once a woman developed bodily communication, her life started to gain the sense of 'prediction'. The women could estimate the interval for the next breastfeeding, and managed other activities with a sense of 'control'. The meaning of 'control' in Japanese is not quite the same as it can be in English. In the women's narratives, the feeling of 'control' was flowing in their life settings, when the woman and her baby were living in 'natural rhythm'. This cultural attitude towards control reflects the Japanese cultural belief that the best state of health is based on living as a part of 'nature' (Jitsukawa 1997). The women perceived that breastfeeding was best, as it is the way of living with natural cycles. In contrast to Western studies, where many women describe a greater sense of control with bottle feeding because the amount of milk fed can be measured (Marshall *et al.* 2007), the woman who shifted on to only bottle feeding in baby's first month did not experience this:

> 'everyone said . . . like it is unusual for babies to get up for night feeding after three months. The amount of milk is . . . still 160 ml for each feeding . . . he only takes 160 ml from the bottle . . . when he took 180 ml, he was unsettled and then vomited. At night, he takes 140 ml, or 120 ml, or sometimes 100 ml. I have to just wait until he stops, it is very tiring . . . He might have not get enough . . .'
>
> Mrs I, interviewed at three months post partum

Mrs I showed her anxiety that her baby was not bottle fed enough. She knew the amount of formula milk was enough by seeing the bottles, and also by knowing her baby showed a good weight gain at each month. The objective measurements and numbers did not give the sense of control in child caring, as Mrs I knew, from seeing other breastfed babies, that 'physical closeness in breastfeeding' and 'cuddling in bottle feeding' were different. As a result, she required more support from her family as well as advice from medical professionals.

Looking at breastfeeding as 'a shift', it was clear that breastfeeding did not form a clear or predictable pattern and 'normal' feeding did not conform to the accounts of textbooks or the patterns and intervals practised in hospitals. The women perceived this as a normal part of breastfeeding, as the natural cycle does not always follow a fixed pattern. For example, Mrs O, a second-time mother stated:

'She started to cry at night . . . maybe the weather is too hot and she is thirsty. I do not like the idea of night feeding at this age, but I think it is easier to latch her on my breasts than giving other liquid from the bottles . . .'

Mrs O, interviewed at six months post partum

Women's practices appeared to change in relation to the seasons, the mother and baby's physical condition, and maternal stress levels. For example, during rainy seasons, complementary food was sustained and breastfeeding practised more to prevent the baby from contracting diarrhoea.

When the women attended their baby's three to four months' follow-up clinic, the public health nurses checked their infant feeding, and taught when and how to introduce complementary food. Following the professional advice, the women tried complementary food. However, if they found their babies did not eat, they simply put aside the medical advice and continued their breastfeeding. This 'baby-centred manner' was based on their bodily communication, which the women used as the best resource to guide their way of living with the baby.

The idea of bodily communication is also found in the process of cessation of breastfeeding, in which mothers tried to respect the baby's wish as well as their wish:

'I would like to wait the time . . . my daughter tells like, . . . thank you, mum, I do not need breastfeeding! . . . I believe . . . I feel it will happen . . . I can hear the child's crying, he is a bit older than mine . . . I know the mother is trying to finish breastfeeding. . . . But . . . I do not like the idea . . .'

Mrs M, interviewed ten months post partum

The women experienced a pressure to cease breastfeeding by 12 months from friends and medical professionals:

'I would like to breastfeed as long as I can, as long as he likes . . . maybe two years old . . . I was advised by other breastfeeding mothers. . . . Do not mention about breastfeeding to any medical professionals after 12 months . . . otherwise I would be labelled as a difficult mother . . .'

Mrs K, interviewed ten months post partum

Concerning the medical advice, the timing of finishing breastfeeding was still found to vary considerably. Moreover, the women were advised that it would be better to cease breastfeeding within a year as it would become more difficult to stop after 12 months. Somehow the idea that long-term breastfeeding spoils children appeared as a common idea among Japanese medical professionals. As a result, the women ceased to talk about their breastfeeding after 12 months, which they described as a way of avoiding unnecessary conflicts with medical professionals. In this context, bodily communication took a salient role for making the process of 'stopping breastfeeding' a negotiation process with their babies.

Overall, from the six women's narratives, the women and their babies required around five months for fully developing bodily communication with their baby. In the case of the second-time mothers, they also needed to develop bodily communications with a new baby while they were looking after their elder child, which meant they spent five months becoming 'a whole family in tune'. The process of breastfeeding required an environment where the woman and her baby could spend their time and space in their own accord. In addition, other people's roles of 'being with a new mother' appeared with the sense of 'sharing the responsibility about child caring with her', which is captured in the Japanese concept of '*mi-mamoru*'. Looking at the hospital environment, when the hospital midwives supported women's breastfeeding with the sense of '*mi-mamoru*', that is less teaching but more supportive in their attitudes, this seemed to facilitate the early development of women and their baby's bodily reflections and bodily communications.

4.4.3   Bodily limitation

Mrs H, who had talked about the difficulty 'to learn' breastfeeding, continued breastfeeding, using additional bottles, until her baby's eighteenth month. The elements that hindered her bodily reflection could be identified from her hospital experience. At the first postnatal visit, she had almost given up breastfeeding, even though her breast condition was not as poor as she perceived. She said:

'I enjoyed talking to other mothers in the feeding room. I can see other women, especially second or third babies' mothers, had masses of breast milk from the beginning . . . I checked her weight and then breastfed. After that, the midwife came to each of us and hand expressed our breasts in turn. I saw my breasts gave only one or two drops. The midwife said, "Nothing . . ."; on the day of leaving the hospital, my baby gained 20 g after breastfeeding, and I was excited, but the midwife said to me, "It is nothing". I just came to believe that, I needed mixed feeding. It is "shikata-ga-nai" . . .'

Mrs H, interviewed at two months post partum

In the women's narratives, the hospital midwives appeared to hinder the woman and her baby's ability to immerse themselves in breastfeeding. In Mrs H's case, the midwife telling her 'nothing' stopped her and her baby from entering into the process of 'bodily reflection'. The Japanese phrase of '*shikata-ga-nai*' (the feeling that 'things do not always happen as the natural law tells') was also commonly used among mixed feeding women. It again relates to the Japanese cultural belief of 'going with the natural rhythms'. People know that nature follows a certain cycle, but it always gives exceptions such as the delay of rainy seasons, a cold summer, typhoons and earthquakes. The concept of 'shikata-ga-nai' represents the Japanese people's wisdom of living with the uncertain nature of life. When the women perceived they did not have enough breast milk, they accepted it as a part of natural law, which does not make possible for all things to happen by their wish.

The women who introduced formula feeds required time to accept mixed feeding as their feeding method. The early stage of mixed feeding was described as problematic, especially as most women in the study went back to their parents' home ('sato-gaeri') for one month after birth, where their mothers cooked the best local food, which was believed to help produce enough breast milk of a good quality. The women were told to breastfeed as many times as they could, which was understood as the best approach to establish breastfeeding. Conflict was experienced when a woman's own mother experienced breastfeeding without any problems; the mother could not make sense of why her daughter did not have enough breast milk. The mixed feeding women's narratives in the first month were characterised by 'tiredness' and 'unhappiness', with considerable energy being used on establishing breastfeeding. The concept of 'shikata-ga-nai' contained a feeling of 'sadness', as the women practically and also theoretically know that breastfeeding was best for babies. At the same time, it is the women's pragmatism (Lock & Kaufert 1998) to remain on partial breastfeeding, even though the usage of bottles in hospital practice and midwives' comments and attitudes sometimes had a negative impact on breastfeeding. Some of the women have the strength to overcome the negative impact, which seemed to be dependent on women's perceptions towards their own as well as others' bodies. The experience of the breastfeeding room in hospital or with other mothers in children's public playrooms was described as the time when the women learnt about 'individual bodily differences' such as the size of breasts, the shape of nipples and the character of the baby.

Mixed feeding appeared as a result of the efforts of the women as well as other family members, to live close to 'natural rhythms' despite the introduction of formula milk. In fact, when the women developed their way of mixed feeding using bodily reflections, the sense of bodily communication appeared, thus the woman's life also gained the sense of being 'in tune' with one's baby.

In the women's narratives, the relationship among new mothers was described as equal. The meaning of equal in this Japanese context means that they tried not to advise or to interfere with each other's breastfeeding practice or any other childcare issues, which seemed to exist as a tacit rule among new mothers. The women actively exchanged general information, but not about individual matters. They interpreted the information based on 'individual bodily differences' and 'bodily limitation', or information could be exchanged only when the women felt that they shared the sense of 'individual differences' in any issues of child caring. In other words, any advice given by a person who could not understand 'bodily limitation' was not considered. Within the Japanese culture, sharing the concept of 'shikata-ga-nai' the women were able to understand or accept the uncertain nature of breastfeeding; thus mixed feeding was considered and supported as a different way of breastfeeding practice.

4.5 Discussion and implications

From the women's narratives it was clear that breastfeeding in public was not practised. However, the women breastfeed with other mothers comfortably in their own space, which was used as a chance to learn more about breastfeeding by 'seeing other people's practice'. In addition, all the women experienced their breasts being touched by hospital midwives either in breast massage or in the process of latching-on practice. The women were sensitive enough to know who was a skilled midwife through sensing their feeling of being touched by the midwife's hands. The women used all those experiences to enhance their process of 'self-reflections'. The women also use local and theoretical knowledge and fellow-mothers' experiences as well as their own mother's experience, and their feeling and intuitions. This suggests that breastfeeding is not guided by theoretical knowledge or theoretical principles alone. In anthropology, it is explained as 'cosmology'; which means how people view the nature of the universe, and through the concept of habitus. In the case of Japanese society, even though Westernised ideas have influenced the traditional Japanese cosmology, the best state of health is viewed as given by living with natural cycles, and the current generation of new mothers still maintain or develop their ability of bodily reflections and also their practicality to live with bodily limitation, in other words, 'the uncertain nature of human life'. Therefore the role of support within the family means giving a sense of 'sharing the uncertain nature of child caring'.

In addition, the women's narratives demonstrated the women's pragmatic ability to work between the traditional Japanese notions of motherhood and the Western ideas of child caring. Their stories also revealed that, in the modern Japanese context, breastfeeding is still embodied knowledge of infant feeding, which is supported by the process of 'self-reflecting', in other words, the time and space used for listening to the messages from their own body as well as their babies. Japanese women's embodied knowledge of breastfeeding supports 'women's perseverance to get on with breastfeeding'. The women's early stage of breastfeeding included the experience of breast engorgement, night breastfeeding, or baby's crying. However, the women did not describe it as a problem or a difficulty, and they just accepted it as a normal part of early breastfeeding. In this situation, the women did not seek the reason behind why breast is best, which is unconsciously learnt through living in Japanese culture. As a result, even though early introduction of formula milk is common, and is encouraged by hospital routines and professional practices and atti tudes, women often continue with mixed feeding rather than ceasing breastfeeding altogether.

In this chapter, we have discussed the differences between theoretical and experiential knowledge, through the narratives of women's everyday lives, and using the concept of embodiment. The women's stories demonstrate the idea of 'to know' as conceptually and practically different from 'to learn' in that the latter represents a more theoretical concept, while 'to know' suggests a more embodied one, which combines bodily experience, bodily reflection and bodily communication with more theoretical forms of learning, such as instruction on 'how' or 'why' to engage in a practice. This has implications for how support is offered for infant feeding, by professionals and in informal social networks. Challenging the disjuncture between such forms of knowledge also has parallels in concepts of research and evidence. It challenges the oppositions between objective and subjective, and between phenomenological or objectivist and practical forms of knowing.

The study discussed here showed that Japanese society has been able to maintain embodied knowledge of breastfeeding, despite rapid social change and modernisation and the impact of medical approaches which have effectively undermined exclusive breastfeeding. Various features of Japanese culture have contributed to this, including cosmology – the view of humans' relationships with the world and nature, and the desire for harmony with natural cycles – the concept of 'kokoro' (a form of bodily and self-reflection) and 'mi-mamoru' – giving support through the time and space for a woman's 'kokoro'. We have seen how in the 1960s and 1970s, the move to hospital birth, introduction of mass produced infant formula, the influence of US culture and paediatric beliefs led to the introduction of widespread formula feeding. As a result it could be possible to describe current Japanese society as having a 'mixed feeding' approach. However, we do not choose the term 'mixed feeding culture' since breastfeeding remains a cultural norm and expectation, not a matter of consumer choice. When women feel they cannot fully breastfeed, they tend to view it as 'shikata-ga-nai', and accept the use of formula milk. This is seen very much as a way of working with the natural order, which includes bodily limitations, and so Japanese women, unlike women in many modernised societies, seem able to maintain breastfeeding practice after formula supplements have been introduced.

The prevalent attitudes are reflected in the language of infant feeding, where the Japanese word 'bo-nyuu' translates as 'mother's milk' – the emphasis is not on the mechanical or nutritive aspects so much as the relationship. We have described the process of coming 'to know' breastfeeding as a process of becoming 'a mother and her baby in tune', a process which involves bodily performance and reflection, of both the mother and her baby. It is also a process of developing a sense of control through learning to live with uncertainty, as well as finding the rhythms of the body and natural cycles.

The concept of embodiment has been used increasingly in sociology in recent years, yet it is not highly developed, and is used surprisingly little in health-related research. We suggest this may be because there is some discomfort, or lack of fit with dominant Western epistemologies – how we come to know what knowledge (or evidence) is and how knowledge is conveyed. This has particular implications for the ways in which international health policies are enacted, including the work of bodies such as UNICEF and the WHO seeking to promote public health through information, education and professional support.

We suggest the anthropological concept of *habitus* may help to illuminate further the issues raised by the narratives of the women in this study. Bourdieu (1987, p. 17) described *habitus* as:

> '*schemes of perception and appreciation deposited, in their incorporated state, in every member of the group*'

'Incorporated' (translated from the original French) means a state of being both known and enacted by the body, or being in a 'merged' state. *Habitus* is thereby both an 'organising principle of actions' (1987, p. 18) and a way of viewing and acting in the world. Bourdieu saw *habitus* as enabling people to deal with uncertain situations. This is very different from a mechanical view of practice, since it operates in terms of both structure and agency or flexibility. People don't simply function automatically in terms of pre-established 'models' or 'roles', but nonetheless dispositions guide practices, generating regulated improvisations. In other words, *habitus*, which is rooted in both culture and interaction with the world produces patterns of practice, which respond to existing beliefs, environment and experiences, and so are capable of flexibility and adaptation. There is continual movement and iteration between objective structures (such as conditions of existence, and pre-existing knowledge and beliefs) and interactions. This implies that humans are never simply pure 'subjects' nor simply products of a structure. This is reflected well in the analysis of the women's narratives in our study. Breastfeeding, in itself, is a biopsychosocial activity, and understanding it requires an appreciation of all these aspects. Similarly, the women's coming to know breastfeeding, and the process of the mother and her baby becoming 'in tune' involve a negotiation of elements which are both philosophical and pragmatic: cosmology and beliefs, cultural norms and expectations, relationships with professionals, family, peers, child, and developing and integrating both embodied, experiential knowledge, and theoretical or formalised knowledge. This theoretical approach has significant pedagogical implications, and the analysis helps to illuminate some of the difficulties experienced, despite decades of research and public health practice, in understanding how to support breastfeeding effectively.

This chapter has argued that developing breastfeeding involves a shift from 'to learn' to 'to know'. The shift was not experienced in a swift manner, and for the women studied here it required around five months for them to come to really know breastfeeding. Therefore here we will introduce three issues which have been largely dismissed in the currently dominant breastfeeding promotion paradigm that appears to advocate the notion that 'teaching the right skills and knowledge enables all women to breastfeed'. We suggest that professional initiatives to promote and support breastfeeding are less likely to be effective without attention to these three issues.

- *The lack of attention to the physical presence and physical energy required for breastfeeding.* While breastfeeding promotion policies such as the *Global Strategy for Infant and Young Child Feeding* emphasise that it is rare for women, even in resource-poor countries, to be unable to produce sufficient breast milk, many studies show that women commonly experience breastfeeding as physically demanding (Britton 2001; Dykes 2005; Kelleher 2006). In this study the feature was described in terms of 'bodily experience' and we pose the question of why this bodily nature of breastfeeding has been missing from so many of the previous breastfeeding discussions.
- *The support of breastfeeding requires a profound understanding of human life, and so it requires a philosophical approach, and reflection to be integrated with*

an evidence-based approach. In this study, the Japanese concept of '*mi-mamoru*' was used to explain the meaning of breastfeeding support as 'a philosophical act', in which the women perceived feelings of 'relaxing and protecting', when other people provided support with the sense of 'sharing the uncertain nature of breastfeeding'. In this study, we became aware that this was also perceived in the researcher's attitudes of 'being with the woman' and 'just listening to her'. It requires an appropriate engagement with the women's life. In our study, the women's narratives illuminated breastfeeding as a behaviour which could not simply be controlled by women's wish, echoing a number of studies of breast-feeding difficulties (Mozingo *et al.* 2000; Shakespeare *et al.* 2004; Kelleher 2006; Marshall *et al.* 2007). The biophysical aspects of breastfeeding need to be understood in relation to the social and cultural environment, and this com-plexity and wholeness is a key to understand breastfeeding as 'a biocultural activity'. Modern maternity care is based on the expectation of 'swift transition of motherhood' or 'back to normal as quickly as possible'. Miller (2002) argued that women experience problems in living within the expectation of 'swift transition' in motherhood in the UK. The women were too afraid to be named as 'a difficult mother' while they could not make a good transition into a new role, to seek support. They tried not to show their uncertain feeling to medical profes-sionals, thus the medical professionals could not fully appreciate the nature of biophysical and emotional transition in motherhood (Miller 2002; Shakespeare *et al.* 2004). This and other studies indicate that the framework of support should be considered for a longer time period, of about five months, which is a challenge in the current Japanese maternity care context. The *Global Strategy for Infant and Young Child Feeding* advocates long-term support for women but few countries have identified means of providing such support.

- *The concept of choice in breastfeeding promotion and women's pragmatism needs consideration.* Current breastfeeding promotion remains heavily based on concepts of health education where teaching the right ideas leads women to choose breastfeeding. In this study, the women's narratives illuminated the complex nature of breastfeeding, which did not happen by women's choice or wish alone, whereas the prevalent health promotion framework assumes that successes are largely dependent on each patient's choice and determination. The women's narratives also illuminated their pragmatism in their process of choice. In this context, some tacit manners and rituals bound women's decisions, which are found in the unspoken part of women's communications, what Lock (1987) has called 'soft rules'. Social expectation is often conveyed by the form of 'soft rules', which are not considered as part of formal knowledge. Lock and Kaufert (1998) argued that women often had to get on with their lives, with no time to examine their own resources or even to collect information. As a result, the women have limited choice or just lived in their everyday life fol-lowing their practical decision; therefore the consumerist concept of 'choice' was just illusion or could be applied for a very limited number of women, as it was more influenced by social environment and cultural belief (Lock & Kaufert 1998).

To connect the biophysical and sociocultural nature of breastfeeding together, to bridge the commonly found dichotomies of art or science, culture or nature, reason or emotion, we finally introduce the sociological concept of 'craft'. The concept of 'craft' here can integrate the time elements and the nature of 'bodily experience', which includes the elements we have discussed: bodily reflection, bodily communication and bodily limitation. Adapting the concept of craft, the nature of breastfeeding could be described as follows:

- Breastfeeding is practised using the common skills and knowledge but is developed for each woman and her baby as a unique couple, where each woman and her baby develop their pattern of breastfeeding using their bodily reflections
- Breastfeeding is practised in a flexible manner, and no fixed pattern is found in each performance. Thus 'bodily communications' are used as the best resource to know the way of breastfeeding and weaning practice. Nonetheless, patterns and rhythms are found, which enable women and their babies to develop a sense of prediction and control, being able to live with uncertainty.

Breastfeeding needs to be understood therefore as 'a craft work', and this enables midwives or other medical professionals to develop the concept of their work as involving craft. We suggest that a craft approach among professionals, combining the different elements we have discussed, and the different forms of knowledge and learning, may help them to support breastfeeding more effectively.

4.6 Conclusion

In modernising societies, people are likely to embrace scientific or theoretical knowledge as they are seen to represent advance and offer the best solutions. However, as Yamamoto (1983) argued, in the context of breastfeeding, increasing promotion of theoretical knowledge could mean the loss of embodied knowledge of breastfeeding from the society. This Japanese study suggests that breastfeeding requires a different paradigm of legitimating knowledge, which needs to be more learnt from women's experiences and also requires a framework with which to view social and cultural elements, and biophysical function and dysfunction as a whole. Although this ethnographic study seems to succeed in conceptualising general approaches to increase the effectiveness of supporting breastfeeding, the concepts of bodily reflection, bodily limitation and bodily communication also illuminated the importance of understanding breastfeeding in relation to women's social and cultural environment.

Since Western societies shifted into a bottle feeding culture, the embodied knowledge of breastfeeding, which is stored in people's everyday life, has also been lost. In order to preserve and utilise this cultural knowledge, it is important for practitioners to be clear that their everyday practice also helps to constitute women's breastfeeding. Those narratives will influence the future practice of breastfeeding as well as constructing the future cultural knowledge. This chapter has introduced an alternative framework to view breastfeeding as 'a craft' and highlighted the timeframe that is required for women to 'come to know' breastfeeding. The supporters' role of 'sharing the uncertain nature of breastfeeding' was experienced as a philosophical one, rather than just a skill or technique. The embodied knowledge and craft of breastfeeding needs to be explored and interpreted within each cultural setting and through practitioners' reflection on their own practice; for midwives and medical professionals, the narratives help to re-think one's own philosophy of 'listening to women and babies' experience'. Although macro-level strategies such as the *Global Strategy for Infant and Young Child Feeding* are vital to underpin and ensure appropriate national policies, and ensure that health services do not continue to actively undermine breastfeeding, as occurred in post-war Japan, these policies need to be enacted through appropriate forms of professional support. The narratives can help professionals to understand individual bodily difference and bodily limitation, and to reconsider the meaning of support. For theoretical researchers, women's narratives help to seek the way of developing a cross-cultural discussion in human experience, filling the gap between Western notions and other cultural notions of breastfeeding.

References

Battersby, S. (2006) Dissonance and competing paradigms in midwives' experience of breast-feeding. Unpublished thesis. University of Sheffield, Sheffield.

Bourdieu, P. (1987) *Outline of a Theory of Practice.* Cambridge University Press, Cambridge.

Britton, C.J. (2001) *Women's Experiences of Early and Long-term Breastfeeding in the UK.* Ph.D. thesis. University of Durham, Durham.

Dykes, F. (2005) Supply and demand: breastfeeding as labour. *Social Science and Medicine,* **60**: 2283–2293.

Ericksen, H.T. & Nielsen, S.F. (2001) *A History of Anthropology.* Pluto Press, London.

Fukuda, M. (1996) Rooming-in, breast milk and breastfeeding. *Shyuusanki-Igaku,* **26** (4): 521–524. [In Japanese.]

Hachiya, S. (1998) Promoting rooming-in: the case of Kitami red cross hospital. *Jyosanpu-Zattushi,* **52** (10): 59–63. [In Japanese.]

Hamlyn, B., Brookers, S., Oleninikova, K. & Wands, S. (2000) *Infant Feeding.* The Stationery Office, London.

Japan Breast Feeding Association (2008) Information about baby friendly hospital At: http://www.bonyuweb.com/shoukai/about_bhf.htm (accessed 13 October 2008). [In Japanese.]

Japan Ministry of Health, Labour and Welfare (2000) *Sukoyaka Oyako 21 kentoukai houkokusyo gaiyou* [*Report from the discussion: National Plan of early 21 century for the health of mothers and children 2001–2010*]. At: http://www/mhlw.go.jp/topics/sukoyaka/tp1117–1_b_18.html (accessed 11 October 2008). [In Japanese.]

Japan Ministry of Health, Labour and Welfare (2006) *Jyunyuu, Rinyuu n no shien gaido sakutei ni kansuru kenkyuukai gijiroke 2006, 10, 11* [The first discussion meeting about infant feeding and weaning guideline]. At: http://www.mhlw.go.jp/shingi/2006/10/txt/s1011–2/txt (accessed 13 October 2008). [In Japanese.]

Japan Ministry of Health, Labour and Welfare (2007) *Jyunyuu, Rinyuu no shien gaido* [Guideline for infant feeding and weaning 2007]. At: http://www.mhlw.go.jp/shingi/2007/s0314–17.html (accessed 15 October 2008). [In Japanese.]

Jitsukawa, M. (1997) In accordance with nature: what Japanese women mean by being in control. *Anthropology and Medicine,* **4** (2): 177–199.

Jordan, B. (2003) Birth in Four Cultures. A Crosscultural Investigation of Childbirth in Yucatan, Holland, Sweden and the United States. 4th Edition. Waveland Press, Prospect Heights, Illinois.

Kelleher, C.M. (2006) The physical challenges of early breastfeeding. *Social Science and Medicine*, **63** (10): 2727–2738.

Kiriyama, K. (2004) *Edo-Ucyuu* [Cosmology in Japanese Edo period]. Shinjinbutsu Ouraishya, Tokyo. [In Japanese.]

Lock, M. (1987) Introduction: health and medical care as cultural and social phenomena. In: Norbeck, E. & Lock, M. (eds) *Health, Illness, and Medical Care in Japan*. University of Hawaii Press, Honolulu, pp. 1–23.

Lock, M. & Kaufert, A.P. (1998) *Pragmatic Women and Body Politics*. Cambridge University press, Cambridge.

Macfarlane, A. (1997) *The Savage Wars of Peace*. Oxford: Blackwell.

Maher, V. (ed.) (1992) The anthropology of breast-feeding: natural law or social construct. Berg, Oxford.

Marshall, J.L., Godrey, M. & Renfrew, M. (2007) Being a 'good mother': managing breastfeeding and merging identities. *Social Science and Medicine*, **65**: 2147–2159.

Miller, T. (2002) Adapting to motherhood: care in the postnatal period. *Community Practitioner*, **75** (1): 16–18.

Mothers' and Children's Health and Welfare Association (2004) *Maternal and Child Health Statistics of Japan*. Mothers' and Children's Health Organisation, Tokyo.

Mozingo, J.N., Davis, M.W., Droppleman, P.G. & Merideth, A. (2000) It wasn't working. Women's experiences with short-term breastfeeding. *American Journal of Maternal Child Nursing*, **25** (3): 120–126.

Nezu, Y. (1992) A new instruction for breastfeeding (Japanese). *Shyuusanki Igaku*, **22** (1): 47–51.

Nishikawa, S. (1992) *Osan no Chie* [Wisdom of Japanese childbirth and child caring]. Koudan-Shya, Tokyo. [In Japanese.]

Oketani, S. (1983) Breast massage. In: Kato, H. (ed.) *Bonyuu-Hoiku*. Medica Science, Tokyo, pp. 468–489. [In Japanese.]

Oobayashi, M. (1985) *Jyosanpu-no-Sengo* [Japanese midwifery after the Second World War]. Keisou-Syobou, Tokyo. [In Japanese.]

Parkes P. (2005) Milk kinship in Islam. Substance, structure, history. *Social Anthropology* **13**: 307–329.

Pearse, J. (1990) Breast-feeding practices in Japan. *Midwives Chronicle and Nursing Notes*, **103**: 310–315.

Sawada, K. (1983) An anthropological view of breastfeeding. In: Kato, H. (ed.) *Bonyuu-Hoiku*. Medica Science, Tokyo, pp. 34–45. [In Japanese.]

Senoo, T., Nanba, M., Kouoto, E., Matushisge, Y., Makabe, F. & Kouzu, T. (1995) The management of breast care and protocol for child caring in the baby friendly hospital. *Perinatal Care*, **14** (11): 1025–1032. [In Japanese.]

Shakespeare, J., Blake, F. & Garcia, J. (2004) Breast-feeding difficulties experienced by women taking part in a qualitative interview study of postnatal depression. *Midwifery* **20** (3): 251–60.

Sueshige, K., Nakao, A. & Ito, Y. (1998) Promoting rooming-in: in a hospital context of breast-feeding practice. *Jyousanpu-Zattishi*, **52** (10): 55–58. [In Japanese.]

Takahashi, E. (1996) The social background of breastfeeding. *Shyuusanki Igaku*, **26** (4): 459–464. [In Japanese.]

Takei, T. (1998) Breast feeding and Breast care in the Soka-city hospital (Japanese), Jyosanpu-Zattushi, 52 (10): 38–43

WHO (2003) *Global Strategy for Infant and Young Child Feeding*. WHO, Geneva.

Yamamoto, K. (1983) *Bo-nyuu* [Breastfeeding]. Iwanami-Shinsyo, Tokyo. [In Japanese.]

5 Breastfeeding and Poverty: Negotiating Cultural Change and Symbolic Capital of Motherhood in Québec, Canada

Danielle Groleau and Charo Rodríguez

5.1 Introduction

In response to the World Health Organization (WHO) global call to adopt health policies protecting, promoting and supporting exclusive breastfeeding, health officials in many Western countries have come to agree that breast milk is the ideal nutrition for newborns, providing important protection against viruses, bacteria, allergies, diabetes, and a variety of cancers and gastrointestinal and respiratory infections (Organisation Mondiale de la Santé et Fonds International de Secours à l'Enfance des Nations Unies (OMS/FISE) 1989; WHO/UNICEF 1989; American Academy of Pediatrics 1997, 2005; Society *et al.* 2005). In addition, the scientific evidence regarding the protective qualities and nutritional superiority of breast milk has convinced many Western nations to follow the recommendations in the *Global Strategy for Infant and Young Child Feeding* (WHO 2003).

The province of Québec (Canada) has followed this international movement since 1997 by including in its health policy the objective of increasing breastfeeding rates as one of its five public health policies (Québec Ministère de la Santé et des Services Sociaux MSSS 1997). Updated in 2001, the policy aims to attain, by 2007, rates of 85% for the initiation of breastfeeding and subsequent duration rates (any breastfeeding rates) of 70%, 60%, 50% and 20% at two, four, six and 12 months post partum, respectively (Ministère de la Santé et des Services sociaux (MSSS) 2001, p. 29). Following these policy goals, a series of provincial surveys have shown a steady increase in breastfeeding initiation rates at birth from 47% (Levill *et al.* 1995) to 54% (Santé Canada 1999), to 72% (Dubois *et al.* 2000) and more recently, to the desired goal of 85% (Neill 2006). These positive results are encouraging and demonstrate that health policies and public health programmes that promote breastfeeding can have a major impact on population breastfeeding rates. Nevertheless, a shadow looms over these results. Although the breastfeeding initiation rate of mothers living in poverty has also recently increased to 83% (non-exclusive breastfeeding), the sustainability of breastfeeding continues to remain low, with duration rates for non-exclusive breastfeeding of 44%, 34% and 27% at two, four and six months post partum, respectively (Neill 2006). These rates remain systematically lower than the general population of Québec, which have duration rates for non-exclusive breastfeeding of 66% at 2 months, 56% at 4 months and 46% at 6 months (Neill 2006).

We have known for some time about the critical importance of reaching this socioeconomic group of mothers because babies born into poverty are more vulnerable to many diseases and have limited access to a nutritional diet (Baker *et al.* 1998). Considering the protective effects of breastfeeding on babies' health and the unique nutritional qualities of breast milk, babies born into low-income families constitute, by far, the social group benefiting the most from breastfeeding (Giugliani *et al.* 1996). However, Québec is not the only Western region finding it difficult to convince disadvantaged women to adopt exclusive breastfeeding for the periods aimed by their health policies. Disadvantaged populations of Western countries such as Canada, the USA, many European countries and Australia, are characterised, in general, by a very low prevalence of exclusive breastfeeding (Raisler 1993). The influence of poverty on infant feeding choices varies by mothers' ethnicity, suggesting that economic factors interact with the cultural context in the genesis of infant feeding decisions and duration of breastfeeding (Groleau *et al.* 2006, 2009; Groleau & Cabral 2009).

Studies have long shown that other contextual factors, such as social support, may influence women's decisions regarding infant and young child feeding. Certain individuals in the mother's social network, as well as health professionals, are known to influence the mother and support her in her decision to breastfeed (Sikorski *et al.* 2003; Britton *et al.* 2007). Several maternal psychological characteristics have also been associated with breastfeeding initiation and duration. For example, a positive attitude toward breastfeeding is a characteristic of breastfeeding mothers whereas the opposite is true for non-breastfeeding mothers (Dix 1991). We know that such attitudes are influenced by whether or not one was breastfed oneself and by the degree of exposure to other nursing mothers at an early age (Riva *et al.* 1999). However, since breastfeeding is not common practice among poor non-immigrant populations in the West, young mothers are, from the outset, much less exposed to other nursing mothers. Maternal depressive symptoms are also associated with a lower preference for and shorter durations of breastfeeding (Misri *et al.* 1997; Galler *et al.* 1999), but these studies have not been able to explain the nature of this relationship. We must be cautious about presenting such tautological findings as determinants of, or barriers to, breastfeeding. Indeed, focusing on individual or psychological characteristics of mothers with regard to their infant feeding choices can promptly shift the blame onto those who choose not to breastfeed or abandon breastfeeding early on, without taking into account important contextual barriers.

In the wake of WHO's various calls to promote breastfeeding, research on breastfeeding has been dominated by an epidemiological-biomedical approach, reducing the ontological status of breastfeeding to its purely biological or performative aspects. Breastfeeding has been mainly studied, and therefore defined, by both its health performance, i.e. how it affects the physical health of the baby and mother, and by the socio-demographic and maternal psychological factors associated with it. But positivistic knowledge of this kind prevents us not only from understanding why these mothers choose not to breastfeed but also from planning and implementing policies and programmes promoting breastfeeding that more effectively meet the needs of disadvantaged mothers. For example, in Québec a longitudinal epidemiological study has shown lower prevalence of breastfeeding initiation among low-income mothers, mothers with depressive symptoms, Québec-born and French-speaking mothers (versus immigrants), and those who reported poor health (Dubois *et al.* 2000). These results demonstrate that mothers having these psychosocial characteristics are less likely to breastfeed. In other words from a public health perspective, we have identified a group 'at risk'. However, such associations, even if they are generalisable to the population of Québec, are still insufficient for understanding the complexity of contextual barriers that such mothers face.

Over the past 20 years, studies have attempted to explore the experiences of mothers in relation to their infant-feeding choices within their social contexts (e.g. Groleau 1998; Mahon-Daly *et al.* 2002; Dykes 2005, 2006; Groleau *et al.* 2006; Groleau & Cabral 2009). These studies have investigated the social processes and cultural contexts related to the decisions and experiences associated with infant feeding. By doing so, they have re-situated the ontological status of breastfeeding to include its dialogical dimension. In other words, they have considered breastfeeding beyond its merely performative or biological dimension to include an understanding of the practice as not only a bodily experience but also one that is related to the collective voices and asymmetry of the social relations in which infant feeding choices are embedded (Van Esterik 1989; Blum 1993; Hermans 2001).

The apparent difficulties of public health programmes to change the infant feeding behaviours of disadvantaged mothers indicate that the related psychosocial and cultural processes in the context of poverty need to be better understood. Qualitative research, often associated with the constructivist paradigm, aims to discover and explore complex phenomena using a transactional/subjectivist epistemology interested in experience and context (Schwandt 2001). The application of this type of research approach may reveal hitherto hidden social processes that hold potential in guiding breastfeeding policies and programmes tailored to this vulnerable population. The study described in this chapter followed this approach by aiming to explore the psychosocial and cultural experiences of French-Canadian mothers who initiated breastfeeding within a context of poverty in Québec. Using the results from our study, we will discuss and illustrate how social process and cultural representations of infant feeding can constitute barriers for the implementation of the *Global Strategy for Infant and Young Child Feeding* (WHO 2003) in a Western context of poverty where breastfeeding does not constitute the norm. Our results will also highlight the adverse implications to be expected if promotional activities are not accompanied by tangible and well-planned contextual strategies that aim to support and protect low-income mothers in a Western context of poverty. Thus we will propose strategies to help bridge the gap between recommendations in the WHO *Global Strategy for Infant and Young Child Feeding* and the actual local infant feeding practices. To do so, we will first discuss the ontological and theoretical position of biomedical knowledge on breastfeeding to help understand adjustments needed to maximise the implementation of this policy.

5.1.1   Ontological and theoretical background

Quantitative studies related to breastfeeding have inherent limitations that can be partially explained by the fact that health behaviours, in general, are linked to subjective experiences and cannot, therefore, be fully appreciated through quantitative analysis alone (Groleau *et al.* 2006). Recent qualitative studies suggest that infant feeding choices represent health behaviours embedded in the social spaces of mothers, their culture, and the representations they hold with regard to illness and health (Mahon-Daly *et al.* 2002; Groleau *et al.* 2006).

Given that breastfeeding is an embodied health behaviour, an interpretative approach from medical anthropology seems particularly useful in shedding light on how culture influences representations of body, health and illness in relation to breastfeeding experiences. Influenced by Geertz's theory of culture (Geertz 1973), the interpretative approach stipulates that illness and health representations are part of a cultural theory of health governed by explanatory models of diseases (Kleinman 1980), illness prototypes (Young 1981) and semantic networks (Good 1994). In an interpretative approach, Young has shown that prototypical experiences related to health, as well as explanatory models of health, have in common the fact that they are often used to confirm popular theories of health shared by people of the same cultural community. Subsequently Groleau (1998) demonstrated and confirmed the usefulness of taking into account the prototypical experiences of mothers with regard to infant feeding, as well as the explanatory models associated with maternal and infant health, to identify the sociocultural determinants of low breastfeeding rates among a given group. Thus, understanding an embodied health behaviour such as breastfeeding requires a corresponding understanding of how associated health and bodily representations are embedded in popular theories of health produced by various sociocultural systems (familial, educational, political, etc.).

Although critically engaged social science research has contributed significantly to our understanding of the politics of women's bodily and reproductive experiences, they have historically produced relatively little critical discussion regarding initiation and duration of breastfeeding of Western born women living in a context of poverty (Van Esterik 1989; Blum 1993; Carter 1995; Dykes 2006). In medical anthropology, such research is interested in representations of illness and health as networks of meaning that reflect social relations of power. Since the population in the present study is economically disadvantaged, certain concepts developed by Bourdieu (Bourdieu 1984, 1985, 1989) were particularly helpful in interpreting our qualitative data. Given that, first, breastfeeding is an embodied experience often performed in social spaces, second, mothers of our study were living in a context of poverty, and, third, having a baby involves a change in identity and status, Bourdieu's concepts of *habitus*, *fields* and *symbolic capital* were particularly helpful in understanding the underlying social processes involved in the abandonment of breastfeeding by Western-born mothers living in poverty. According to Bourdieu (1989, p. 14):

> *'There is a twofold social genesis, on the one hand, of the schemes of perception, thought, and action which are constitutive of what I call habitus, and on the other hand, of social structures, and particularly of what I call fields and of groups, notably those ordinarily we call social classes.'*

Thus, in Bourdieu's social theory, habitus refers to the disposition of agents or:

> *'the mental structures through which they apprehend the social world are essentially the product of the internalization of the structures of that world.'*
>
> Bourdieu (1989, p. 18)

Thus, the social world is neither totally structured nor totally chaotic, and representations held by agents vary according to their position, disposition, or habitus.

According to Bourdieu, the social power of agents is determined by the totality of their capital and the relative weight of their different types of capitals (Bourdieu 1977, 1984, 1985). Capital, according to Bourdieu, is not limited to economic capital but includes cultural, social and symbolic capital (Bourdieu 1985). *Symbolic capital*, as defined by Bourdieu, is a form of power that comes with social position, affords prestige, and leads others from the same field to pay attention to the agent holding such capital. Symbolic capital thus engenders a sense of duty and inferiority in others who look up to those who have that power. This concept is particularly relevant for poor mothers because, as stated by Attree (2005, p. 236), poor women have 'few alternative sources of capital and ways of legitimizing their role in society.' For these mothers, therefore, the rearing and health of children are key sources of symbolic capital and must be seen as a context in which infant feeding decisions and experiences take place. Thus, an interpretative critical approach inspired by the post-structuralist critical concepts of *habitus*, *symbolic capital* and *fields* (Bourdieu 1984, 1989), and the interpretative concepts of *explanatory models* and *prototypes* (Kleinman 1980; Young 1981; Good 1994) were used in this study to interpret how French-Canadian mothers living in poverty introduced breastfeeding and negotiated this cultural change within the context of their lives.

5.1.2 Our study

We conducted ethnographic interviews among 42 disadvantaged French-Canadian mothers between 2004 and 2007, to explore their experience of breastfeeding. We recruited mothers from urban, suburban, and rural areas of the province of Québec to account for different social contexts.

A total of 42 mothers were interviewed twice, first at one month post partum and then at six months' post partum. The majority who participated in the study were young with the vast majority being under 26 years of age (31/42; 74%). Nearly half of mothers (19/42, 45%) were parenting their first child. At one month post partum, most mothers (31/42, 74%) were living with a partner. The mothers came from different geographical regions, with 12/42 (28%) living in urban areas, 14/42 (33%) in suburban areas, and 16/42 (38%) in rural areas. Of these, 11/42 (26%) had breastfeeding durations of between one hour and one week, 9/42 (21%) of between one week and one month, and 22/42 (52%) of more than one month.

Recruitment took place over two years using a theoretical sample that included the following restrictive criteria: low socioeconomic status according to local norms established by regional public health agencies; self-declared as born in Canada with French as their first language (the majority in Québec); and equal distribution of mothers across geographical regions (urban, rural and suburban). Mothers who participated in this project were referred to us by numerous community organisations and local community clinics from across the province. Through their cooperation, we were able to draw a sample of 111 mothers – some intending to breastfeed, others not – from which 42 who eventually initiated breastfeeding were selected.

Three data collection tools were used in this study: a semi-structured ethnographic interviews; a short socio-demographic questionnaire; and the Edinburgh Postnatal Depression Scale (EPDS) (Cox et al. 1987). The most important method used to generate data was the ethnographic semi-structured interview used to interview every mother at one and six months post partum. Through these interviews, mothers were able to generate their narratives related to pregnancy, childbirth and the postpartum period, as well as their representations related to their health and that of their babies with regard to breastfeeding, their social experiences, as well as their values and concerns during the perinatal period.

For the purpose of better describing the socio-demographic characteristics of mothers, a standard closed-question socio-demographic questionnaire was used in an initial telephone conversation with mothers during their pregnancy. The EPDS, a quantitative assessment of distress that has been validated for Québec French (Des Rivières-Pigeon et al. 2000), was administered three times after birth – at one, three, and six months post partum – to identify those women likely to have psychological distress.

Interviews of all mothers were recorded and transcribed in full. The various themes that emerged from mothers' narratives, as well as those corresponding to the interpretative critical framework outlined above, were coded using the software Atlas.ti (Muhr 1991). Triangulation of codes was carried out by three different people – two research assistants and the first author – who were either present or not during the interviews. Prior to the interviews, we had entertained no specific preconception regarding the values, representations or barriers to prolonged breastfeeding for disadvantaged French-Canadian mothers because: their social environment was little known to researchers; and sociological and anthropological literature on the subject was virtually non-existent. After each interview was coded and analysed individually, we conducted transversal analyses of the interviews to identify representations and recurring collective experiences of mothers. The coded transcripts were then analysed according to the interpretative-critical approach explained above.

5.1.3   The findings of our study

In this section, we will examine duration of breastfeeding in relation to distress and reasons given by mothers in their narratives to explain why they abandoned breastfeeding prematurely. We will then explore their social experience of breast-feeding in relation to the discourse they encountered in various environments, namely, their families, their social milieu, and that of healthcare professionals. Compared with the general population's rate for postpartum depression (13%) (O'Hara & Swain 1996), our purposeful sample presented a high proportion of mothers with psychological distress at one month post partum (8/38, 21%), three months post partum (6/34, 18%), and six months post partum (12/31, 39%)[i]. Although our sampling was theoretical and presented higher rates than in the general population, it remained comparable with the prevalence of depression at six months post partum (38.2%) found by another study on low-income women in Québec (Séguin *et al.* 1999). This underscores the importance of understanding the role played by distress in mother's decision to abandon or continue breastfeeding while taking into account their social context. We will first explore the reasons mothers evoked, in their narratives, for abandoning breastfeeding.

5.1.3.1   *Mothers who abandoned breastfeeding within one week*

Nearly half of the mothers in our sample (20/42) abandoned breastfeeding in the first postpartum month, and half of these did so within the first week (12/20). Only one of these 12 mothers did not give a reason during the interview for why she had abandoned breastfeeding. Almost all the other mothers (11/12) spontaneously explained why they had abandoned breastfeeding prematurely. Of these, almost all cited technical difficulties, of which the most prevalent was 'the baby doesn't want to take the breast'. Several mothers also cited not having enough milk, which was an explanation for why their baby did not take the breast correctly. In all cases, urgency to feed the baby, whom mothers qualified as 'starving', was what persuaded them to formula feed after a few days and often within a few hours of unsuccessful breastfeeding attempts.

> 'The baby had a hard time taking the breast. It was hard, because the baby tried to get milk, take the breast, for hours – maybe two or three – but it wasn't working. The baby was crying so much he was getting hysterical. I was feeling so bad. I told myself, "It's already hard enough with the baby. Now you can't even feed him".'
>
> Annie, interviewed at one month post natal

> 'I cried a lot. I returned to my room and I cried – I cried like a baby. I felt so low. Because, in my mind, it was clear: I wanted to breastfeed, but the baby didn't

---

[i] Edinburgh Postnatal Depression Scale data were not available for some mothers at one, three and six months postnatal, which explains why *n* is lower than our actual sample of 42 mothers.

want to. He was having problems . . . he wasn't using his tongue properly to
suck. I took it personally. I told myself I wasn't a good mother.'

Nathalie, interviewed at one month post natal

These mothers were alone and had no one in their family, social or professional milieu to help them with their technical problems related to breastfeeding. Two of the mothers said they were exhausted and had stopped breastfeeding to 'conserve energy'. As stated before, a quarter of these mothers were still in distress after one month, which leads us to consider whether lack of support in the face of so many difficult problems did not contribute to their high levels of distress.

'I wanted to breastfeed from the start. I was thinking that it was good for the
baby, that he would be less sick. It will be good for me because he will heal sooner
(baby was sick at birth). It will be more practical, no need to heat and sterilise
the milk. That is what I wanted, from the start of my pregnancy. But it didn't
work. My baby could not take the breast well. It was hard. . . . Because the baby
tried and tried for hours to take the milk, the breast. For two or three hours and
then it would not work. He would be in crisis, he would scream and scream. I
felt so bad, I would say to myself "you already have problems with your baby
[being sick] and on top of it you can't feed him". I took it personally. . . . I cried
so much, I would come back to my room and cry and cry . . . like a baby. I felt
completely down, because in my mind it was obvious, I wanted to breastfeed
and the baby, he didn't want to breastfeed. I was telling myself I am not a
good mother.'

Lianna, interviewed at one month post natal

As seen in the excerpt above, the narratives of these mothers consistently make reference to strong feelings of guilt about not being up to the task of breastfeeding; such feelings also made them doubt their abilities as mothers.

5.1.3.2 *Mothers who abandoned breastfeeding between one week and one month*

The reason most often cited by nearly half of mothers who stopped breastfeeding between one week and one month was related to conserving their energy level (1/9). The problem seemed to be more pronounced for mothers who continued breast-feeding beyond the first postpartum week than for those who stopped breastfeeding in the first few days after the birth. This suggests a cumulative effect of fatigue during the first postpartum weeks coupled with the importance mothers place on their ability to care for their babies. However, technical problems such as breast pain were a problem for a third of these mothers. Mothers seem to indicate in their narratives that they associated pain with thrush or cracked nipples. Exhaustion and painful breasts seem to have been greater barriers for these mothers than for those who abandoned breastfeeding in the first few days following childbirth.

'The baby had thrush, and then I got it. It hurt so much I stopped nursing. I stopped the baby before he finished drinking'
                                    Jade, interviewed at one month post natal

Again, the cumulative effect of breastfeeding problems, combined with the absence of social and professional support for resolving them, seems to have played an important role in the abandonment of breastfeeding.

5.2   Social experience of breastfeeding

5.2.1   Negotiating conflicting values in the family environment with respect to infant feeding choices

It is clear from the mothers' narratives that the more they were exposed to conflicting messages in their family environment with respect to breastfeeding the sooner they abandoned the practice.

'My mother didn't breastfeed – but my mother-in-law did a bit, so I had her to help me a little. My own parents were more reluctant. They didn't want me to breastfeed. But for me it was important. So I haven't had a lot of support from them.'
                                    Marianne, interviewed at one month post natal

'I know there are a lot of my aunts and uncles who find breastfeeding too much trouble. They were all bottle fed, and they seem to know exactly how many ounces they drank. Some of them are saying, "I don't know how you do it . . . it's so hard". They see it as this huge problem, because that's their mentality – they weren't brought up that way.'
                                    Camille, interviewed at one month post natal

Thus, some mothers who chose to breastfeed felt negatively judged or stigmatised by relatives.

'My mother-in-law asked me to go feed my baby in another room so I wouldn't embarrass my father-in-law. I just went; I was so humiliated. I stayed there for a long time during the whole Christmas party because my baby drinks all the time. It's hard . . . you just feel like quitting.'
                                    Camille, interviewed at one month post natal

A large majority of mothers (10/12) who abandoned breastfeeding within the first week reported having been exposed to anti-breastfeeding discourse from relatives. Among mothers who breastfed between one week and one month, somewhat fewer (5/8) received mixed discourses from family members regarding breastfeeding. Finally, women who breastfed for more than one month were the least exposed to anti-breastfeeding discourses from their significant others (10/22), notably from their mothers and spouses.

Family members who were pro-formula often referred to their own experience or that of relatives as prototypes of healthy people who were formula fed. Such pro-formula discourse was often used by women in the family as evidence that formula feeding is not harmful for the baby's health.

'My mother told me "My daughter, you were fed with formula and well . . . you are a healthy girl no?". So OK, breastfeeding is healthy, but bottle also is correct for your baby's health. It won't harm your baby. Look at me, I am healthy and I was bottle fed. You have to think about your own self, your own energy.'

Magalie, interviewed at one month post natal

In addition, all mothers had been told by family members how difficult and exhausting breastfeeding could be.

'When I stopped giving the breast, everybody [referring to her family] was satisfied because they considered it too complicated . . . You know now [since she stopped breastfeeding] everybody can help while I rest. It is better for my health. The baby was too strong, he would pull so hard on my breast that they would bleed.

Alice, interviewed at one month post natal

As mentioned earlier, mothers who quickly abandoned breastfeeding had experienced technical problems for which they received little help. They had to deal with these problems themselves, in addition to having received conflicting messages from their relatives regarding their infant feeding choice. In other words, by choosing to breastfeed when most of the older women in their family had not done so, they were exposed to disapproving discourse that consequently took on greater significance and contributed to feelings of guilt when breastfeeding problems arose.

In addition, anti-breastfeeding discourse referred to breastfeeding as causing excessive fatigue and undermining the mother's ability to care for her baby. Many mothers were forced to manage, simultaneously, unresolved breastfeeding problems, fatigue, emotional distress and isolation. As stated above, the insecure economic situation of all mothers in our study continuously added to their stress. For those who abandoned breastfeeding early, this only compounded their strong sense of guilt. Therefore, for mothers who were already vulnerable, conflicting discourse within the family environment had the combined effect of reducing access to emotional support, undermining their perceptions of their own competence as mothers, and causing an overwhelming sense of failure and guilt.

5.2.2   Negotiating breastfeeding in public places

In Québec, the promotion of breastfeeding usually begins in prenatal courses. Not all participants in our study attended prenatal courses, since such courses are generally not popular among French-Canadians mothers living in a context of poverty. For those who did attend, some felt a certain amount of pressure from nurses to adopt breastfeeding. They felt there was an attempt to convince rather than encourage and support them. The second encounter with breastfeeding promotion indicated by mothers in their narratives was in the hospital setting after childbirth, where nurses responsible for promoting breastfeeding discussed with them the importance of breastfeeding. The usual hospital stay after giving birth in Québec is very short, typically 24 hours. With respect to support received at the hospital, there was a clear difference between mothers who abandoned breastfeeding within one week and those who continued for longer. Mothers who breastfed beyond one week tended not to report a lack of support in hospital. In contrast, nearly 10/12 of mothers who abandoned breastfeeding within the first week reported not having received sufficient help from nurses. For example, one mother who attempted and then abandoned breastfeeding talked of failure and emphasised, in particular, the lack of support she received at the hospital for persevering.

'Well, maybe they could have insisted a little more, knowing that I wanted to breastfeed . . . So you end up giving a bottle to your baby yourself. As for breast-feeding, I would have liked them to help me out a little more, to explain it to me, to show me how to do it. I didn't know how to do it . . .'

Laurence, interviewed at one month post natal

Most breastfeeding mothers felt that nurses in the hospital tended to give them inconsistent and conflicting information about breastfeeding techniques and dealing with such problems as painful breasts and insufficient milk. In addition, many mothers who shared their hospital room with a formula-feeding mother were displeased by the way, in their opinion, ward nurses judged or stigmatised these mothers for their infant feeding choice.

'The nurse told her, "Maternal milk is best for your baby. Don't you want the best for your baby?". I imagine if I was not breastfeeding, I would have had to deal with that. . . . It also happened during the prenatal class . . . you know . . . those who intended not to breastfeed were looked down by others.'

Clara, interviewed at six months post natal

Breastfeeding mothers explained that, although their infant feeding choice shielded them from the pressure and stigmatising comments of hospital staff, most faced negative comments and attitudes on returning to their social and familial spaces. Mothers who continued to breastfeed for more than one week were those who were most comfortable breastfeeding in social and public spaces (22/30) reflecting not only their state of being but also the reaction of other people in their environment. Several of these mothers talked in terms of respect for others. Particularly, they were aware that some people might feel uncomfortable seeing a mother breastfeed in public and that this requires a certain amount of discretion and respect on their part. Asking the person in the room if they are comfortable with breastfeeding or bringing a small blanket to a store or restaurant to hide the breast were notable examples.

'It depends . . . it depends on what you consider breastfeeding in public. I wear a sweater so no one can see; at least it's covered. There are women who breastfeed. . . . They don't care if everyone can see their breasts. As far as I'm concerned, I don't care if people see my breasts – but it's out of respect for those who see me breastfeed. If the person is uncomfortable with me breastfeeding, then I'm not respecting them if I do it in front of them.'

Frédérique, interviewed at six months post natal

'If that's what you mean by breastfeeding in public, well, yes, but with a certain respect – respect for others, respect for my own body, respect for myself. I wouldn't breastfeed in front of 500 people – not without covering myself . . . I'm discreet. It's my body. It's not everyone else's. You don't want to make other people uncomfortable by breastfeeding in front of them. If your breast is exposed, it can make people uncomfortable.'

Stéphanie, interviewed at one month post natal

Most women who abandoned breastfeeding within one week were embarrassed to breastfeed in front of others.

'When I see women breastfeeding openly in a restaurant, I tell myself that they could do it in the washroom.'

Camille, interviewed at one month post natal

'I think it's unacceptable. It's something you do in private.'

Clara, interviewed at one month post natal

Breastfeeding mothers also mentioned experiencing this problem when they breastfed in family or public spaces and sometimes had to face judgemental or disparaging looks from strangers, or when they had to defend their choice for breastfeeding before older-generation family members who made negative comments in their presence. Defending this choice in the face of negative family, social, and public discourses created additional emotional challenges for mothers already feeling exhausted, distressed or isolated.

Likewise, as mentioned earlier, mothers who had significant technical problems breastfeeding while holding a crying baby in the middle of the night were not only deprived of technical and emotional support but also had to negotiate conflicting discourse from family members who indirectly blamed them for undermining their own capacity to be competent mothers. Discourse of family members and close peers unequivocally stated that formula feeding would make things easier for the mothers, help them conserve their energy, and was a *sine qua non* condition for being a 'good mother' in the challenging context of their lives.

5.3   Contextualising our study

Beyond the clearly physiological dimension of breastfeeding, our results demonstrate, as other studies have done in the past (Dykes 2005, 2006; Groleau *et al.*

2006; Groleau & Cabral 2009), that breastfeeding cannot be reduced to merely biological or performative ontologies. Breastfeeding, like formula feeding, is a behaviour profoundly linked both to cultural representations related to the health of mothers and infants and to social processes, especially social relations of power, reciprocity and interdependence.

Our individualist worldview can bring us to take for granted that the breastfeeding social unit is rooted in the mother–child dyad and biological unit. In fact, our results reveal that even in an individualist society, such as Québec society, infant feeding experiences involve a much larger social unit that includes family, friends, community, and health professionals, with whom mothers exchange knowledge on infant feeding choices while engaging in power relationships. Foucault argues that power and knowledge are inseparable, mutually dependent and reinforcing (Foucault 1977). Furthermore, he states that power is 'diffuse, diverse, ambiguous, and located everywhere in day-to-day relationships and encounters, with everyone being caught up in mechanisms of power' (p. 176). Bourdieu (1985) argues that power is exercised according to the overall capital a person holds (economic, social, cultural, symbolic) in a specific social space.

With this in mind, we can argue that choosing to breastfeed in a social environment where formula feeding is the norm has implications for power relationships. As for other Western populations living in a context of poverty, formula feeding has become the norm for disadvantaged French-Canadians. In other words, it has become a habitus, the 'normal' or even 'natural' way to feed a baby. The promotion of breastfeeding is therefore an incentive for disadvantaged mothers to deviate from this habitus and adopt a feeding method perceived by many of their close ones as 'unnatural'. The introduction of breastfeeding is therefore an agent of cultural change that has an impact on power relationships of mothers within the various fields they engage in.

Power relations between mothers and nurses at the hospital were not the same as those within their family or social environments. At the hospital, several mothers in our study felt they were treated like children or judged negatively because of their young age. Interestingly, none mentioned that this was due to their low socioeconomic status. The majority of mothers (31/42) were 26 years of age and under. Another recent study (Whitley and Kirmayer 2008) found that young non-immigrant English-speaking mothers in Montréal (Québec, Canada) also experienced social stigmatisation because of their young age. This qualitative study theorised that, since the average age of mothers at first birth has recently risen to 28 years, with close to half of births occurring to women 30 years and older, 'anglophone Euro-Canadian mothers in their 20s may be facing some of the social exclusion traditionally associated with "teenage mothers"' (p. 346). Similarly, many mothers in our study were exposed to stigmatising comments and disapproving gazes because they had given birth at a 'young' age. However, back in their family and social environments, i.e. with people of a similar socioeconomic background, it was considered quite normal and 'natural' to be a young mother. In the context of their own socioeconomic milieu, becoming a mother for these women was not stigmatising, but rather a key source of symbolic capital, earning them respect among their peers and family.

Where the situation of mothers living in poverty differs from that of middle- or higher-income women is in the former's limited access to other sources of symbolic capital besides maternal competence and status. As stated in the introduction, the rearing and health of children of mothers living in poverty constitute key sources of symbolic capital within the mothers' *field* of family and peers. However, in the social space of the hospital, a *field* in which medical knowledge affords authoritative power, these mothers have little symbolic capital and feel, for the most part, negatively judged, stigmatised, or considered 'at risk' because of their age or other psychosocial stereotypes (some were followed by a social worker for psychosocial or drug-related problems). Many mothers living in a context of poverty soon felt disempowered by stigmatising discourses of health professionals such as 'Don't you want the best for your baby?' even when such messages were not directed at them but at the formula-feeding mothers with whom they shared a hospital room. Many mothers were aware that, in the hospital context, they were not perceived as competent mothers. In this field, therefore, their symbolic capital was poor, and few mothers were capable of defying the authoritarian discourse of health professionals, in particular, hospital nurses. In some instances, this discourse took the form of behaviour by some nurses towards the mothers. For example, some mothers mentioned that they had felt disrespected, even overpowered, by nurses who touched their breasts without asking permission while giving breastfeeding advice. Mothers who were distressed, single or experiencing psychosocial or medical difficulties (i.e. an important proportion of these mothers) felt especially vulnerable to this kind of overpowering discourse and associated behaviour.

However, mothers who received respectful, appropriate technical support for breastfeeding during their hospital stay, and who did not experience distress or the stress of having to take care of their baby alone, were more likely to be able to overcome technical problems related to breastfeeding during the first week after discharge. As a result, these mothers were more likely to breastfeed beyond the first postpartum week. However, mothers who did not receive appropriate technical support during their hospital stay returned home to face the same lack of support when breastfeeding problems arose. Consequently, these mothers rapidly replaced breastfeeding by formula feeding. As evoked in mothers' narratives, this change had much to do with lack of support from healthcare professionals, community and family. The *Global Strategy for Infant and Young Child Feeding* (WHO 2003, p. 8) states that mothers should:

> *'have access to skilled practical help from, for example trained workers, lay and peer counsellors and certified lactation consultants, who can help to build mothers' confidence, improve feeding techniques, and prevent or resolve breastfeeding problems.'*

Our study has illustrated that this support becomes essential to secure the sustainability of breastfeeding in a poverty context where breastfeeding is not the norm. Dealing alone with technical problems related to breastfeeding was not the only barrier these mothers had to face. Many of them also had to negotiate conflicting discourses from family members who disapproved of their choice of breastfeeding.

Whereas high levels of reported hospital support helped mothers cope with technical problems related to breastfeeding within the first few days after discharge, such support seems to have had less impact beyond the first postpartum week when mothers were increasingly exposed to and affected by conflicting family and social discourse. Such discourse was not only critical of breastfeeding but also reinforced the normative idea that, by breastfeeding, mothers were jeopardising their own energy levels and undermining their ability to take care of their babies, i.e. to be competent mothers. When the *Global Strategy for Infant and Young Feeding* states that 'implementing the strategy thus calls for increased political will, public invest-ment, awareness among health workers, and involvement of families and commun-ities' (WHO 2003, p. 7), we cannot simply assume that communities and family members, as key agents, will readily accept the scientific evidence that breastfeeding is better than formula feeding. The conflicting discourse and accompanying stigma regarding breastfeeding experienced by a majority of mothers in our study within their family or social milieus had a negative impact on many of them and may have contributed to their feelings of inadequacy, guilt, and distress both while breast-feeding and once they had abandoned the practice. Health professionals also need to be aware – perhaps through training programmes – of the effect of their own promotional discourse on mothers who are particularly vulnerable and rapidly stigmatised and disempowered by such discourse. Such training would help hospital and postpartum home nurses avoid, on one hand, risking damaging mothers' self-esteem by trying to convince them to breastfeed, and on the other hand, failing to meet their professional objectives by not convincing mothers to breastfeed. In addition, conflicting family and community discourses against breastfeeding need to be addressed by health professionals to ensure that future mothers are not burdened by such negotiations when they encounter breastfeeding problems and/or fatigue during the postpartum period. Our study data indicate that the more mothers' families and social environments are characterised by anti-breastfeeding discourses, the sooner mothers abandon breastfeeding after hospital discharge. Our study also suggests that community and accessible lay support, as highlighted as important in the *Global Strategy for Infant and Young Child Feeding*, must be addressed well in advance, such as during the prenatal period, involving key persons in the mother's milieu. Interventions that challenge a habitus so closely related to the symbolic cap-ital of mothers must be planned early on and go beyond the mother–child social unit by involving key members of the mother's family and social units during pregnancy.

The *Global Strategy for Infant and Young Child Feeding* states that 'families in difficult situations require special attention and practical support to be able to feed their children adequately' (WHO 2003, p. 10). This is particularly relevant to mothers living in the context of poverty where breastfeeding is not the norm. Indeed, our data lead us to argue that poverty makes women more vulnerable to social stigma both at home and in the hospital setting, although, as we have seen, for different reasons. Not only must mothers cope with chronic stress related to their economic situation, but may also have to take care of their babies alone, thus constituting an additional source of stress and fatigue. Their symbolic capital is more closely linked to the notion of their own 'parental competency', all the more significant since it is one of the only sources of symbolic capital accessible to them. This situation is very different from that of middle- and upper-income women, who are generally more educated and more likely to derive symbolic power from their profession, social status or other achievements besides motherhood. The training of health professionals to understand this social reality is all the more essential in order to prevent their discourse from contributing to the disempowerment of mothers living in poverty.

Our data suggest, therefore, that mothers living in the context of poverty have a greater need for continuously accessible emotional and technical support in the perinatal period to cope with: social stigma; family, social and professional reprobation linked to their 'controversial' infant feeding choice; and technical problems related to breastfeeding. Breastfeeding a child in a formula-feeding environment represents a kind of challenge by these mothers to the established order, notably, of older women in their family and social milieu. Their health behaviour becomes a reflection of the discourse and practices related to health that they must negotiate within their sociocultural environment. In this respect, the emphasis placed by the *Global Strategy for Infant and Young Child Feeding* on the importance of community networks of trained counsellors and mother-to-mother breastfeeding supporters, becomes as a central strategy to adopt in a poverty context where formula feeding constitutes a cultural norm. For French-Canadian women living in a context of poverty, this strategy is essential for preventing breastfeeding promotion from having a harmful effect on the emotional wellbeing and symbolic capital of mothers. Lay support becomes essential in providing opportunities for mothers to learn from 'positively deviant' (Sternin *et al.* 1998) peers about strategies to overcome local cultural barriers to breastfeeding.

Our research indicates that breastfeeding, like any normative infant feeding practice, is not neutral. In fact, attempting to change a normative infant feeding practice may have a negative impact on mothers' lives and wellbeing. In other words, if breastfeeding policies are adopted without the financial means and systemic strategic planning necessary to ensure support, community links and continuity of care, detrimental effects can be expected. Thus as stated in the *Global Strategy*, 'providing sound and culture-specific nutrition counselling to mothers of young children' (WHO 2003 p. 9) is essential. But this counselling must take into account not only the 'local foodstuffs' but should also assess the local systemic and ideological barriers breastfeeding mothers have to face.

5.4 Conclusion

At present, in Québec and elsewhere in the West, programmes promoting breast-feeding do not always benefit infants from the social group that needs it most, i.e. those born in the context of poverty (European-Commission 2006; Neill 2006). Many mothers in our study chose to abandon breastfeeding and adopt formula feeding to protect their physical and emotional wellbeing in the face of socioeconomic hardship and stigma. By breastfeeding, they challenged the local infant feeding habitus and social order, while jeopardisng their perceived competence as mothers, a key element of both their symbolic capital and self-esteem. If national and international breastfeeding policies and guidelines fail to take into account the particular circumstances and needs of low-income women, as well as the disempowering discourse they must negotiate in different social spaces, health promotion interventions are likely to have a detrimental effect on populations that have the greatest need for the health benefits of breastfeeding.

Acknowledgements

The authors wish to thank Jeffrey Freedman for his revision and translation of part of this chapter as well as the Fond de Recherche en Santé du Québec (FRSQ) for the salary awarded to both authors as well as the Fond Québécois de Recherche Sur La Société et la Culture (FQRSC) for funding the project.

References

American Academy of Pediatrics (1997) Breastfeeding and the use of human milk. *Pediatrics*, **100**: 1035–1039.
American Academy of Pediatrics (2005) Breastfeeding and the use of human milk. *Pediatrics*, **115** (2): 496–506.
Attree, P. (2005) Low-income mothers, nutrition and health; a systematic review of qualitative evidence. *Maternal and Child Nutrition*, **1**: 227–240.
Baker, D., Taylor, H. & Henderson, J. (1998) Inequality in infant morbidity: causes and consequences in England in the 1990s. ALSPAC Study Team. Avon Longitudinal Study of pregnancy and Childhood. *Journal of Epidemiology and Community Health*, **52** (7): 451–458.
Blum, L.M. (1993) Mothers, babies and breastfeeding in late capitalist America: the shifting contexts of feminist theory. *Feminist Studies: FS*, **19**: 291–311.
Bourdieu, P. (1977) Sur le pouvoir symbolique. *Annali*, **32** (3): 404–411.
Bourdieu, P. (1984) *Distinction*. Harvard University Press, Cambridge, MA.
Bourdieu, P. (1985) The forms of social capital. In: Richardson, G. (ed.) *Handbook of Theory and Research for the Sociology of Education*. Greenwood, New York.
Bourdieu, P. (1989) Social space and symbolic power. *Sociological Theory*, **7** (1): 14–25.
Britton, C., McCormick, F.M., Renfrew, M.J., Wade, A. & King, S.E. (2007) Support for breastfeeding mothers. *Cochrane Database of Systematic Reviews*, (**1**): CD001141.
Carter, P. (1995) *Feminism, Breast, Breastfeeding*. Macmillan, London.
Cox, J.L., Holden, J.M. & Sagovsky, R. (1987) Detection of postnatal depression: development of the 10-item Edinburgh Postnatal Depression Scale. *British Journal of Psychiatry*, **150**: 782–786.
Des Rivières-Pigeon, C., Séguin, L., Brodeur, J.M., Perreault, M., Boyer, G., Colin, C. & Goulet, L. (2000) The Edinburgh Postnatal Depression Scale: the validity of its Quebec version for a population low socioeconomic status mothers. *Canadian Journal of Community Mental Health*, **19** (1): 201–214.
Dix, D.N. (1991) Why women decide not to breastfeed. *Birth*, **18** (4): 222–225.
Dubois, L., Bedard, B., Girard, M., & Beauchesne, É. (2000) L'Alimentation. Dans Etude longitudinale du development des enfants du Quebec (ELDEQ 1998–2002). Institut de la statistique du Québec, Québec.
Dykes, F. (2005) Supply and demand: breastfeeding a labour. *Social Science and Medicine*, **60** (10): 2283–2293.
Dykes, F. (2006) *Breastfeeding in Hospital. Mothers, Midwives and the Production Line*. Taylor & Francis Group, Routledge, New York.

European-Commission (2006) *Protection. Promotion and support of breastfeeding in Europe: A Blueprint for Action.* European Commission, Dublin Castle, Ireland.

Foucault, M. (1977) *Discipline and Punish – the Birth of the Prison.* Penguin, Harmondsworth.

Galler, J.R., Harrison, R.H., Biggs, M.A., Ramsey, F. & Forde, V. (1999) Maternal moods predict breastfeeding in Barbados. *Journal of Developmental and Behavioral Pediatrics*, 20 (2): 80–87.

Geertz, C. (1973) *The Interpretations of Cultures.* Basic Books, New York.

Giugliani, E., Issler, R., Kreutz, G., Meneses, C., Justo, E., Kreutz, E., *et al.* (1996) Breastfeeding pattern in a population with different levels of poverty in Southern Brazil. *Acta Paediatrica*, 85 (12): 1499–1500.

Good, B.J. (1994) *Medicine Rationality, and Experience. An Anthropological Perspective.* Cambridge University Press, Cambridge.

Groleau, D. (1998) Déterminants culturels et l'approche écologique: le cas de la promotion de l'allaitement chez les immigrantes vietnamiennes. Ph.D. thesis. In: *Département de Médecine Sociale et Préventive.* Faculté de Médecine, Université de Montréal, Montréal.

Groleau, D. & Cabral, I.E. (2009) Reconfiguring insufficient breast milk as a sociosomatic problem: mothers of premature babies using the kangaroo method in Brazil. *Maternal and Child Nutrition*, 5 (1): 10–24.

Groleau, D., Soulière, M. & Kirmayer, L.J. (2006) Breastfeeding and the cultural configuration of social space among Vietnamese immigrant woman. *Health and Place*, 12 (4): 516–526.

Groleau, D., Zelkowitz, P. & Cabral, I.E. (2009) Enhancing generalizability: moving from an intimate to a political voice. *Qualitative Health Research*, 19 (3): 416–426.

Hermans, H.J.M. (2001) The dialogical self: toward a theory of personal and cultural positioning. *Culture Psychology*, 7 (3): 243–281.

Kleinman, A. (1980) Patients and healers in the context of culture. An exploration of the borderland between anthropology, medicine and psychiatry. University of California Press, Berkeley.

Levill, C., Hanvey, L., Avard, D., Chance, G. & Kaczorowski, J. (1995) Enquête sur les pratiques et les soins de routine dans les hôpitaux canadiens dotés d'un service d'obstétrique. Santé Canada et Institut Canadien de la Santé Infantile, Ottawa.

Mahon-Daly, P., Gavin, J. & Andrews, B. (2002) Liminality and breastfeeding: women negotiating space and two bodies. *Health and Place*, 8: 61–76.

Misri, S., Sinclair, D.A. & Kuan, A.J. (1997) Breast-feeding and postpartum depression: Is there a relationship? *Canadian Journal of Psychiatry*, 42 (10): 1061–1065.

MSSS (1997) Priorités nationales de santé publique 1997–2002. In: *Direction générale de la santé publique.* Ministère de la Santé et des Services sociaux, Gouvernement du Québec, Québec.

MSSS (2001) *L'allaitement maternel au Québec. Lignes directrices.* Ministère de la Santé et des Services sociaux, Gouvernement du Québec, Québec.

Muhr, T. (1991) ATLAS/ti – a prototype for the support of text interpretation. *Qualitative Sociology*, 14 (4): 350–371.

Neill, G., *et al.* (2006) *Recueil statistique sur l'allaitement maternel au Québec, 2005–2006.* Institut de la statistique du Québec, Gouvernement du Québec, Québec.

O'Hara, M.W. & Swain, A.M. (1996) Rates and risk of postpartum depression – a meta-analysis. *International Review of Psychiatry*, 8 (1): 37–54.

OMS/FISE (1989) Protection, encouragement et soutien de l'allaitement maternel. Le rôle spécial des services liés à la maternité. Suisse, Organisation Mondiale de la Santé/FISE, Genève.

Raisler, J. (1993) Promoting breast-feeding among vulnerable mothers. *Journal of Nurse-Midwifery*, 38 (1): 1–4

Riva, E., Banderali, G., Agostoni, C., Silano, M., Radaelli, G. & Giovannini, M. (1999) Factors associated with initiation and duration of breastfeeding in Italy. *Acta Paediatrica*, 88 (4): 411–415.

Santé Canada, Statistique Canada et le Centre canadien d'information sur la santé (1999) Rapport Statistqiue sur la santé de la population Canadienne. Enquête Nationale sur la santé de la Population 1996–1997. Gouvernement du Canada, Canada.

Schwandt, T.A. (2001) *Dictionary of Qualitative Inquiry.* Sage Publications, Thousands Oaks, California.

Séguin, L., Potvin, L., St-Denis, M. & Loiselle, J. (1999) Depressive symptoms in the late postpartum among low socioeconomic status women. *Birth*, 26: 157–163.

Sikorski, J., Renfrew, M.J., Pindoria, S. & Wade, A. (2003) Support for breastfeeding mothers: a systematic review. *Paediatric and Perinatal Epidemiology*, **17** (4): 407–417.

Society, Canadian Paediatric, Dietitians of Canada and Health Canada. (2005) *Nutrition for Healthy Term Infants*. Minister of Public Works and Government Services, Government of Canada, Ottawa.

Sternin, M., Sternin, J. & Marsh, D.R. (1998) Field guide: designing a community-based nutrition education and rehabilitation program using the 'positive deviance' approach. Save the Children and BASICS, Westport, Conn., USA.

Van Esterik, P. (1989) *Mother Power and Infant Feeding*. Zed Books, London.

Whitley, R. & Kirmayer, L.J. (2008) Perceived stigmatisation of young mothers: an exploratory study of psychological and social experience. *Social Science and Medicine*, **66**: 339–348.

WHO (2003) *Global Strategy for Infant and Young Child Feeding*. WHO, Geneva.

WHO/UNICEF (1989) Protecting, promoting and supporting breastfeeding. The special role of maternity services. WHO and UNICEF, Geneva, Switzerland.

Young, A. (1981) When rational men fall sick: an inquiry into some assumptions made by medical anthropologists. *Culture, Medicine and Psychiatry*, **5**: 317–335.

6 Achieving Optimal Infant and Young Child Feeding Practices: Case Studies from Tanzania and Rwanda

Lucy Thairu

6.1 Introduction

The promotion of optimal infant feeding practices entails the provision of accurate and complete information to relevant stakeholders while respecting beneficial cultural traditions (World Health Organization (WHO) 2003a). In order to achieve optimal infant health, the WHO *Global Strategy for Infant and Young Child Feeding* recommends exclusive breastfeeding for the first six months of life, and thereafter the infant should receive nutritionally adequate and safe complementary foods with breastfeeding continuing for up to 2 years of age or beyond.

Over the past decade, ambiguity in defining breastfeeding patterns made it difficult to demonstrate the significance of exclusive breastfeeding in averting infant mortality, as compared to predominant breastfeeding (Labbok & Coffin 1997). The infant feeding pattern can be defined as (WHO Collaborative Study Team on the Role of Breastfeeding on the Prevention of Infant Mortality 2000):

- Exclusive breastfeeding – if the infant receives breast milk only and, with the exception of medical prescriptions, does not receive water
- Predominant breastfeeding – if the infant receives water or water-based drinks in addition to breast milk
- Partial breastfeeding – if the infant receives breast milk and some artificial feeds, either milk or cereal, or other food
- Replacement feeding – if the infant is exclusively fed a breast milk substitute (i.e. does not breastfeed at all).

A recent study from Ghana showed the importance of early and exclusive breastfeeding in reducing deaths from infectious diseases in the first month of life (Edmond *et al.* 2007). The study explored the odds of newborn death from tetanus, meningitis, pneumonia, diarrhoea or septicaemia according to the timing of breastfeeding initiation and the exclusivity of breastfeeding. Results showed that the odds of dying were almost three times higher when breastfeeding was initiated more than a day after delivery versus within an hour. Furthermore, in contrast with exclusive breastfeeding, the odds of death were almost 1.5 times higher when breastfeeding was predominant, and almost six times higher when breastfeeding was partial. The Ghanaian results emphasise the relevance of international 'best practice' recommendations for breastfeeding, including: initiating breastfeeding within an hour of delivery; breastfeeding 'on demand'; and exclusive versus predominant or partial breastfeeding.

6.1.1   Breastfeeding in the context of HIV/AIDS

According to the *Global Strategy for Infant and Young Child Feeding* (WHO 2003a), special attention is needed for supporting infant feeding when infants are born to human immunodeficiency virus (HIV)+ women. Vertical or mother-to-child transmission of HIV (MTCT) was first documented in 1983 (Ammann 1983). By the mid-1980s, there was convincing evidence that the virus could be transmitted through breast milk (Thiry *et al.* 1985). By the end of the decade, HIV+ mothers in the developed world were advised to avoid breastfeeding to reduce the risk of transmission (Logan Stuart 1988). However, there was already concern about the danger of similar guidance for HIV+ mothers in resource-poor settings. By 2003, research had confirmed that, in conditions of poverty and limited hygiene, the risk of infant morbidity and mortality due to artificial feeding was greater than the potential benefit of preventing HIV transmission through breastfeeding avoidance (Coutsoudis *et al.* 2003).

Parallel to investigations about breastfeeding versus replacement feeding, the impact of the *breastfeeding pattern* on MTCT had gained recognition by the end of the 1990s. The risk of HIV was found to be lower if breastfeeding was exclusive rather than mixed (Coutsoudis 2000). Given the potential danger of mixed feeding, HIV+ mothers were advised to cease breastfeeding 'rapidly' or 'abruptly', 'keeping the period of transition as short as possible' in order to reduce the risk of HIV transmission during breastfeeding cessation (Piwoz 2001). With respect to the *timing* of breastfeeding cessation, until recently HIV+ mothers were advised to discontinue breastfeeding 'as soon as was feasible' in order to reduce infant exposure to the virus (WHO 2003b). However, research from the past two years indicates that early breastfeeding cessation (i.e. before six months post partum) compromises infant health and survival (Thea *et al.* 2006; Athena Kourtis 2007; Kafulafula 2007; Onyango 2007; Sinkala 2007), and this practice is now discouraged. Nevertheless, the optimal timing of breastfeeding cessation remains unclear, and perhaps it should be determined based on individual circumstances (WHO 2006).

Current research has provided convincing evidence that, in resource-poor settings: breastfeeding is preferable to replacement feeding; exclusive breastfeeding is superior to predominant or partial breastfeeding; and breastfeeding should begin within a few hours of delivery, continue for at least six months and be complemented with other foods until breastfeeding cessation is feasible. These optimal infant feeding practices, in conjunction with the provision of anti-retroviral therapy (ART) to HIV+ mothers during delivery and lactation, reduce the risk of MTCT and promote child health and survival (Thior *et al.* 2006; Kafulafula 2007).

In this chapter I describe the results of two investigations on infant and young child feeding practices in Tanzania and Rwanda. I discuss current practices in breastfeeding initiation and exclusivity during the neonatal period based on the research conducted in Tanzania. In the Rwandan study, I discuss infant and young child feeding practices in the context of HIV/AIDS. Based on these local assessments, I conclude by discussing the practices that appear to promote optimal infant and young child nutrition, and those which require improvement.

6.2   Infant feeding practices among mothers of unknown HIV status in Tanzania

This study[i] was conducted with women from one small rural community in the south of Pemba Island, one of the two major Zanzibar islands situated off mainland Tanzania. The main economic activities include subsistence agriculture (mostly cloves and coconuts) and fishing. Reflecting long historical ties with the Muslim world, more than 99% of Pembans are Muslim. Kiswahili, the main language, is predominantly African with many words borrowed from Arabic (Goldman 1996). The study was preceded by ethnographic observation and key informant interviewing, which was used to obtain background information on infant feeding practices. This information was used to inform the study described here. The study was conducted in three phases:

(1)   Women were asked about their expectations about infant feeding, including breastfeeding initiation, breastfeeding pattern and details of what liquids and foods they intended to feed their baby and when they intended to give them.

(2)   Four specific recommendations with the aim to support early and exclusive breastfeeding were provided to each woman (Box 6.1). We made it clear that these were proposals for 'good practice' and that we were interested in finding out what each woman, as a prospective mother, thought about them. We asked each woman whether she was interested in trying out the advice, and why she thought she would/would not attempt the behaviour.

(3)   Subsequent interviews were conducted with the women to assess whether they had followed our recommendations. Interviews were conducted on average 5.5 (3.7 SD) days post partum.

All pregnant women who had visited the primary health care unit (PHCU) in the community were contacted. To ensure inclusiveness, we asked for referrals to pregnant friends and relatives who lived in the same community. To be eligible, women had to be in the last month of pregnancy, reside within the community and plan to remain there during 'postpartum seclusion'. The practice of postpartum

---

[i] The results of this study are partially published in: Thairu, L. & Pelto, G. (2008) Newborn care practices in Pemba Island (Tanzania) and their implications for newborn health and survival. *Maternal and Child Nutrition*, 4: 194–208. They are also presented in a dissertation submitted to Cornell University: Thairu, L. (2006) Ethnography of infant feeding in Sub-Saharan Africa: case studies in the context of HIV/AIDS and newborn care. Division of Nutritional Sciences, Cornell University, Ithaca, NY, USA.

Box 6.1   Good practice recommendations

- Begin breastfeeding immediately after the baby is born, before two hours are over. Newborn babies are unable to keep themselves warm. This is why, immediately after the baby is born, he needs to get warmth from his mother. During breastfeeding, the baby is close to his mother's body, this allows him to get warmth.
- Feed the baby frequently, at night and during the day. People think that the newborn should eat at the same time as adults eat. But you shouldn't give the baby food only when you are eating. Babies have smaller stomachs and they cannot store a lot of food. That is why they need to be fed very frequently, even at night.
- Do not to give the baby cow's milk, porridge, or other foods. People give the newborn cow's milk or porridge because they think their milk is not enough and that the baby is still hungry. But you shouldn't give the baby these feeds when he is still very young. When the baby breastfeeds, he is satisfied, he has already got enough to eat, so there is no need to give him these feeds.
- Do not to give the baby any water to drink. People give the newborn water to drink because they believe he is thirsty. But you shouldn't give the baby water when he is still very young. When the baby breastfeeds, he is satisfied, he has already got enough water, so there is no need to give him water.

seclusion is based on the belief that new mothers are a source of 'ritual pollution', requiring them to abstain from sex and to be secluded from the rest of the community. Some women return to their parents' home (sometimes located in another community), whereas others remain in their own compounds.

Data were collected between December 2004 and March 2005. All interviews were conducted in the mother's home in Kiswahili by four female interviewers (myself, and three Pemban interviewers). Interviews were tape-recorded and transcribed. Each Kiswahili transcript was reviewed in consultation with the other interviewers and additional items and discrepancies noted. To ensure accurate translation into English, we consulted two dictionaries (Akida 1981; Johnson 1939) and discussed locally specific terms. All open-ended responses were coded in order to classify each woman's pre-delivery intentions and post-delivery experiences.

Study approval was obtained from the research ethics committees of the Pemba Public Health Laboratory, the Zanzibar Ministry of Health and Cornell University. Informed consent was sought from each respondent prior to each interview.

6.2.1   Findings

There were no refusals among the eligible women, which yielded a sample of 30. Two women dropped out after the first interview. Two of the remaining 28 dropped out after delivery (one had a still birth, one relocated for postpartum seclusion). Of the 26 who completed the study, 85% were referred by the PHCU. The characteristics of the sample are shown in Table 6.1.

6.2.1.1   Breastfeeding intention

All 26 women intended to breastfeed. The women perceived breast milk as a 'natural food' for infants and breastfeeding as a 'normal' behaviour that transmits good

Table 6.1   Tanzanian mothers' demographic characteristics (n = 26)

Maternal age in years, mean (SD)	30 (6.7)
Number of children, mean (SD)	5 (3)
Newborn age in days at the time of the third interview, mean (SD)	5.5 (3.7)
Women who had one or more children die, %	35
Home delivery, %	46
Person who assisted with this delivery, %:	
Traditional birth attendant	35
Doctor or nurse	54
Family member	4
Other/don't know	8
Spent postpartum seclusion in natal home, %	23
Number of individuals living in household, mean (SD)	6 (2.6)
Type of roof, %	
Roofing made of dried coconut leaves	58
Roofing made of corrugated iron sheets	42
Transportation, %	
No means of transportation	50
Owned bicycle	38.5
Owned motorcycle and/or car	12
Access to water, %	
From communal tap	84
From a well	16
Level of education, %	
No schooling	50
Primary school	50
Literate, %	50

health and nutrition to newborns. Their statements about breast milk and breast-feeding included: 'breast milk is his right'; 'I will breastfeed the baby because he will be hungry, and he needs to grow'; and 'a baby is not able to eat anything else.' Using the strict definition of exclusive breastfeeding, only two women intended to avoid any other infant nutrition apart from breast milk.

6.2.1.2   *Timing of initiation of breastfeeding*

Information on when women intended to initiate breastfeeding were fully available for 13 mothers. Two of the 13 intended to initiate breastfeeding shortly after delivery. The remaining 11 women mentioned other time periods such as 'after I have taken a shower' or 'the next day.' Of the 11 mothers who had not planned on early breastfeeding initiation, all agreed to try out our advice. Their motivations for agreeing to our recommendations included: 'when babies are born they want to eat immediately' or 'it is our tradition to breastfeed the baby as soon as he is born'.

Eight of the 11 mothers who had agreed to initiate breastfeeding immediately after giving birth, successfully implemented our advice (Figure 6.1). Three women felt unable to follow through with their decision. The first, a 42-year-old woman who had experienced prolonged labour reported: 'he did not breastfeed on the day that he was born [. . .] he was tired because he took a long time before he was born, I thought he would be born dead.' In justifying her lack of adherence, a 20-year-old

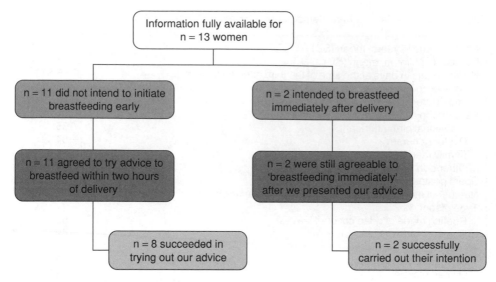

Figure 6.1   Timing of breastfeeding initiation: prepartum intentions, decisions to try recommended best practices and post-delivery outcomes.

mother alluded to 'ritual uncleanliness' following childbirth and to the need to 'wash away the filth'. The third woman described the severe postpartum haemorrhage she experienced during delivery as follows: 'at the time I was having problems so I could not breastfeed, my health was not good, I was feeling faint, I was losing a lot of blood . . .'. We observed that, even during the interview, the woman did not appear to be doing so well.

6.2.1.3   Breastfeeding on demand

The majority of women (n = 21) intended to breastfeed 'on demand,' the remaining five planned on breastfeeding 'according to a schedule'. All five mothers who had expected to follow a feeding schedule agreed to 'breastfeed on demand'. Their willingness did not relate to scheduling but focused on positive features of breast milk as 'baby's food' or 'breast milk is his fruit, he was created with it' as well as concerns for the newborn's wellbeing, including 'because the baby is not old enough to eat or drink anything else'.

Four of the five women who had agreed to breastfeed 'on demand' succeeded in implementing their choice (Figure 6.2). A 42-year-old woman who did not follow the advice had experienced prolonged labour.

6.2.1.4   Feeding the baby non-breast milk foods

Eighteen mothers intended to give solid or liquid nutrition to their newborn. Porridge (n = 11) and cow's milk (n = 11) were the most common items. Justifications for feeding their babies with porridge and cow's milk included: 'I will give him

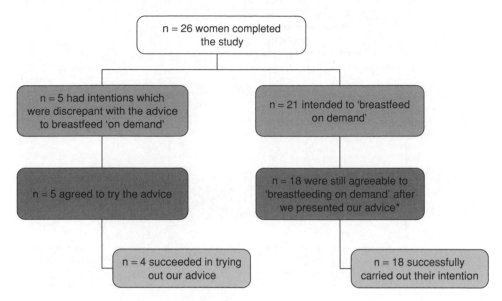

Figure 6.2   Breastfeeding on demand: prepartum intentions, decisions to try recommended best practices and post-delivery outcomes.

*Three women changed their minds between the first interview and the second. Two reported breastfeeding on demand at the third interview, the third had experienced severe postpartum haemorrhage.

cow's milk because he will be hungry and because I have nothing in my breast' or 'it will help him, I cannot afford anything else'. Biscuits (n = 7) were justified by the belief that they are 'foods for young infants' or '[biscuits] will allow the mother to rest a little' or that they will help soothe a baby who is crying. Motivations for less common items such as juices, cassava, eggs, tea, soup, powdered milk and mangoes were related to the perception that the infant would be 'hungry' that the mother would 'not have enough' milk or that the substitutes would 'build the baby's body'.

Thirteen of the 18 women who had intended to give their infants solid and fluid nutrition chose to try our recommendation to avoid this practice. The women appealed to the concept of the infant's developmental stage to explain their willingness to adopt this new behaviour, for example, 'because the baby's stomach is small, and he cannot yet digest heavy foods'. The mothers also believed that breast milk is 'the ideal food for baby' and that it is 'enough for the baby'.

Eleven of the 13 women who had agreed to avoid other foods and fluids (Figure 6.3) were successful in implementing their choice. However, two introduced cow's milk, biscuits or infant formula to their newborn's diet by days 3 and 5. In justifying their behaviour, these two women recounted stories related to the newborn's cues, such as crying or being hungry. A 42-year-old woman explained that her baby was too 'tired' and since he was crying she had to give him cow's milk and water. The other woman, who was 20 years old, reported that her newborn was 'thirsty' (to justify water), 'hungry' (to justify biscuits) and 'crying a lot' (to justify cow's milk).

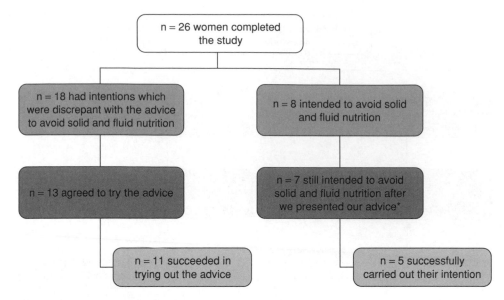

Figure 6.3 Feeding the baby non-breast milk foods: prepartum intentions, decisions to try recommended best practices and post-delivery outcomes.

*One woman had changed her mind between the first interview and the second.

6.2.1.5   Feeding the baby water

Fourteen women planned to give their newborns water. Examples of motivations for water included: 'if you do not drink water, you cannot be a human being' or 'in the same way that I feel thirsty, I think he is also thirsty'. Ten of the 14 women chose to try avoiding water for the baby to drink. Among the five who rejected the advice, a pervasive theme was the belief that 'human beings need water to survive'. The women also stressed the extreme nature of their infants' thirst. Examples given by mothers to justify rejecting our advice included: 'eating and drinking go together, for this reason, if he breastfeeds, he eats, so he must drink water' or 'my heart tells me that babies cannot go for long periods without being given water to drink' or 'breast milk is salty and it makes the baby thirsty'. Those who agreed to try the advice referred to the 'sufficiency' of breast milk in justifying their choice, e.g. 'because my breast milk will be enough'. Another explanation for trying the recommendation was trust in the information provided to them, e.g. 'because this is what you [the professionals] have advised us.'

Six of the ten women who had agreed to try avoiding water (Figure 6.4) adhered to their prepartum choice. Some of their motivations related to beliefs that the 'mother's milk is enough' and their trust in the information we provided to them. The four women who did not follow our advice gave their infants water, on average, five days after birth. In justifying their behaviour, one of the women indicated that, in spite of her desire to do otherwise, she gave her newborn water because she was unable to produce sufficient milk. The second mother highlighted the infant's thirst,

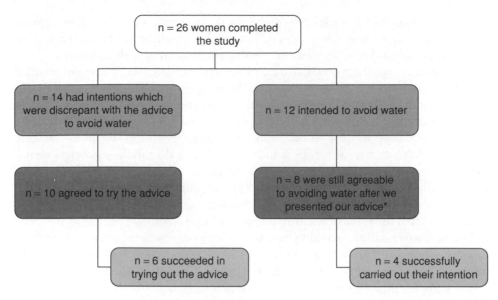

Figure 6.4   Feeding the baby water: prepartum intentions, decisions to try recommended best practices and post-delivery outcomes.

*Five women had changed their intentions when we presented the recommendations. Of these, three reported giving their newborns water at the time of the interview, two had avoided the practice.

the third had experienced prolonged labour, and the fourth noted that 'for a human being, water is life'.

6.2.2   Barriers and opportunities to promoting early and exclusive breastfeeding in Tanzania

The first week post partum is a critical time for initiating and establishing exclusive breastfeeding. Results from our study have highlighted cultural factors that facilitated or constrained the adoption of recommended best practices. For some of the mothers who experienced extreme and unusual difficulties in the early postpartum period, failure to follow the recommendations was not a choice, but was rather an inevitable outcome of traumatic childbirth. It is noteworthy that two of the 26 newborns in our study died some time after the last interview.

It is likely that our style facilitated the women's positive responses. We sought to be courteous, non-judgemental, providers of information and treated women with respect encouraging them to consider behaviour change. Based on prior experience in Pemba, we knew that mothers felt 'talked down to' by health personnel. We therefore made considerable effort to give a rationale for each suggestion, and encouraged women to discuss their reactions and challenge the recommendations.

The results show that early breastfeeding initiation fits easily into pre-existing cultural expectations. Willingness and success in trying out the new behaviour was high as eight of the 11 of those who had chosen to try, succeeded in doing so. With one exception, it was only difficult birth conditions that prevented success. The exception was a young woman who felt she should not touch the baby until she had bathed – a reflection of cultural beliefs about ritual pollution associated with childbirth.

Breastfeeding on demand was also easily accommodated. Many women intended to follow this practice even before they heard our suggestion. Those whose intentions were discrepant agreed to try adopt the behaviour, and four out of five succeeded in behaviour change, the one who failed had experienced delivery problems.

The advice not to give solid foods and fluid nutrition counters cultural expectations. Only two of the 26 women intended to do this. Nonetheless nearly three-quarters of them agreed to try and most (82%) of these succeeded. The positive value that culture places on breast milk was an important supporting factor, but concerns about the insufficiency of breast milk in sustaining infant wellbeing may have obstructed the value of exclusive breastfeeding.

The recommendation to avoid water for the newborn was the most problematic. Results confirm earlier finding (Almroth 1990) that the practice of giving water to infants is based on pervasive beliefs such as 'preventing infant thirst,' or that 'water is necessary for life.' The majority of women expected to give their newborns water, but about a half were willing to reconsider their intention. Of those who indicated a willingness to try, only 55% followed through. The dramatic comment from one woman – 'My heart tells me that babies cannot go for long periods without being given water to drink' – is an indication of the depth of cultural expectations relating to water. Implementation of the *Global Strategy for Infant and Young Child Feeding* will need attention to mothers' difficulty in avoiding water for the newborn, as this behaviour may be more resistant to change. It is possible that providing information about the lack of nutritional value in water and the risk of infection may promote behaviour change.

6.3   Infant feeding practices among HIV+ mothers in Rwanda

By 2005, over 50% of the 386 public healthcare facilities in Rwanda were providing prevention of mother-to-child transmission (PMTCT) of HIV services to women. Specific services varied, but all included HIV counselling and testing for women during pregnancy and, for those found to be HIV+, a single dose of nevirapine during delivery (for the mother and for her infant) as well as an infant HIV test at 15 months. While universal coverage was expected by 2008, the programme has experienced a number of challenges. For example, despite the high acceptance of HIV testing (more than 80% of pregnant women are tested), health staff in 2005 did not feel adequately prepared to address questions related to HIV and infant feeding. This may have been due to lack of training. For example, by 2005, those counsellors who had been trained in HIV and infant feeding had only received a two-hour module devoted to the topic and no nationwide training programme addressing this aspect of PMTCT had been initiated.

In 2005, UNICEF, the Rwandan national Treatment Research and AIDS Center (TRAC) and the Nutrition Working Group in Rwanda commissioned a study on

HIV and infant feeding[ii]. The objective of this study was to describe infant feeding practices among HIV+ mothers in Rwanda, and to use the data to inform the country's policy on PMTCT through breastfeeding. Until January 2006, Rwanda was composed of 12 administrative provinces, including Kigali, the capital city. Three clinics were randomly selected from each province (total of 36 clinics). All mothers who were enrolled in selected PMTCT centres and those who attended the clinic on the day that the interviews were conducted were invited to participate (n = 706). As criteria for eligibility, the mothers had to be HIV+ and to have an infant under 18 months of age. Ethical approval was obtained from the Rwandan National Ethical Committee. The protocol was reviewed and approved by the TRAC and by the Nutrition Working Group in Rwanda. Informed consent was sought from all respondents prior to participation.

6.3.1   Findings

A total of 706 HIV+ women were interviewed and data were fully available for 681 women. Unfortunately we did not document the total number of eligible women who attended the clinics and this is one of the study limitations. Participant characteristics are provided in Table 6.2. The women's infant feeding practices are described in the section that follows.

6.3.1.1   Infant feeding choices

Eighty-four per cent (572/681) of mothers stated that they chose to breastfeed their infants. Of these, 53% justified their choice by explaining that they lacked the financial means to make other choices. Twenty per cent noted that they found breastfeeding to be 'easy'. It is important to note that exclusive breastfeeding is by far the norm in Rwanda, where nearly 80% of all mothers practise exclusive breastfeeding in the first six months of life. This is the highest rate of exclusive breastfeeding both in Africa and the world (Mukuria 2006).

A total of 106 women stated that they chose replacement feeding for their infants. Of these, however, 72% (n = 76) indicated that they did not, in fact, avoid breastfeeding completely. Therefore, a total of 648 mothers actually breastfed their infants and of these, 44% (n = 284) were still breastfeeding their infants at the time of the interview, at a mean infant age of 6 (4.5 SD) months. With respect to initiation, 59% (n = 384) began breastfeeding within half an hour following birth, 22% (n = 145) within an hour of birth and 16% (n = 102) within a day of birth (the remainder indicated an 'other' time period).

[ii] Thairu, L. (2005) Evaluation des pratiques d'alimentation des nourrissons et des jeunes enfants dans le contexte du VIH/SIDA au Rwanda. Kigali, UNICEF.

Table 6.2   Rwandan human immunodeficiency virus (HIV)+ mothers' demographic characteristics (n = 706)

Age in years, mean (range)	30.0 (17–49)
Number of children, mean (range)	3.2 (1–10)
Infant age in months, mean (range)	9.0 (0.1–18)
Religion, %:	
Protestant	36
Catholic	35
Muslim	7
Adventist	11
Other	11
Mother's level of education, %	
Never gone to school	32
Primary school	57
Post primary	9
Other	2
Mean weekly household income, Rwandese francs (US dollars)	3000 (5.6)
Proportion of income destined used to purchase food for household, %	
All	28
Three-quarters	45
Half	20
Less than half	7
Source of water, %	
Electrogaz	10
Margot	10
River	7
Communal tap	48
Well	22
Other	3

6.3.1.2   Cessation of breastfeeding

Over half (52%; n = 340) of HIV+ mothers thought that infants should be taken off the breast at six months of age, and 45% (n = 293) thought that cessation was possible at 10 months or older, which was the oldest response category in the survey. Participants were asked to describe what their most important motivations for ceasing to breastfeed were (see Table 6.3). Just over a quarter of mothers (n = 172) believed that either a new pregnancy or resuming menstrual periods was the most important motivation for stopping breastfeeding.

6.3.1.3   Infant feeding counselling

The majority of mothers (93%) recalled receiving some information about breast-feeding from their PMTCT counsellors. However, the quality of the information was inconsistent. With respect to other infant feeding options, only 42% (n = 272) of the mothers were aware of the use of infant formula as an option for infant nutri-tion, and 33% (n = 225) were aware of the use of cow's milk as a replacement food. Seventeen per cent of the mothers (n = 116) both felt that they should not breastfeed and had not received any information about a suitable breast milk substitute.

Table 6.3   Rwandan human immunodeficiency virus (HIV)+ mothers' most important stated motivation for ceasing to breastfeed*

Motivation	Frequency	Per cent
When the infant begins to speak	40	6
When the infant begins to walk	23	3
When the infant refuses breast milk	103	15
If the mother becomes pregnant again	147	22
If the infant begins to teethe	32	5
If the infant expresses interest in eating with adults	142	21
Six months after birth	74	11
When the mother begins to have her menstrual period	25	4
Other reasons	95	14
Total	681	100

*Mothers could only choose one option. However, it is not inconceivable that a number of 'events' could culminate in her decision to stop breastfeeding. For example, an infant could begin to lose interest in breast milk around the same time that the mother realises she is pregnant. This would lead to her decision to terminate breastfeeding.

6.3.2   Promoting optimal infant feeding practices in the context of HIV/AIDS

Over the past two and a half decades, the uncertainty and the complexity of the scientific information about breastfeeding and HIV transmission, which has frequently changed and evolved, has confounded attempts to provide mothers with consistent and accurate information regarding optimal infant feeding practices (Chopra *et al.* 2002; de Paoli *et al.* 2002). Now that research is increasingly unequivocal (Coovadia & Kindra 2008), there is a need to assess mothers' infant feeding behaviour and to use this 'grassroots' knowledge to identify gaps and design future interventions.

Three chronological levels are useful in situating the results of the Rwandan study within recent epidemiological research on HIV and infant feeding. The first level is the infant feeding decision that the mother makes, ideally in an informed manner with a skilled counsellor prior to delivery. The second is the actual pattern in which she feeds her infant post partum. The third level is the time at which the mother ceases to breastfeed her infant. At each of these chronological levels, the infant outcome of interest, where it can be measured, is HIV-free survival. Alternatively, some studies use HIV infection and malnutrition, illness due to infectious diseases other than HIV, hospitalisation or mortality in infant and young children as proxy indicators.

6.3.2.1   *Type of infant feeding method (any breastfeeding versus replacement feeding from birth)*

By 2005 the global public health recommendation for HIV-infected mothers who choose to breastfeed was to breastfeed exclusively from birth for the first few months (WHO 2001). Recent investigations confirm the soundness of this recommendation and further specify that exclusive breastfeeding for the first six months is preferable. With respect to diarrhoea and acute respiratory infections, a study from Côte d'Ivoire showed less favourable outcomes by 24 months among infants who were replacement fed in comparison to those who were breastfed (Becquet *et al.* 2007). Estimated hazard ratios for formula feeding were 1.4 and 1.7 for diarrhoea and acute respiratory infections, respectively. In that study, malnutrition and mortality were not significantly associated with the mode of infant feeding. There was no significant difference in infant survival by 12 and by 24 months with ART prophylaxis. Similar findings were observed in Botswana by 18 months and with ART prophylaxis (Thior *et al.* 2006). Neither of these studies reported on relative rates of HIV-free survival if breastfeeding was exclusive. Taken together, the two investigations indicate that when the mother is HIV-infected, replacement feeding from birth does not improve HIV-survival compared with breastfeeding, even in a better-off African country such as Botswana. Another study from South Africa (Coovadia *et al.* 2007) indicated that if breastfeeding is exclusive there is a significant difference in cumulative mortality at three months (6% in exclusive breastfeeding versus 15% in replacement feeding).

Since mortality is estimated to be more than nine times higher for infected versus uninfected infants (Mbori-Ngacha *et al.* 2001; Nduati *et al.* 2000; Becquet *et al.* 2007), it is important to assess the proportion of infants who are alive and HIV-negative at a given time point (i.e. 'HIV-free survival') (Nduati *et al.* 2000). In the Botswanian study, there was no significant difference between breastfed and replacement-fed infants when mothers received highly active ART (HAART) and when zidovudine prophylaxis was provided to both mothers and infants (Thior *et al.* 2006). Further, confirming these results, the study from South Africa (Coovadia *et al.* 2007) did not show any significant differences in HIV-free survival between infants who were breastfed and those who were replacement fed (75% in both cases by six months of age).

In the Rwandan study, various factors may have influenced some of the 81% of mothers who chose to breastfeed and the 70% who breastfed exclusively. These may include the stigma of replacement feeding in a predominantly breastfeeding culture, the common practice of exclusive breastfeeding in the general population, and the high cost of replacement feeding. This suggests that, since most mothers prefer breastfeeding, as the cost of ART decreases and as drugs become increasingly accessible in this part of the world, efforts should be directed to making breastfeeding 'safer' in order to reduce the risk of postnatal transmission. It was reduced in the Botswana study when eligible mothers were put on HAART.

6.3.2.2 *Pattern of breastfeeding: exclusive breastfeeding versus mixed feeding*

Several studies have shown that exclusive breastfeeding protects against postnatal transmission better than mixed feeding patterns (Coutsoudis *et al.* 1999). Recent additional persuasive evidence supports the advice to breastfeed exclusively for the first six months (Coovadia *et al.* 2007). Infants fed solid foods in addition to breast milk were at higher risk of HIV transmission than those fed infant formula and breast milk (hazard ratio of 10.87 versus 1.82, respectively, compared with exclusive breastfeeding). In fact, in ZVITAMBO (Zimbabwe Vitamin A for Mothers and Babies Project), the highest risk of transmission was observed in mothers who partially breastfed (thus primarily replacement fed their infants), compared with those who exclusively or predominantly breastfed their infants (Iliff *et al.* 2005). This finding is important because PMTCT services often give the message on mixed feeding only to those women who choose to breastfeed, whereas it is equally or more important to stress in women who choose to replacement feed.

Results from Rwanda draw attention to the very high prevalence of exclusive breastfeeding. We found no indication that mothers who mixed fed did so because they believed their breast milk was insufficient. This finding is encouraging. It suggests that even higher rates of exclusive breastfeeding can be achieved if mothers are educated about the need to avoid feeds other than breast milk and, if they are supported, to have faith that their milk is adequate for their babies, even if their health and nutritional status are less than ideal.

6.3.2.3 *Cessation of breastfeeding*

Early cessation of breastfeeding (prior to six months) was previously believed to be the safest alternative for HIV+ mothers (Kuhn & Stein 1997). Because of concerns about the increased risk of postnatal transmission due to mixed feeding in comparison with exclusive breastfeeding, the 'period of transition' was to be 'kept as short as possible' (UNICEF 1997). This formed the basis for the practice of cessation at or before six months of age ('early') and over a short period of time ('rapidly' or 'abruptly'). Early breastfeeding cessation (before or at six months) has recently been shown to lead to worse overall outcomes (increased mortality, decreased rates of HIV free survival) compared to longer periods of breastfeeding (Athena Kourtis 2007; Onyango 2007). Gastroenteritis was also more frequent in infants who ceased breastfeeding early (Onyango 2007), even when infants were given ART prophylaxis (Kafulafula 2007). Controlling for HIV-status and when all mothers received HAART, early cessation has shown to be associated with higher mortality in infants and young children (Homsy 2006). Investigators in the Zambia Exclusive Breastfeeding Study found no significant differences in HIV-free survival between a group of mothers who had been randomised to a group given advice to stop breastfeeding at four months and a group that continued breastfeeding as long as they wanted to (Sinkala 2007). Thirty-five per cent of the mothers assigned to stop breastfeeding at four months did not comply with the advice and continued breastfeeding. An analysis based on actual practice (regardless of the group to which mothers had been randomised) also showed no significant difference in HIV-free survival for early versus late breastfeeding cessation.

Since higher levels of cell-free HIV in breast milk are associated with a higher risk of postnatal transmission (Roussea *et al.* 2004), viral loads can be used as a surrogate marker to assess the risk of postnatal transmission. Levels of virus in breast milk were found to be almost ten times higher in women who were trying to stop breastfeeding rapidly, in comparison to those who were intending to continue breastfeeding in the Zambia study (Thea *et al.* 2006). This finding suggests that abrupt cessation may not be advisable.

Based on these recent findings, early and abrupt breastfeeding cessation is no longer recommended. According to a WHO consensus statement (WHO 2006): 'At six months, if replacement feeding is still not Affordable, Feasible, Acceptable, Safe and Sustainable (AFASS), continuation of breastfeeding with additional complementary foods is recommended, while the mother and baby continue to be regularly assessed. All breastfeeding should stop once a nutritionally adequate and safe diet without breast milk can be provided.'

We found that mothers in Rwanda lacked funds to purchase infant foods that would be adequately nutritious to replace breast milk. Modified cow's milk could be used as a replacement food for non-breastfed infants in Rwanda. Because of cow's milk lower concentrations of iron, vitamin A, vitamin C and folic acid, infants fed with cow's milk had to be supplemented with these and other micronutrients. Modification of cow's milk for infant consumption would have included dilution with water (to reduce its greater concentration in protein, sodium, phosphorous and other salts) and the addition of sugar (to compensate for the energy lost during dilution). Because of the difficulty of accessing the supplementary micronutrients required for the infant, and of safe and appropriate modification of cow's milk, cow's milk does not appear advisable before the infant is six months of age. However, it could be crucial for older infants once breastfeeding stops if suitable commercial breast milk substitute are not accessible or affordable. At these older ages, cow's milk is easier for the infant to digest and no longer causes gastrointestinal bleeding, which leads to iron deficiency anaemia.

When complementary feeding begins and when breastfeeding ends, mothers could be supported by providing some of the ingredients needed for preparing infant foods, fuel and other equipment. The new WHO guidance (WHO 2003b) specifies that if foods are provided for replacement fed infants or for those who stop breastfeeding, an equivalent should be provided to those who continue to breastfeed, so as not to coerce women towards one option. Of course, the long-term solution would be to build mothers' capacity to purchase high-quality complementary feeds by improving their financial situation. For example, creating associations for HIV-infected mothers that promote income-generating activities, such as the health centre in Gihundwe funded by UNICEF, where members are involved in income-generating activities such as making soap and weaving baskets.

6.3.2.4   *Infant feeding counselling*

Although the success of PMTCT sites depends on their ability to help mothers make informed decisions and then to implement them, at the time of the study Rwandan counsellors were not adequately prepared for this task. The finding that some mothers had heard that they should not breastfeed, but they had not received any information about a suitable breast milk substitute, highlights the lack of training of counsellors in Rwanda. With regard to the safety of replacement foods, we found that mothers lacked knowledge about their preparation. Clearly, there is an urgent need for a comprehensive curriculum on infant feeding for counsellors in Rwanda.

In congruence with the new WHO guidance (WHO 2003b), mothers should be assisted in deciding when to stop breastfeeding sometime between six and 24 months rather than being told to do so at exactly six months of age. Infant feeding counsellors need to be trained in conducting postnatal assessment of whether replacement feeding meets the AFASS criteria at various points post partum beginning at six months. Unlike AFASS evaluation done prenatally, this postnatal AFASS assessment can also take the mother's health status into account.

In training healthcare providers on HIV and infant feeding, practitioners may consider partnering the older, more experienced sites with the recent ones. This will allow recent sites to learn from the more experienced ones. Another approach is to have a core group of highly trained trainers who would go around to the sites. This would guarantee that training is standardised across sites and ensure that spin-off training sessions are accurate.

6.4   Conclusion: bridging the gap between policy and actual practice to promote optimal infant feeding practices

Both of the studies described here provide a window into understanding how flexible or constraining cultural expectations are from the perspective of initiating and maintaining exclusive breastfeeding, while respecting the social and cultural environment. The strength of specific facilitators and constraints for optimal infant feeding practices could be different in other settings in sub-Saharan Africa than those examined here, and require additional research.

The findings from both of the studies are encouraging. First, in both settings, the majority of women chose to breastfeed, even when they were aware of their HIV+ status. Second, early initiation and breastfeeding on demand do not appear to require special interventions, apart from providing women with information. According to the *Global Strategy for Infant and Young Child Feeding* (WHO 2003a) the promotion of optimal infant feeding practices requires the provision of accurate and complete information to relevant stakeholders while respecting beneficial cultural traditions. Over the past 25 years, it has been difficult to provide HIV+ mothers in resource-poor settings with accurate information as recommended in the *Global Strategy*. This is due, in part, to the complexity of the scientific information. Now that there is increasing consensus about the appropriate course of action in resource-poor settings, PMTCT programmes need to revise the infant feeding information they provide.

The high prevalence of exclusive breastfeeding in Rwanda is encouraging and perhaps it indicates that HIV+ mothers are now aware of the danger of mixed feeding. However, the study highlights the need to educate HIV+ mothers about the danger of early weaning and to promote appropriate complementary foods. As shown in the Tanzania study, many women are willing to try improving their infant feeding behaviour, and, with the exception of avoiding water for the newborn, when such mothers agree to try a new behaviour, they generally succeed.

References

Akida, H., Alidina, M., Abdalla, A., Massamba, D., Mganga, Y., Mhina, G., et al. (1981) Kamusi ya Kiswahili Sanifu. Walton Street, Oxford. Reprinted in Kenya by permission of Oxford University Press.

Almroth, S.B. & Bidinger, P.D. (1990) No need for water supplementation for exclusively breast-fed infants under hot and arid conditions. *Transactions of the Royal Society of Tropical Medicine and Hygiene*, **84**, 602–604.

Ammann, A.J. (1983) Is there an acquired immune deficiency syndrome in infants and children? *Pediatrics*, **72**: 430–432.

Athena Kourtis, D.F., Hyde, L., Tien, H.C., Chavula, C., Mumba, N., Magawa, M., Knight, R., Chasela, C., Van der horst, C. & the Ban Study Team (2007) Diarrhea in uninfected infants of HIV-infected mothers who stop breastfeeding at 6 months: the BAN study experience. Fourteenth Conference on Retroviruses and Opportunistic Infections (CROI). Los Angeles, 25–28 February 2007.

Becquet, R., Bequet, L., Ekouevi, D.K., Viho, I., Sakarovitch, C., Fassinou, P., et al. (2007) Two-year morbidity-mortality and alternatives to prolonged breast-feeding among children born to HIV-infected mothers in Cote d'Ivoire. *PLoS Medicine*, **4**: e17.

Chopra, M., Piwoz, E., Sengwana, J., Schaay, N., Dunnett, L. & Saders, D. (2002) Effect of a mother-to-child HIV prevention programme on infant feeding and caring practices in South Africa. *South African Medical Journal*, **92**: 298–302.

Coovadia, H. & Kindra, G. (2008) Breastfeeding to prevent HIV transmission in infants: balancing pros and cons. *Current Opinion in Infectious Diseases*, **21**: 11–15.

Coovadia, H.M., Rollins, N.C., Bland, R.M., Little, K., Coutsoudis, A., Bennish, M.L., et al. (2007) Mother-to-child transmission of HIV-1 infection during exclusive breastfeeding in the first 6 months of life: an intervention cohort study. *Lancet*, **369**: 1107–1116.

Coutsoudis, A. (2000) Influence of infant feeding patterns on early mother-to-child transmission of HIV-1 in Durban, South Africa. *Annals of the New York Academy of Sciences*, **918**: 136–144.

Coutsoudis, A., Pillay, K., Spooner, E., Kuhn, L. & Coovadia, H.M. (1999) Influence of infant-feeding patterns on early mother-to-child transmission of HIV-1 in Durban, South Africa: a prospective cohort study. South African Vitamin A Study Group. *Lancet*, **354**: 471–476.

Coutsoudis, A., Pillay, K., Spooner, E., Coovadia, H.M., Pembrey, L. & Newell, M.L. (2003) Morbidity in children born to women infected with human immunodeficiency virus in South Africa: does mode of feeding matter? *Acta Paediatrica*, **92**: 890–895.

De Paoli, M.M., Manongi, R. & Klepp, K.I. (2002) Counsellors' perspectives on antenatal HIV testing and infant feeding dilemmas facing women with HIV in northern Tanzania. *Reproductive Health Matters*, **10**: 144–156.

Edmond, K.M., Kirkwood, B.R., Amenga-etego, S., Owusu-agyei, S. & Hurt, L.S. (2007) Effect of early infant feeding practices on infection-specific neonatal mortality: an investigation of the causal links with observational data from rural Ghana. *American Journal of Clinical Nutrition*, **86**: 1126–1131.

Goldman, H. (1996) A comparative study of Swahili in two rural communities in Pemba, Zanzibar, Tanzania. Anthropology Department, New York University, New York.

Homsy, J., Moore, D., Barasa, A. & Mermin, J. (2006) Mother-to-child HIV transmission and infant mortality among women receiving highly active antiretroviral therapy (HAART) in rural Uganda. *The President's Emergency Plan for AIDS Relief Annual Meeting. The 2006 HIV/AIDS Implementers' Meeting. Building on Success: Ensuring Long-Term Solutions*. Durban, South Africa.

Iliff, P.J., Piwoz, E.G., Tavengwa, N.V., Zunguza, C.D., Marinda, E.T., Nathoo, K.J., Moulton, L.H., Ward, B.J. & Humphrey, J.H. (2005) Early exclusive breastfeeding reduces the risk of postnatal HIV-1 transmission and increases HIV-free survival. *AIDS*, **19**: 699–708.

Johnson, F. (1939) *A Standard English-Swahili Dictionary*. Walton Street, Oxford. Reprinted in Kenya by permission of Oxford University Press.

Kafulafula, G.T.M., Hoover, D., Li, Q., Kumwenda, N., Mipandol Taha, T., Mofenson, L., & Fowler, M. (2007) Post-weaning gastroenteritis and mortality in HIV-uninfected african infants receiving antiretroviral prophylaxis to prevent MTCT of HIV-1. Fourteenth Conference on Retroviruses and Opportunistic Infections (CROI). Los Angeles, 25–28 February 2007.

Kuhn, L. & Stein, Z. (1997) Infant survival, HIV infection, and feeding alternatives in less-developed countries. *American Journal of Public Health*, 87: 926–931.

Labbok, M.H. & Coffin, C.J. (1997) A call for consistency in definition of breastfeeding behaviors. *Social Science and Medicine*, 44: 1931–1932.

Logan, S., Newell, M., Ades, T., Peckham, C., Brierley, J., Roth, C. & Warwick, C. (1988) Breastfeeding and HIV infection. *Lancet*, 331: 1346.

Mbori-ngacha, D., Nduati, R., John, G., Reilly, M., Richardson, B., Mwatha, A., *et al.* (2001) Morbidity and mortality in breastfed and formula-fed infants of HIV-1-infected women: a randomized clinical trial. *Journal of the American Medical Association*, 286: 2413–2420.

Mukuria, A.G., Kothari, M.T. & Abderrahim, N. (2006) *Infant and Young Child Feeding Up-date*. USAID, Washington DC.

Nduati, R., John, G., Mbori-ngacha, D., Richardson, B., Overbaugh, J., Mwatha, A., *et al.* (2000) Effect of breastfeeding and formula feeding on transmission of HIV-1: a randomized clinical trial. *Journal of the American Medical Association*, 283: 1167–1174.

Onyango, C., Mmiro, F., Bagenda, D., Mubiru, M., Musoke, P., Fowler, M., Jackson, J. *et al.* (2007) Early breastfeeding cessation among HIV-exposed negative infants and risk of serious gastroenteritis: findings from a perinatal prevention trial in Kampala, Uganda. Fourteenth Conference on Retroviruses and Opportunistic Infections (CROI), Los Angeles, 25–28 February 2007.

Piwoz, E., Huffman, S.L., Lusk, D., Zehner, E.R. & O'Gara, C. (2001) *Issues, Risks and Challenges of Early Breastfeeding Cessation to Reduce Postnatal Transmission of HIV in Africa*. US Agency for International Development and Academy for Educational Development, Washington DC.

Roussea, C.M., Nduati, R.W., Richardson, B.A., John-Stewart, G.C., Mbori-Ngacha, D.A., Kreiss, J.K., *et al.* (2004) Association of levels of HIV-1–infected breast milk cells and risk of mother-to-child transmission. *Journal of Infectious Diseases*, 1880: 1880–1888.

Sinkala, M., Kankasa, C., Kasonde, P., Vwalika, C., Mwiya, M., Scott, N., *et al.* (2007) No benefit of early cessation of breastfeeding at 4 months on HIV-free survival of infants born to HIV-infected mothers in Zambia: The Zambia Exclusive Breastfeeding Study. Fourteenth Conference on Retroviruses and Opportunistic Infections (CROI), Los Angeles, 25–28 February 2007.

Thairu, L. (2005) Evaluation des pratiques d'alimentation des nourrissons et des jeunes enfants dans le contexte du VIH/SIDA au Rwanda. UNICEF, Kigali.

Thairu, L. (2006) Ethnography of infant feeding in sub-Saharan Africa: case studies in the context of HIV/AIDS and newborn care. Division of Nutritional Sciences, Cornell University, Ithaca, NY.

Thairu, L. & Pelto, G. (2008) Newborn care practices in Pemba Island (Tanzania) and their implications for newborn health and survival. *Maternal and Child Nutrition*, 4: 194–208.

Thea, D.M., Aldrovandi, G., Kankasa, C., Kasonde, P., Decker, W.D., Semrau, K., *et al.* (2006) Post-weaning breast milk HIV-1 viral load, blood prolactin levels and breast milk volume. *AIDS*, 20: 1539–1547.

Thior, I., Lockman, S., Sineaton, L.M., Shapiro, R.L., Wester, C., Heymann, S.J., *et al.* (2006) Breastfeeding plus infant zidovudine prophylaxis for 6 months vs formula feeding plus infant zidovudine for 1 month to reduce mother-to-child HIV transmission in Botswana: a random-ized trial: the Mashi Study. *Journal of the American Medical Association*, 296: 794–805.

Thiry, L., Sprecher-Goldberger, S., Jonckheer, T., Levy, J., Van de Perre, P., Henrivaux, P., *et al.* (1985) Isolation of AIDS virus from cell-free breast milk of three healthy virus carriers. *Lancet*, 2: 891–892.

UNICEF (1997) HIV and infant feeding: a policy statement developed collaboratively by UNAIDS, UNICEF and WHO.

WHO (2001) New data on the prevention of mother-to-child transmission of HIV/AIDS and their implications: Technical consultation. UNFPA/UNICEF/WHO/UNAIDS Inter-Agency Team – Conclusions and recommendations. WHO, Geneva.

WHO (2003a) *Global Strategy for Infant and Young Child Feeding.* WHO, Geneva.

WHO (2003b) *HIV and Infant Feeding: Framework for Priority Action.* WHO, Geneva.

WHO (2006) WHO HIV and infant feeding technical consultation held on behalf of the Inter-agency Task Team (IATT) on prevention of HIV infections in pregnant women, mothers and their infants. WHO, Geneva.

WHO collaborative study team on the role of breastfeeding on the prevention of infant mortality. (2000) Effect of breastfeeding on infant and child mortality due to infectious diseases in less developed countries: a pooled analysis. *Lancet*, 355: 451–455.

7 Bodies in the Making: Reflections on Women's Consumption Practices in Pregnancy

Helen Stapleton and Julia Keenan

7.1 Introduction

Pregnancy and early family formation may be seen as opportunities for pregnant women, family and friendship networks to examine and revise habitual behaviours, attitudes and expectations, including those relating to food and other consumption practices. Current debates about rising levels of obesity and binge drinking, together with changing understandings of 'healthy' eating, increasingly ascribe consumption practices with a moral weighting, particularly within family settings. Furthermore, more than two decades of research examining the relationship between the intrauterine environment and health outcomes in later life (Barker 1992) have highlighted the significance of pregnancy-related behaviours and decisions. In contrast to more traditional understandings of pregnancy as a 'natural' event in the lifecycle and a time of relaxed control, particularly around food and eating, such emphases have implications for pregnant women. Hence, infant feeding cannot be considered to begin at birth. In recognition of this, the *Global Strategy for Infant and Young Child Feeding* (World Health Organization (WHO) 2003, p. 3) states:

> '*Mothers and babies form an inseparable biological and social unit; the health and nutrition of one group cannot be divorced from the health and nutrition of the other*'.

The strategy also emphasises a need for health professionals and policy makers to focus on women's health status throughout the life course (assuming all women become mothers) as a means of improving health outcomes for children:

> '*Improved infant and young child feeding begins with ensuring the health and nutritional status of women, in their own right, throughout all stages of life and continues with women as providers for their children and families*'
> WHO (2003, p. 5).

This chapter reports on findings from a longitudinal study, conducted with women living in a large city in the north of England. More broadly, our research explored ways in which food and eating practices were manifested and negotiated within diverse and dynamic family settings, including those where some participants had concerns about food and body shape which pre-existed pregnancy and mother-hood. In this chapter, we discuss participants' understandings of, and responses to, general food and consumption-related advice and information in the context of pregnancy, and examine the origins and 'palatability' of this within the context of their personal biographies and social relationships. Finally, we discuss whether, and to what degree, consumption-related information is understood to be enabling or limiting. In support of our theoretical arguments, we draw on antenatal interviews with 30 pregnant women, from across the age and social class spectrum, undergoing the transition to motherhood for the first time. A third of the study participants were of normal weight, another third were overweight/obese and the last third were managing diabetes[i]. Hence, a significant number of participants might be expected to have some concerns about control over food intake, both during pregnancy and in the context of raising children. We draw directly on our empirical data to discuss theoretical perspectives and analyse *a priori* understandings underpinning terms such as 'health/y' and 'balance'. We show how such understandings intersect with lay and expert perceptions and discuss how they may impact on participants' concerns about diet and body image. We also describe participants' relationships with 'expert' and lay knowledges, and how parental roles may be (re)negotiated in the ongoing process of 'making' an infant.

7.2 Background

7.2.1 Consumption and weightiness in pregnancy: current context, advice and practice

Public health concerns surrounding the economic and social costs associated with rising levels of obesity and associated co-morbidities, including diabetes, have resulted in a plethora of UK policy-related documents (e.g. Wanless 2004; Department of Health 2006; National Institute for Health and Clinical Excellence (NICE) 2006)[ii]. The global increase in these conditions over the past decade has been such that they are no longer considered the exclusive preserve of industrialised nations with prevalence rates in industrialising nations also rapidly increasing (Seidell 2000; Batnitzky 2008; WHO 2008). Inequalities in health, such as low birth weight, are strongly associated with adult adiposity (Kuh *et al.* 2002) and research confirms that obesity in adulthood is more pronounced in children of lower socioeconomic status (Parsons *et al.* 1999; Stamatakis *et al.* 2005). The literature linking breastfeeding

---

[i] Within the limits of this chapter, it is not possible to address some of the specificities of specialist diabetes management advice and support in the context of pregnancy. It is anticipated such findings will be discussed in further publications.

[ii] This is not to ignore the considerable volume of literature exploring contestations of obesity. For example, see: Cooper, 1997, 1998; Gard & Wright, 2001; Campos, 2004; Rich & Evans, 2005; Aphramor, 2005; Evans, 2006; Monaghan, 2007.

with obesity in later life is equivocal with a number of studies reporting some protective effects (Dewey 2003; Owen *et al.* 2005; Shields *et al.* 2006) and others reporting no such benefits (Li *et al.* 2003; Victora *et al.* 2003).

Although the practice of routinely monitoring maternal weight throughout pregnancy has been discontinued in the UK – largely because, as a screening procedure it lacks sensitivity and specificity as well as simultaneously holding significant potential to generate anxiety (Farrar & Duley 2007) – appropriate weight gain in pregnancy is nonetheless strongly associated with satisfactory fetal and maternal outcomes and ongoing epidemiological research links intrauterine wellbeing with health outcomes over the life course (Acheson 1998; Parsons *et al.* 2003). The current UK clinical recommendation (NICE 2008) is for women's weight to be recorded as a one-off measurement at the first antenatal 'booking' appointment for the purpose of calculating body mass index (BMI) with those measuring over 35 (30 = obese) placed under consultant care but, as with average weight women, not routinely weighed again in pregnancy. Obese status is also associated with a range of co-morbidities including pre-eclampsia, gestational diabetes and pregnancy induced hypertension (Villamor & Cnattingus 2006; Walsh & Murphy 2007) and has been found to restrict care options and choices in pregnancy (Heslehurst *et al.* 2007), although this is not to suggest that such limitations are appropriate or acceptable. Although our data would support the fact that women defined as being medically obese do not necessarily experience any such clinical complaints or reduced choice or compromised care, the lack of monitoring of weight gain/diet in pregnancy is interesting in the light of research suggesting that changes in body shape and composition (% of fat, bone, muscle, etc.) resulting from pregnancy can also be triggers for later obesity and risk of type 2 diabetes (Soltani & Fraser 2000).

Any pregnancy, although perhaps especially a first, is increasingly viewed by institutions at a variety of levels, be they local, national/state (NICE 2003) and trans-state (WHO 2003), as a significant 'window of opportunity' within which to promote healthier lifestyles and encourage expectant women/mothers to take responsibility for safeguarding – or improving – their own health and that of their future child/ren. The dietary regimes, weight gain and consumption habits of pregnant women, and subsequently of their infants, are thus of interest to maternity and related professionals seeking to optimise fetal outcomes and address inequalities in maternal and child health, hence pregnancy as a significant lifecycle stage for maximising family-focused public health opportunities. In the UK, women are currently encouraged to continue eating a nutritionally balanced diet with recommended (increased) levels of certain essential vitamins and minerals (particularly folic acid), to exercise caution in respect to a variety of food safety issues and not to consume alcoholic drinks. Pregnant women are also advised that they do not require additional calories for the first six months of pregnancy and only about 200 extra calories per day for the last three months; guidelines for appropriate weight gain in relation to pre-pregnant BMI are widely available[iii]. The public health role of

---

[iii] See http://www.eatwell.gov.uk/agesandstages/pregnancy/whenyrpregnant/ and http://www.eatingfor pregnancy.co.uk/

health practitioners in maternal and child health in disseminating policy-related information to pregnant and post-natal women has, consequentially, become more pronounced (Ö Lúanaigh & Carlson 2005).

More intense discussion and scrutiny of everyday eating routines has arguably transformed consumption practices into highly politicised arenas with pregnant women increasingly self-critical and self-conscious about what and how they consume. The increasing emphasis on individual accountability for health outcomes imbues food and related consumption practices with a heavy moral weighting. Yet, in making decisions about the 'right' kinds of food to eat in pregnancy, particularly when faced with new physiological states, many women – especially those pregnant for the first time – have little personal experience to draw upon and social/support networks may also be restricted due to changes in family and kinship structures, and living arrangements (Silva & Smart 1999; Smart *et al.* 2001; May 2004). Furthermore for many women, especially those who have delayed entry into motherhood, the experiences of their own mothers and other female family and friends may be construed as less relevant due to changing scientific research around nutrition, exercise and weight gain in pregnancy. Such attitudes are not universal, however, as younger women (Stapleton 2006) and those from lower socioeconomic groups (Kirkham & Stapleton 2001) are often still heavily reliant on, and value, the advice provided by their mothers and grandmothers.

7.2.2   Regulating and monitoring in pregnancy: self and other

Whereas health professionals closely monitor fetal growth and development, they generally do not monitor the nutritional status, consumption habits, and/or weight management practices of pregnant women with the same intensity, unless specialist support for a pre-existing, or current pregnancy-related, condition (such as diabetes) is required. Mechanistic views of pregnant women as mere fetal containers in need of close medical surveillance have been extensively debated (Murphy-Lawless 1998; Ettorre 2000), however, as Castel (1991) indicates, there are screening systems in place which effectively 'filter' pregnant women into 'high' and 'low' risk categories, thereby identifying the minority perceived to be in need of intensive monitoring.

If maternal food-related consumption practices and/or weight are not routinely monitored in a formal way for the 'normal' majority, nor enshrined in law (i.e. with punitive legislation in place for women exhibiting consumption behaviours deemed to be dangerous), informal regulation nonetheless operates through strong moral imperatives to manage the self 'responsibly' in preparation for motherhood. Focusing less on structural or political factors, which significantly determine inequalities in infant and young child health, public health documents such as the *Global Strategy for Infant and Young Child Feeding* (WHO 2003) prefer to 'tap into' such moral imperatives, emphasising deficiencies in caregivers' knowledge;

'ever keen to ensure that they have accurate information to make appropriate feeding choices, parents nevertheless are limited by their immediate environment.

Since they may have only infrequent contact with the health care system during a child's first two years of life, it is not unusual for caregivers to be more influenced by community attitudes than by the advice of health workers'

WHO (2003, p. 22).

While clearly emphasising the need for caregivers (and pregnant women) to be well informed, this document also positions healthcare systems as repositories of 'expert' information, and thus fails to acknowledge community attitudes and family and kinship networks as legitimate and credible sources of alternative information. Furthermore, although there is passing reference to sociocultural factors as significant influences on women's nutrition decisions in pregnancy, there is no recognition of the impact of physiological disruption on consumption choices, for example, in the context of diabetes/obesity when women may be managing significant metabolic and/or weight fluctuations. Although the analysis of empirical data presented in this chapter emphasises cultural practices and embedded norms, which make optimal nutrition and weight gain difficult to achieve for many pregnant women, we do not uncritically accept scientific information as objective or neutral 'truths' (Foucault 1970), nor seek to denigrate what women themselves understand as optimal. Furthermore, the *Global Strategy for Infant and Young Child Feeding* assumes a 'rational subject' model of information transmission in which professionals in maternal and infant health are invested with authority, and where individual women's embodied, and enculturated, understandings and experiences tend to be discredited and/or discounted. At the same time, pregnant women are assumed to be autonomous social actors, in full knowledge and control of their changing physiology and free to make and justify their nutritional and consumption choices. Indeed, some commentators assert that a defining feature of neoliberal public health policies, such as the *Global Strategy for Infant and Young Child Feeding* (WHO 2003), is this central assumption of a discrete, autonomous, self-monitoring subject that will seek out and act on 'expert' advice (Petersen & Lupton 1996), i.e. there is an underlying assumption that access to information translates into effective self-regulation. Individuals and caregivers are expected to willingly engage in reflexive techniques and/or practices of subjectification and to exercise responsibility in the choices they make, and will often provide (unprompted) 'accountancy talk' to explain their behaviours/choices to others assumed to be monitoring them and, perhaps more significantly, are validated for doing so. That said, it should be remembered that 'choice' and indeed 'autonomy' are both socioculturally constructed, potentially coercive, and limited 'through intersections of class, race . . . ideology and resources' (Edwards 2004, p. 2).

Given the pressures towards heightened self-management and/or reflexivity, some authors are concerned that contemporary motherhood is becoming increasingly intensive (Hays 1996; Furedi 2001). Indeed, it has been argued that perceived levels of risk have become inflated to the extent that parents have been moulded into 'paranoid risk managers' (Furedi 2001). Whether intensive or not, self-monitoring practices are supposedly freely exercised and indeed many pregnant women in this respect willingly collaborate with those whom they regard as experts. For example, Tina Miller's (2005) recent research on British higher socioeconomic women's transitions to first-time motherhood found that they obtained advice from a range of sources but regarded that provided by health professionals as the most reliable. In order to manage perceived risks, many women in Miller's study wanted to be told what to do and emphasised their own non-expert status. Other studies, however, have suggested that health professionals play an important role in facilitating their clients to subvert institutional norms, often to secure their own preferences (Hutchinson 1990; Stapleton *et al.* 2002). Hence, although much emphasis has been placed upon the anxiety-provoking nature of the heightened reflexive subjectification engendered by such policies (Furedi 2001), rather less has been made of the validatory possibilities of 'doing everything right', nor the uneven playing field in this respect, which favours well-educated, white nationals, whose personal 'sacrifices' could also be seen as future investments in upward social mobility. We return to this point in our conclusion.

7.3   Study aims, design and methodology

The findings shared in this chapter were generated in the context of a larger qualitative study[iv] that investigated food and consumption practices among pregnant women and how their understandings of these events were subsequently enacted (or not) in mother–child, food-related, relationships. The findings presented in this chapter focus on the transition to parenthood among first-time mothers.

The study sought to identify whether, and to what degree, maternal understandings about food-related issues were transmitted to children, and the extent to which these were influenced by external agents. The perceptions of women were central to the study aims because as we have previously stated, fetal wellbeing, and indeed health outcomes throughout the life course, are increasingly linked with pregnancy-related behaviours, and because women-as-mothers are usually the primary carers within the family domain.

The wider study sample comprised 60 women recruited to two cohorts. We sought to recruit women from across the social class (higher to lower socioeconomic groups) and age range and to include a diversity of family forms. Cohort one, whose accounts inform this chapter, comprised 30 women who, at the point of recruitment, were anticipating motherhood for the first time. Cohort two comprised a further 30 women who were already mothers with at least one child aged between 9 months and 2 years. As we wished to explore a variety of personal trajectories underpinning notions of balance and control with regard to consumption practices, each cohort included:

[iv] The larger study 'Changing Habits? Food, family and transitions to motherhood' was one of 17 individual projects contributing to the 'Changing Families Changing Food' programme, based at the University of Sheffield and funded by the Leverhulme Trust . See: http://www.shef.ac.uk/familiesandfood/

- Ten women living with diabetes (type 1, type 2 or gestational)
- Ten women who were seen by themselves and/or others to be overweight/obese (BMI[v] >30)
- Ten women of 'normal' weight, with 'normal' eating practices[vi].

We conducted 120 in-depth, semi-structured interviews to generate data. Pregnant women were interviewed on three occasions (approximately three months before giving birth, and when their infants were approximately 3 and 9 months of age, respectively). Cohort two participants were interviewed on one occasion only. Interviews lasted between one and one and a half hours. Demographic data were collected across a range of variables including household composition and income, education and employment, and housing and relationship status. The software package NVivo7 was used to mechanise the more clerical and administrative tasks associated with data analysis: coding, retrieval, interrogation and archiving activities. Data were analysed thematically (Attride-Stirling 2001) in accordance with the method of cross-sectional, categorical indexing outlined by Mason (2002). The longitudinal element of the study was invaluable for drawing out the contested and processual nature of consumption practices, as well as highlighting individual concerns about body image and weight, and intentions regarding childrearing.

Ethical approval and governance was granted by the local National Health Service (NHS) research ethics committee and the appropriate hospital trust. Consent was recognised to be an ongoing process and hence, participants in the longitudinal element of the study, were asked to re-consent prior to each episode of data collection.

By way of enlivening the text and illustrating theoretical points, we have included verbatim, but anonymised, quotations derived from interview transcripts. The 'identifier' following each quotation indicates whether participants were recruited to an overweight/obese (O), diabetic (D) or 'normal' weight (N) cohorts. Text in square brackets within quotations indicates the voice of the interviewer.

7.4 Consumption in pregnancy: socioeconomic grouping and autonomy

7.4.1 A new regime?

When invited to discuss dietary intake during pregnancy, including any changes made, many of our more educated participants (such as Betty, below) presented

[v] BMI = weight in kilograms divided by the square of height in metres (kg/m^2). A cut-off point of 25 kg/m^2 is recognised internationally as a definition of adult overweight, and 30 kg/m^2 for adult obesity (British Medical Association (BMA) 2005). Although BMI does not measure body fat directly, it is considered an inexpensive, relatively unobtrusive, and easily recorded alternative for measuring adiposity. Factors such as age and gender can be taken into consideration, and BMI status is, not unproblematically, widely used as a screening device.
[vi] Interestingly, BMI calculations for a number of women in this cohort, including those from professional and medical backgrounds, defined them as overweight/obese. The BMI range for participants in this study was 17 (under weight) to 45.2 (obese).

themselves as having made (self)conscious nutritional choices. They described strategies used to ensure the consumption of a 'healthy' (science-based) diet which emphasised 'balance' between food groups and the need for a daily intake of fruit and vegetables, occasionally enhanced by additional vitamin and mineral supplements.

'I think you do eat healthily [in pregnancy] but I always have done anyway . . . I eat fresh vegetables and fruit every day. . . . I'm quite conscious of eating, of food impulses . . . So, so yeah I think I have been quite conscious of it through the pregnancy.'

Betty, age 23 (N)

Betty's statement, 'I think you do eat healthily', may be read as alluding to normative expectations that pregnant women will automatically exercise an increased sense of responsibility with respect to monitoring, and regulating, dietary intake. The motivation for such participants' dietary changes was primarily to maximise benefits for the developing fetus, but also to 'programme' the fetus to accept a healthy diet – and as wide as possible a variety of foods – when weaned onto solids:

'Just . . . eat a healthy diet 'cause of the baby really.'

Danielle, age 31 (O)

And they do say try and stick to a lot of fruit and veg and vary your diet because your baby needs a variation of diets.

Amanda, age 26 (D + O)

Participants' narratives often emphasised the role of an external, 'expert' agent – a 'they', usually a health/childcare professional or media source.

For some women, maximising health benefits on behalf of their fetus also involved eating foods that they had previously disliked or had avoided, sometimes because they impacted adversely on their own health, especially digestion:

'I have also begun eating cheese which is something that I don't usually eat. Because of the calcium and, and that mainly. . . . I usually avoid it because I've been always very constipated myself.'

Alejandria, age 31 (N)

For others, this also meant rationalising, and over-riding, taste or digestive aversions experienced as a result of the physiological changes of pregnancy. Whereas some women invested faith in such aversions as their body's way of defending against harmful foods, Elsie was concerned about calcium availability:

'At first anything creamy I couldn't really stand so I really went off cheese though I did make myself eat it. I really went off milk I couldn't stand it so I'd, I'd have

yoghurt which at least was sweet you know, because I was very conscious of the calcium.'

Elsie, age 31 (N)

As well as being appreciated by some participants for its neutralising benefits, milk was widely considered to be a dietary substance invested with health giving properties and hence it was often ascribed an elevated status during pregnancy. We will return to this issue later in the chapter.

Some participants viewed pregnancy as an ideal opportunity to introduce changes in partners, and household, diets:

'I didn't eat tomatoes until I became pregnant so I [laugh] think 'cause I started, he [partner] should start as well'.

Betty, age 23 (N)

We [self and partner] did try to be a bit more healthy, you know, during the pregnancy and not just me, you know, we 'cause now we always if, even if I make like a pasta dish we'd always make a big salad with it and, you know, we'll always try to have loads of fruit . . .

Sandra, age 30 (N)

Indeed, Sandra and her partner, who had altered their purchasing patterns in recent years in favour of organic food, extended the range of foods they purchased during pregnancy to include dairy produce in addition to fruit and vegetables.

With respect to making changes, some participants voiced concerns about the lack of individually specific advice and information available from midwives:

'We found with our midwife that you, if you ask the right questions you get the answer. If you don't ask anything you don't get told anything. She's very nice and she's very good but you need to know what you're asking for really.'

Betty, age 23 (N)

This concurs with ongoing debates (Petersen & Lupton 1996) that suggest that a self-monitoring, self-regulating, subject is *assumed* by health professionals, who generally do not routinely volunteer non-standard information to seemingly 'educated' clients unless they specifically request it. Indeed, participants who shared Betty's higher socioeconomic status tended to seek additional information, most commonly from the internet or books, to supplement that provided by health professionals. They frequently discussed the concept of dietary 'balance' as part of a discourse which emphasised the importance of imposing, but also of maintaining, self-regulating strategies, and as this being something which did not necessarily begin in pregnancy, but which stemmed from ongoing embodied practices or beliefs about the relationship between food, diet, weight and the environment. In this respect, vegetarian or vegan regimes, which pre-dated pregnancy for all women who volunteered this information, were framed not as limiting, but as conferring distinct health advantages because they stressed the need for fruit and vegetable consumption, and adequate protein intake on a daily basis. Adhering to such diets required a considerable investment of time and energy to acquire, and maintain, a secure knowledge base. To that end, their appeal was limited to more educated women.

7.4.2   Eating for health

Monitoring personal dietary intake in order to maximise benefits for the developing fetus was prevalent in the more highly educated participants. This contrasted with attitudes expressed by participants from less educated backgrounds:

> 'No, I didn't think, "Oh I've got to have my five-a-day[vii] now" [laugh] I'm pregnant.'
>
> Anne, age 29 (D)

This was especially so for teenage participants who were more likely to invoke the power of transmitted maternal advice and experience to counter perceptions of the scientific evidence provided by midwives:

> 'I mean my Mum's always ate whatever she wanted to with us, and all of us are all right.'
>
> Kelly, age 18 (N)

The four teenagers in our study were mostly living in parental homes throughout pregnancy and the early postpartum period and hence consumed food provided, and prepared, by parents – notably their mothers. Their autonomy to implement food-related changes was thus seriously constrained. The one teenager who was living independently appeared to be eating very little, mostly because of concerns about excess weight gain:

> 'I've been to the hospital a few times in the last couple of weeks to check whether it (the fetus) seemed to be growing all right and that. [Because you were saying it wasn't growing so well?] No I weren't 'cause I weren't, I weren't eating much at first 'cause I were getting paranoid about my weight and that [Like what, what were you eating?] Like a sandwich or something like that. Not even that [laugh]. [For the whole day?] Yeah.'
>
> Stacey, age 17 (N)

---

vii The £10m UK '5-a-day' initiatives were set up to help families on low incomes to access fruit and vegetables. For information about how the schemes evaluated, see: http://www.biglotteryfund.org.uk/er_eval_5aday_report_evaluation.pdf

Previous research has identified adolescence as a particularly vulnerable period in the female lifecycle for disordered patterns of eating to become established (Tiggemann *et al.* 2000).

As the following quotations attest, participants on limited incomes tended to continue their established patterns of eating rather than introduce dietary changes in response to pregnancy.

'I were never like that through my pregnancy, it's not been, "Oh I'll eat this because it's healthy".'

Kelly, age 18 (N)

'I think really because I tend to have quite a healthy diet anyway it's not really had a bearing on what I've decided to eat or not eat.'

Amely, age 38 (N)

Many poorer women intimated that while there was room for improvement – and their diets might have been 'healthi*er*', most refuted any inference that what they ate was *un*healthy, or that their diets were significantly lacking in nutrients or needed reassessing. This assertion is particularly interesting in the light of a recent survey which suggested that poorer women eat more restricted diets, including fewer than recommended amounts of fresh fruits and vegetables (National Diet and Nutrition Survey (NDNS) 2004); poverty is also associated with obesity and low weight gain in pregnancy (NICE 2008). The relationship between poverty and restricted access to food in pregnancy is recognised (Food Standards Agency and Welsh Assembly 2003) and the negative impact of poverty on pregnancy outcomes, and as a significant constraint on childhood development, is also well documented (D'Souza & Garcia 2003), especially with respect to pregnant teenagers (Burchett & Seeley 2003). Despite reportage from the tabloid press to the contrary, there is evidence to suggest that the problems that arise in households with inadequate food supplies occur because there is insufficient money available to spend on food, not because money is being spent unwisely (Nelson 2000).

In the following quotation, however, Kelly expresses the limits to her own agency in her efforts (irrespective of financial constraints) to manipulate pregnancy outcome through dietary intervention:

'I've always been told that the baby will take the good out of the food and what's left, you preserve. [So the baby gets first choice?] Yeah, that's what I've always been told and it's what I've always believed, that baby gets the best first.'

Kelly, age 18 (N)

The inference here is that Kelly's own nutritional needs must be satisfied with 'what's left' and that her own health and wellbeing is of rather less importance in comparison with her developing fetus. Also, pregnant women are widely understood, and encouraged by society, to form a 'bonding' relationship with their unborn child, yet during prolonged periods of nausea/vomiting and general feelings of malaise they may also be encouraged, like Kelly, to view the baby as something of a separate entity, which they must feed and nurture despite their own preferences and appetites. Elsewhere in our data, and significantly from women who had prolonged pregnancy-related sickness[viii], midwives, perhaps seeking to appease their concerns for fetal development, were reported to use the word 'parasite' when describing the fetus in relation to its mother.

Kelly's comments further reiterate the sense of 'fatalism' that has long been seen as a defining characteristic of lower socioeconomic populations (Willis 1977; Pill & Stott 1987; Roberts 1996). It also conveys a sense of the culturally embedded, and embodied, nature of belief systems and the challenges health professionals face in overcoming resistance to change such that health promotion messages may be translated into what they see as positive behavioural change.

In summary, although conscious of links between consumption and fetal development (as evidenced in further discussion below), teenagers and mothers in lower socioeconomic groups did not frame food consumption in terms of potential to *maximise* benefits for their unborn child and challenged notions that they ate a diet that was harmful to their fetus. In this sense then, these women did not understand pregnancy as a 'project to be managed', nor exhibit the possibly aspirational intentions of women in higher socioeconomic groups to improve the health and bodies of future generations.

7.5   Consumption in pregnancy: prohibitions and exclusions

7.5.1   'Risky' foods

Discussions about dietary intake during pregnancy not only covered what to eat in pregnancy, but also frequently revolved around what not to eat: foods considered 'risky' with respect to consumption, storage and preparation. Participants from across the socioeconomic spectrum appeared to have internalised certain food-related messages, and hence categories of 'prohibited' foods were referred to in a very matter-of-fact, taken-for-granted manner. Although some women admitted to missing certain foods and joked about ceremoniously requesting them immediately after birth, most were of the opinion that abstinence during pregnancy was necessary because it was protective against possible negative outcomes. Hence, a period of heightened awareness and temporary abstinence was understood to be one of the necessary 'small sacrifices' which mothers-to-be should anticipate in advance of assuming a maternal role.

> *'Especially not since I've been pregnant, but even before no, I'm a bit funny about stuff like that – if it's gone out of date . . .'*

Danielle, age 31 (O)

[viii] Many of the women in this study, particularly those managing diabetes or overweight/obesity linked to polycystic ovary syndrome, experienced more extreme and prolonged periods of sickness and nausea, sometimes resulting in substantial weight fluctuations and challenging diabetic control.

'[So have, have you followed all these things (food restrictions) then?] Oh, yeah. 'Cause I'd just feel terrible [laugh] if something happened. . . . It is a pain but you just get, it just gets engrained into your system just to check things before you buy them, or put them in your mouth.'

Helen, age 30 (D + O)

As with advice about alcohol and occasionally smoking in pregnancy (discussed next), women in this study from across the socioeconomic spectrum questioned, and sometimes dismissed, the food safety advice they were given by midwives, although on notably different grounds. For women in lower socioeconomic groups dietary advice, which focused predominantly on lists of 'foods to avoid', was largely dismissed as irrelevant, often because they did not recognise, or normally eat, the food items referred to. Unlike the higher socioeconomic group participants in Miller's study (2005), the comparable participants in this study frequently contested 'expert' advice, not necessarily on grounds of dietary relevance because it competed with knowledge transmitted by mothers and other sources, but on the grounds that media representations and their own information sources suggested rather more scientific uncertainty around purported risks than indicated by maternity professionals. In the following quotation Betty (vegetarian), who reported being 'told off' for disregarding guidance about soft cheeses, felt confident in continuing to eat these foods as she could not detect any adverse effects on her developing fetus:

'I've been eating feta and goat's cheese which apparently you're not supposed to but I've taken a lot of this kind of, these guidelines with a pinch of salt in pregnancy.'

Betty, age 23 (N)

Participants from higher socioeconomic groups such as Sandra, who had grown up in countries outside the UK where official guidance was reported to be less cautious, reinterpreted 'expert' opinion in the context of their own embodied dietary habits.

'I think it was precautions that I don't need to take. So I haven't . . . I don't eat many, much nuts, you know, in general but I've been having hazelnuts and things like that every so often. Because I don't think there's anything wrong with it I think it's just, you know, pushing it a bit too far 'cause it's about allergies I think.'

Sandra, age 30 (N)

7.5.2   Alcohol consumption

Participants across the age and socioeconomic spectrum vociferously contested current recommendations on alcohol consumption in pregnancy and interpreted available guidance within the context of individual lifestyles and identities.

'I was probably fairly relaxed. I didn't drink anything for the first 12 weeks but after that, . . . I gave myself a rule of a unit a day, which is actually more than

I know you're supposed to have but in practice, it probably worked out at maybe a unit a day three or four days a week. And I, we have a glass of wine with tea most nights.'

Hayley, age 37 (N)

Some higher socioeconomic status participants recognised that a range of politicised stances and expert views on this issue were in circulation and indeed during the course of this research, official guidelines changed a number of times. As will become evident later in this chapter, pregnant participants who continued to drink alcohol were generally able to rationalise their decisions if challenged.

Those who had planned pregnancy often welcomed the opportunity to restrict their alcohol intake, seeing it as a signal of readiness to move on from the more hedonistic lifestyles of their youth, which most considered unsuitable for motherhood:

'I did at one point in my twenties want some kids, but then I was living a far too wild a lifestyle at that point. . . .'

Marianne, age 32 (N)

Decreasing alcohol consumption, however, was sometimes associated with a reduction in opportunities for normal socialising:

'I miss it when I go out because he says, "Are you coming to the pub?" And I say, "Well it's boring now, I'm just sat there with a glass of orange and breathing everybody's smoke in, it's boring." '

Scarlet, age 33 (O)

Although many women were aware that alcohol intake is assessed in terms of 'units', and that an upper limit is recommended, most (and particularly older women from lower socioeconomic groups) considered themselves as 'moderate' drinkers and did not appear overly anxious about measuring their intake in the precise terminology of 'units of consumption'.

Younger women's narratives on alcohol, tobacco, and occasionally 'recreational' drug consumption, reflected pre-pregnant lifestyles which generally emphasised 'hard' or 'fast' living. In contrast to popular stereotyping of young women as ignorant and self-centred, however, all teenagers contributing to the study reported having made strenuous attempts to change their consumption patterns in pregnancy, often with little support from their peers and local cultures. For example, Stacey reported that she had stopped her regular use of cocaine and Ecstasy and that she had reduced her intake of cannabis and alcohol because of concerns for her baby's welfare. Behavioural change of this dimension was a significant achievement for Stacey, particularly given the unresponsiveness of her partner:

'[Have you made a sort of conscious effort to not drink when you're pregnant?] I have, yeah, I don't, like [partner] drinks all the time but I don't. . . . I don't

want it. I don't. There's no point in drinking when I know I can't get drunk so [laugh] [And why can't you get drunk?] 'Cause of the baby. It might harm the baby so . . .'

Stacey, age 17 (N)

Stacey emphasises her belief that vigilance is necessary, not so much for her own health, as to afford protection for her unborn child. The threat of intervention from the 'the social' (social services) acted to incentivise some young women and encourage them to cease engaging in behaviours which could signify them as deviant and/or irresponsible. Peer experiences of continued alcohol consumption and the production of 'intelligent' children, however, reinforced the sense of fatalism referred to earlier in this chapter:

'Well, I [pause] one of my friends . . . she's got two girls. No she's got three now but . . . while she were pregnant with them she drank a lot of vodka and Red Bull. And them two, they've, [pause] being told that they could move up a couple of years each [in school] and they're only like four and six. They're really like classed as intelligent children . . . myself I think it's way you carry them it's either gonna happen for you or it's, it's not.'

Janice, age 27 (O)

Some participants found that drinking alcohol in public when visibly pregnant contravened socially accepted norms. As Betty illustrates in the following quotation, pregnant women who ignore these norms may themselves become the object of criticism and/or hostility by self-appointed 'experts'.

'I've been conscious of what I've drunk. . . . I stuck to . . . two units a week . . . I don't actually think there's very much wrong with that but there are some people I know who are pregnant who wouldn't touch a drop of alcohol. . . . I couldn't go into a pub and drink. The one experience I went in it was shocking . . . This man stared at me for the entire . . . He was staring at me for ages and ages and ages and [when] I got up to go to the toilet [he] deliberately banged into me so all the wine went everywhere. I couldn't believe it. I could not believe it. . . . But that people make judgements probably isn't shocking and probably I would make a judgement [about pregnant women drinking alcohol] if I hadn't experienced being pregnant. So I can't say [pause] that they're wrong to do it '

Betty, age 23 (N)

Despite the physically aggressive intrusion she describes, Betty nonetheless empathises with the man concerned, and with his motives, and hence dismisses his actions. In doing so she affirms society's freedom to judge, and indeed to enforce, perceived norms of behaviour for pregnant women in public spaces. Limitations on the freedom of movement, and hence on an individual's social life and the ongoing project of self-construction, have been previously described in relation to pregnancy (Longhurst 1999), childbirth (Sharpe 1999), and the transition to parenthood

(Aitken 1999). Within these discrete discourses, the totalising processes associated with the 'confinement', to which pregnant women are routinely subjected, becomes ever more real. The word 'confinement' – meaning limit or boundary – is a recurring image and experience for most women; it is also a word which enters the pregnancy vocabulary early on and very powerfully, restricting access to public spaces, curbing indulgence in alcohol and tobacco, and eliminating a range of other previously enjoyed pleasures and freedoms.

7.5.3 Smoking

The few higher socioeconomic group mothers who had smoked prior to pregnancy did not contest scientific assertions that this would damage their fetus, and all quit, or at least drastically cut down, on smoking. In the following quotation, however, teenager Shauna (from a lower socioeconomic group) questioned the validity of the advice she received from health professionals regarding smoking in pregnancy. She made a link between her previous experiences of miscarriage following smoking cessation and hence offered a rational argument to continue smoking in this pregnancy. Her decision was given further credence by the results of her ultrasound scans which revealed that her baby was larger, rather than smaller, for gestational age and hence she (logically?) deduced that her continued tobacco consumption could not be impacting negatively on its growth and development. However, what Shauna (diagnosed with gestational diabetes and having gained a significant amount of weight) failed to appreciate was that her impaired insulin control was likely to result in a larger than average-sized baby, with potentially negative consequences for her own, and her baby's health (Villamor & Cnattingus 2006). Contrary to what Shauna believed, 'bigger' is not 'better'.

> *'I haven't really changed [smoking habits]. I did when, when I were first pregnant . . . I'd had two miscarriages before and I stopped smoking both times. And so I thought well, if anything were gonna happen it were gonna happen either way anyway and so I just carried on smoking . . . it's like when people say smoking makes your baby smaller, in my case it haven't, it's made it bigger [laugh].'*
>
> Shauna, age 19 (D + O)

Kelly, who reported reducing her cigarette consumption, invoked the power of transmitted maternal wisdom and experience to counter what she perceived to be 'fallacious' biomedical evidence and justified her decision not to quit smoking altogether:

> *'She [midwife] came to see me and it were all, "Oh you shouldn't do this and you shouldn't do that . . . and you shouldn't smoke." . . . my Mum, she smoked with us, with all of us . . . she smoked with all of us and we're all fine. . . . I believe it's a fallacy. I know it's probably been proven but . . . I don't believe that. I know it*

can do some harm. I sound really naïve here; I know it can do some harm but I don't believe it can do as much harm [in pregnancy] as what it can when the baby's actually here.'

Kelly, age 18 (N)

Kelly's final point highlights a central issue in debates concerning child safety and protection; that the (in)visibility of the fetus may be a significant barrier to pregnant women adopting healthier behaviours.

Women who were unable to stop smoking, occasionally reported acts of deception designed to deflect unwanted attention from maternity staff, which would invariably attract more intense surveillance:

'When I were first pregnant I used to say, "Oh, I've cut down, and, Oh, I'm gonna stop." But now I just think, Oh, what's the point. There's no point in lying. [laugh] Not gonna say I'm gonna stop 'cause I know I'm not.'

Shauna, age 19 (D + O)

A number of women, especially those who had smoked since early adolescence, reported being able to stop smoking quickly and effortlessly when they first realised they were pregnant. The ease with which they accomplished this behavioural change came as a surprise to most, especially for obese women who were unable to exploit the same control in relation to their eating patterns[ix]. In the following quotation Fiona explains the importance of 'will power' as an invaluable aid in changing established routines:

'It's like before I got pregnant I used to smoke. Really bad. Then as soon as I found out I were pregnant [clicked fingers] stopped smoking like that. . . . And I hadn't smoked all way through my pregnancy. But it's like what [partner] says, he says, "You've got willpower. That's strongest thing to ever stop doing – smoking." He says, "You've got willpower to do that," he says. But it's chocolate and crisps . . .'

Fiona, age 25 (O)

As we have previously mentioned, changing unhealthy patterns 'for the sake of the baby' was reported by participants to be generally less problematic, and more easily accomplished, than if they were attempting to make these changes for their own benefit. This is not to imply that any alteration in behaviour patterns during the course of pregnancy is predictive of long-term change, but it is nonetheless interesting to question why women invoked the health of their baby to support smoking cessation, but why this failed to evoke a similar response in challenging unhealthy or suboptimal eating patterns.

[ix] It is unclear from our data to what, if any, extent participants used smoking to manage weight concerns.

7.6   Consumption in pregnancy: cravings, calories and weight management

More educated women generally dismissed the idea that pregnancy justified an additional caloric intake. Whilst increased dietary requirements were acknowledged, for example in response to 'cravings', the importance of self-restraint was frequently reiterated:

> *'I don't believe in this eating for two, I don't think you eat for two. I think if you're genuinely hungry, yes, you eat but I think there are a lot of people . . . I mean I saw my friend when she were first pregnant and she was like eating bags of mini eggs and cream buns. And I was like, "You don't normally eat that, are you craving it?" And it were like, "No". Why do it then?'*
>
> Jessica, age 34 (D)

Although participants generally denied 'eating for two' many nonetheless conceded a response to increased feelings of hunger, resulting in more snacking behaviour, often of 'naughty' foods (cake and chocolate), rather than healthier options.

> *'[You've not been eating for two then?] Actually I have strong feelings about that. I think that's absolute rubbish . . . Ah, well, pregnancy's completely changed what I snack on. I've absolutely stuffed my face with cake. I've really had cravings for chocolate and cake.'*
>
> Betty, age 23 (N)

Participants from higher socioeconomic groups suggested that snacking behaviour was tolerated providing that neither maternal nor fetal weight gain was adversely affected. By contrast, women from lower socioeconomic groups, especially those who were already overweight with a history of dieting, tended to view pregnancy as a time for relaxing constraints around (over)eating. In the following quotation Fiona describes what might constitute bingeing behaviour:

> *'[And how much chocolate and crisps will you eat in a day?] Oooh, loads . . . Cheese and onion crisps [laugh] . . . And Mars bars [laugh] . . . you sit there though and you have one and then like ten minutes later [laugh] you'll have another one, then another one.'*
>
> Fiona, age 25 (O)

Dieter Janice reconciled a tendency to continue overeating in pregnancy by invoking agency on behalf of her baby:

> *'I haven't been as conscious as like when I were dieting before so if I've just fancied something I've had it. Whereas before if I fancied it I just thought, Oh no that's healthier. I'd have that, but if I've fancied it this time I've sort of had it. I convinced myself it's my baby telling me I need to eat it.'*
>
> Janice, age 27 (O)

Despite relaxing prior constraints, many such overweight/obese participants – who often reported a substantial history of dieting – nonetheless expressed anxieties about weight gain in pregnancy and some would have welcomed an opportunity to discuss their concerns with a health professional. That said, it is suggested that professionals may have felt hampered by a lack of access to information about safe and effective interventions for their obese clients, especially during pregnancy. Although participants were generally aware of the pregnancy-related risks associated with their overweight/obese status, some experienced difficulty on the occasions they sought clarification from maternity care providers.

'Nobody's mentioned my weight. I've asked them if I'm likely to have more trouble in labour or anything because of my weight and they've said no, unless I've been having trouble all the way through, which I haven't, so . . .'

Scarlet, age 33 (O)

'I'm quite scared like because of my weight. I'm quite scared. There could be quite many complications. I can end up in having caesarean rather than having normal delivery. . . . Like I read about all these things and I ask my midwife and she told me it could be a complication, but there could be like you can have normal delivery also.'

Nighat, age 29 (O)

A number of pregnancies were identified by maternity care providers as being 'at risk' because of fetuses being occasionally smaller, but more often larger, in size than expected for their gestational age. These women were subsequently subjected to more intensive monitoring, for example in the form of additional antenatal scans and medical consultations. Despite apparent concern for the consequences of inappropriate fetal growth rate on its healthy development, with the exception of women managing diabetes, participants did not report being questioned about their current diets, nor their weight histories.

Attitudes to body image were similarly not explored within the context of the antenatal consultation. Although the relationship between childbearing and weight gain is complex, research suggests (Öhlin & Rössner 1996; Linne *et al.* 2002) that pregnancy and the postnatal period are vulnerable phases in the lifecycle when women may accumulate excess weight. Overweight status prior to conception and excessive weight gain during pregnancy are both predictors of postpartum weight retention (Ford & Barrowclough 2001; Walker *et al.* 2005); all of these factors are positively associated with further undue weight gain in a future pregnancy (Villamor & Cnattingius 2006).

In a review of the literature examining control over weight gain during pregnancy, Johnson *et al.* (2004) highlighted contradictions in the current knowledge base, with some studies reporting that women exert high levels of control and others suggesting that pregnancy is a time for relaxation of usual control measures. Studies attempting to identify the significance of factors such as weight prior to pregnancy, previous dieting behaviour, and body image concerns, demonstrate similar contradictions (Davies & Wardle 1994; Wiles 1994). Our findings would therefore seem to corroborate research on these issues.

7.7 Autonomy and sociocultural constraints on choice and consumption

Prior to pregnancy, many participants from higher socioeconomic groups indicated that they had experienced relative freedom in decision making about their consumption practices and body weight maintenance. This was also true for many women from higher socioeconomic groups who were overweight/obese but who denied being on diets or that they were seeking to lose weight. Rather, the majority reported eating healthily and feeling physically fit; these women resisted medicalised constructions of their bodies as overweight, obese, or deviant. Although they could recount incidences of discrimination in their youth, such women accepted themselves as 'naturally' larger than average in size, and reported being accepted and respected by family and peers. The ability to retain self-governing status, however, may be seriously challenged in pregnancy when a woman's body – and her body image – become the object of wider scrutiny. Hence, family members, health professionals, and sometimes complete strangers, may pass comment or indeed, make unsolicited and often unwanted, physical contact with the 'bump'.

> '. . . one of my [clients] said to me the other day, "Eh, you must have clapped some weight on with your pregnancy." And I said, "Well, not really, no. I've, I've always been like this" [laugh].'
>
> Elsie, age 31 (N[x])

> 'Cause if anybody ever touched my belly before I were pregnant I'd be like, "What you doing?" [laugh]. Don't touch me fat! [laugh]'
>
> Janice, age 27 (O)

For a number of women, it was clear that their significant others were monitoring their food intake. Although this attention was mostly welcomed and viewed as a positive response indicating concern, some participants resented what they perceived to be intrusive attempts that impinged on their sense of autonomy. In the following quotation, Antonia, who was struggling with sleep deprivation, ongoing nausea, and concerns about body image and 'fatness', signalled her irritation at her father's insistence to eat:

> 'Like the other day, I had a jacket potato. [coughs] And my Dad forced me to have something else because he says, "Oh it won't be growing" . . . like in the

---

[x] Elsie, and a number of other participants including a medical doctor and several nurses, self-defined as being of average weight, although their pre-pregnancy BMI medically defined them as overweight/obese.

morning, this morning he's [dad's] done me some toast. I didn't feel like eating it but I have to eat it for the lecture. I get a lecture if I don't [eat it].'

Antonia, age 17 (N)

Nighat also reported pressure from her husband:

'When I become pregnant I have to eat what my husband say because he's more [laugh] controlling on me now'.

Nighat, age 29 (O)

In this context, attempts to maximise the health/bodies of future generations threatens to usurp women's personal autonomy and the degree of control they exercise over dietary choices.

7.7.1   The magic of milk and other revered food items

Meanings associated with some everyday food items, particularly milk, tended to be inflated during pregnancy and ascribed a 'sacred' status (Douglas 1966). Milk was widely appreciated as a 'healthy' substance, containing calcium and other ingredients considered necessary for adequate growth and development. Even when ingesting milk simulated sensations of nausea, many participants nonetheless reported increasing their consumption because they believed it to be beneficial to maternal and fetal health and wellbeing. For Alejandria, who grew up outside the UK, milk consumption from an early age was perceived as appropriate preparation for future motherhood:

'First it was the argument that I needed to grow, and then you will eventually be a mother so you have to have calcium and things. But it was a healthy thing'.

Alejandria, age 31 (N)

Religious and other non-Western cultural allegiances were also important considerations influencing food choice and autonomy. Shenaz, Anu and Nighat, all qualified health professionals with familial roots in South Asian cultures, expressed concerns about ingesting traditional foods, often because of the unknown effects of these substances on fetal health and wellbeing. These viewpoints clearly articulate the contested nature and meaning of phrases such as 'healthy' with respect to food and eating in pregnancy, especially for participants from non-English cultures.

'If I would be in Pakistan I would be expected to have like more greasy food after having my baby, because in our traditional we take like more greasy food and more not so good [food] after having delivery.'

Nighat, age 29 (O)

'I know that she's [mother in law] you know, got her heart in the right place but I said, "I ain't eating that rubbish [a traditional herbal mixture], not while I'm

pregnant because I don't know what's in it, I haven't got a clue what's in it" and I said, "For all I know, it could be anything." I said, "Yeah, it's herbal and I know it's herbal and I know she wouldn't poison me but you know, you don't know what effect that particular herb or spice has on a baby." I goes, "I'm not going to take that risk." And he [husband] was like, "Yeah but everybody's had it." I said, "I don't care who's had it, I don't care if your mother's had it and she's given birth to ten children or 20 or whatever, and I don't care whether whoever's had it," I goes, "I can't."'

Shenaz, age 30 (D + O)

It is possible that Nighat's overweight status may have increased her concerns about gaining additional weight from consuming 'not so good' symbolically important, but nonetheless, high-calorie foods at a time in her life when she would be taking care of her newborn baby and less able to exercise, rather than being concerned about nourishing a body depleted of energy from childbirth. Pregnant women from non-English backgrounds reported struggling with how best to manage traditional food-related customs and beliefs in which they no longer believed or valued, (indeed, many dismissed them as 'old wives tales'), but with which they were nonetheless expected to comply. In Shenaz's family, the consumption of rich, heavy, 'fattening' foods was considered particularly important following pregnancy. Shenaz, however, was of the opinion that these foods were wholly inappropriate considering she was managing polycystic ovary syndrome, type 2 diabetes and was also seriously overweight (BMI = 39).

Differences in understandings about the (in)appropriateness of ingesting hot/cold foods associated with being a Muslim, and their potential effects on maternal health or fetal development, symbolised another aspect of these tensions. The significance of pregnancy – as an important hiatus in the life cycle – was assumed into food-related events and practices and women were expected to behave in accordance with traditional principles. The pressure to conform was particularly stressful for participants who, through processes associated with enculturation/integration, were more inclined to embrace the values of the host country. Maintaining harmonious relationships with the extended family, especially with elders to whom they were expected to defer, was nonetheless viewed as essential by the majority of participants Customary foods or practices which did not provoke conflict were respected and maintained.

This section has detailed some of the ways in which women's autonomy to make dietary changes/choices is compromised, and highlights women's skill or educational capital in attesting or managing competing claims to their consumption behaviours. This illustrates that the *Global Strategy*'s call to ensure the optimal health and nutritional status of women remains a complex challenge.

7.8   Conclusion

Our analysis emphasises the significance of cultural practices and embedded norms and their impact on pregnancy-related consumption practices. Through the lens of our empirical data we have exposed some of the assumptions made about women's ability to exert control over their pregnant body including dietary intake especially when they have been identified as 'high risk' and in need of additional medical surveillance. The diversity of accounts suggests that childbearing women expend variable degrees of effort and control to achieve a desired 'balance' across a range of consumption-related issues and that 'success' is achieved only within contexts which permit individual women to exercise their autonomy. Thus, expertise and monitoring in pregnancy are experienced as enabling and/or limiting in more socially patterned ways than is currently acknowledged.

Maternal dieting and weight patterns and enculturated nutritional/consumption norms (including smoking and drug use) received little sustained attention and, hence, it is perhaps unsurprising that the advice offered by maternity professionals was often perceived to be of limited relevance to women's everyday lives and individual circumstances (see Kirkham & Stapleton 2001; Stapleton 2007). Furthermore, anxieties about gaining excess weight are not helped by a lack of understanding about the role of exercise and taboos on dieting in pregnancy. Finally, younger participants still living in the parental home exercise very little control over food choices and poorer participants report having insufficient equipment and access to food outlets and lacking basic cooking skills.

Our research also suggests that the pressures associated with 'doing' pregnancy and motherhood in the contemporary late modern era may be interpreted by some women as opportunities for re/deconstructing the body. While the narratives from some participants portrayed them as 'typical' subjects of late modernity who were financially independent, well informed, and experienced decision makers, capable of self-governance, other narratives, especially from younger, poorer women, and some women from lower socioeconomic groups, demonstrated rather less evidence of reflexive self-governance. Whereas accounts from the first group of participants implied that pregnancy was a continuation of a taken-for-granted autonomous condition, flexibly applied to changing physiology, contrasting experiences were also articulated. The amount of accumulated, and embodied, 'capital' (Bourdieu 1986) with which women enter pregnancy and subsequently make the transition to motherhood is clearly important in this respect. Younger women in particular tended to reject dietary-related advice from 'experts' referring instead to mothers and extended family and friendship networks. They also used previously embodied maternal experiences to counter what some perceived as inappropriate advice. This was not without potential consequences, however, as young women whom maternity professionals regarded as disengaged from the project of self-monitoring risked being labelled as irresponsible and subjected to closer scrutiny.

The findings from our study strongly suggest that structural and cultural factors, together with lived and embodied understandings and experiences of control, may work to undermine public health policies such as the *Global Strategy for Infant and Child Feeding* (WHO 2003), which assume and validate a rational actor who is fully informed and willing to exercise self-regulation. In this way we have illustrated that the implementation of a global strategy to ensure the optimal health and nutritional status of women remains a complex challenge.

References

Acheson, D. (1998) *Independent Inquiry into Inequalities in Health*. HMSO, London. At: http://www.archive.official-documents.co.uk/document/doh/ih/ih.htm (accessed 7 April 2008).

Aitken, S.C. (1999) Putting parents in their place. Child rearing rights and gender politics. In: Teather, E.K. (ed) *Embodied Geographies: Spaces Bodies and Rites of Passage*. Routledge, London.

Aphramor, L. (2005) Is a weight-centred health framework salutogenic? Some thoughts on unhinging certain dietary ideologies. *Social Theory and Health*, 3: 315–340.

Attride-Stirling, J. (2001) Thematic networks: an analytic tool for qualitative research. *Qualitative Research*, 1: 385–407.

Barker, D. (ed) (1992) *Fetal and Infant Origins of Adult Disease*. BMJ Books, London.

Batnitzky, A. (2008) Obesity and household roles: gender and social class in Morocco. *Sociology of Health and illness*, 30: 445–462.

British Medical Association (2005) *Preventing Childhood Obesity: A Report from the BMA Board of Science*. British Medical Association Board of Science.

Bourdieu, P. (1986) *Distinction: A Social Critique of the Judgement of Taste*. Routledge and Kegan Paul, London.

Burchett, H. & Seeley, A. (2003) Good enough to eat? The diet of pregnant teenagers. The Maternity Alliance and The Food Commission. At: http://www.foodcomm.org.uk/Too_good_to_eat.PDF (accessed 13 April 2008).

Campos, P. (2004) *The Obesity Myth: Why America's Obsession with Weight is Hazardous to Your Health*. Gotham Books, New York.

Castel, R. (1991) From dangerousness to risk. In: Burchell, G., Gordon, C. & Miller, P. (eds) *The Foucault Effect: Studies in Governmentality*. Harvester Wheatsheaf, London, pp. 281–299.

Cooper, C. (1997) Can a fat woman call herself disabled? *Disability and Society*, 12: 31–41.

Cooper, C. (1998) *Fat and Proud: The Politics of Size*. The Women's Press, London. For information on activist activities, see http://www.charlottecooper.net/index.htm.

Côté, J.E. (1996) Sociological perspectives on identity formation: the culture-identity link and identity capital. *Journal of Adolescence*, 19: 417–428.

Davey Smith, G., Dorling, D. & Shaw, M. (eds) (2001) *Poverty, Inequality And Health In Britain, 1800–2000: A Reader*. The Policy Press, Bristol.

Davies, K. & Wardle, J. (1994) Body image and dieting in pregnancy. *Journal of Psychosomatic Research*, 38: 767–799.

Department of Health (2006) *Forecasting Obesity to 2010*. HMSO, London. At: http://www.dh.gov.uk/en/Publicationsandstatistics/Publications/PublicationsStatistics/DH_4138630 (accessed 13 April 2008).

Dewey, K.G. (2003) Is breastfeeding protective against child obesity? *Journal of Human Lactation*, 19: 9–18.

Douglas, M. (1966) *Purity and Danger*. Routledge, London.

D'Souza, L. & Garcia, J. (2003) *Access to Care for Low Income Childbearing Women. Limiting the Impact of Poverty and Disadvantage on the Heath of Low-Income Pregnant Women. New Mothers and Their Babies: a Scoping Exercise*. National Perinatal Epidemiology Unit and Maternity Alliance, Oxford and London.

Edwards, N. (2004) Why can't women just say no? And does it really matter? In: Kirkham, M. (ed) *Informed Choice in Maternity Care*. Palgrave MacMillan, Basingstoke, pp. 1–29.

Ettorre, E. (2000) Reproductive genetics, gender and the body: Please Doctor, may I have a Normal Baby? *Sociology*, 34: 403–420.

Evans, B. (2006) 'Gluttony or sloth': critical geographies of bodies and morality in (anti)obesity policy. *Area*, 38: 259–267.

Farrar, D. & Duley, L. (2007) Commentary: but why should women be weighed routinely during pregnancy? *International Journal of Epidemiology*, 36: 1283–1284.

Food Standards Agency Wales and Welsh Assembly (2003) *Food and Well Being. Reducing Inequalities Through a Nutrition Strategy for Wales*. Food Standards Agency Wales & Welsh

Assembly Government, Cardiff. At: http://www.food.gov.uk/multimedia/pdfs/foodandwellbeing. pdf (accessed 13 April 2008).

Ford, F. & Barrowclough, D. (2001) Weight gain during pregnancy – does it contribute to the rising rate of obesity in women in the UK? *Nutrition and Food Science*, 31: 183–188.

Foucault, M. (1970) *The Order of Things: An Archaeology of the Human Sciences*. Pantheon Books, London.

Furedi, F. (2001) *Paranoid Parenting: Abandon Your Anxieties and be a Good Parent*. Allen Lane, The Penguin Press, London.

Gard, M. & Wright, J. (2001) Managing uncertainty: obesity discourses and physical education in a risk society. *Studies in Philosophy and Education*, 20: 535–549.

Hays, S. (1996) *The Cultural Contradictions of Motherhood*. Yale University Press, Yale.

Heslehurst, N., Lang, R., Rankin, J., Wilkinson, J.R. & Summerbell, C.D. (2007) Obesity in pregnancy: a study of the impact of maternal obesity on NHS maternity services. *BJOG International Journal of Obstetrics and Gynaecology*, 114: 334–342.

Hutchinson, S.A. (1990) Responsible subversion: a study of rule-bending among nurses. *Scholarly Inquiry for Nursing Practice*, 4: 3–17.

Johnson, S., Burrows, A. & Williamson, I. (2004) Does my bump look big in this? the meaning of bodily changes for first-time mothers-to-be. *Journal of Health Psychology*, 9: 361–374.

Kirkham, M. & Stapleton, H. (2001) *Informed Choice in Maternity Care: An Evaluation of Evidence Based Leaflets*. University of York, NHS Centre for Reviews and Dissemination, York.

Kuh, D., Hardy, R., Chaturvedi, N. & Wadsworth, M.E.J. (2002) Birth weight, childhood growth and abdominal obesity in adult life. *International Journal of Obesity*, 26: 40–47.

Li, L., Parsons, T.J. & Power, C. (2003) Breast feeding and obesity in childhood: cross sectional study. *British Medical Journal*, 327: 904–905.

Linne, Y., Barkeling, B. & Rossner, S. (2002) Long-term weight development after pregnancy. *Obesity Reviews*, 3: 75–83.

Longhurst, R. (1999) Pregnant bodies, public scrutiny: 'giving advice to pregnant women'. In: Teather, E.K. (ed) *Embodied Geographies: Spaces, Bodies and Rites of Passage*. Routledge, London.

Mason, J. (2002) *Qualitative Researching*. Sage, London.

Miller, T. (2005) *Making Sense of Motherhood*. Cambridge University Press, Cambridge.

Monaghan, L.F. (2007) Body Mass Index, masculinities and moral worth: men's critical under-standings of 'appropriate' weight-for-height. *Sociology of Health and Illness*, 29: 584–609.

Murphy-Lawless, J. (1998) *Reading Birth and Death: A History of Obstetric Thinking*. Cork University Press, Cork.

NDNS (2004) National Diet and Nutrition Survey: adults aged 19 to 64 years Volume 5. Office for National Statistics, London.

Nelson, M. (2000) Childhood nutrition and poverty. *Proceedings of the Nutrition Society*, 59: 307–315.

NICE (2003) *Routine Antenatal Care for Healthy Pregnant Women: Understanding NICE Guidance – Information for Pregnant Women, Their Families and the Public*. Clinical Guideline 6. The Stationary Office, HMSO.

NICE (2006) *Obesity. Guidance on the Prevention, Identification, Assessment and Management of Overweight and Obesity in Adults and Children*. Clinical Guideline 43. National Institute of Clinical Excellence, London. At: http://www.nice.org.uk/nicemedia/pdf/CG43quickrefguide2. pdf (accessed 7 April 2008).

NICE (2008) *Improving the Nutrition of Pregnant and Breastfeeding Mothers and Children in Low-income Households*. Public health guidance 11. National Institute of Clinical Excellence, London. At: http://www.nice.org.uk/nicemedia/pdf/PH011quickrefguide.pdf (accessed 4 May 2008).

Ö Lúanaigh, P. & Carlson, C. (eds) (2005) *Midwifery and Public Health: Future Directions, New Opportunities*. Churchill Livingstone, Edinburgh.

Öhlin, A. & Rössner, S. (1996) Factors related to body weight changes during and after pregnancy: the Stockholm pregnancy and weight development study. *Obesity Research*, 4: 271–276.

Owen, C.G., Martin, R.M., Whincup, P.H., Smith, G.D. & Cook, D.G. (2005) Effect of infant feeding on the risk of obesity across the life course: a quantitative review of published evidence. *Pediatrics*, **115**: 1367–1377.

Parsons, T., Power, C. & Manor, O. (2003) Infant feeding and obesity through the lifecourse. *Archives of Disease in Childhood*, **88**: 793–794.

Parsons, T.J., Power, C., Logan, S. & Summerbell, C.D. (1999) Childhood predictors of adult obesity: a systematic review. *International Journal of Obesity*, **23**: S1–S107.

Petersen, A. & Lupton, D. (1996) *The New Public Health: Health and Self in the Age of Risk*. Sage, London.

Pill, R.M. & Stott, N.C.H. (1987) The stereotype of 'working-class fatalism' and the challenge for primary care health promotion. *Health Education Research*, **2**: 105–114.

Rich, E. & Evans, J. (2005) Fat ethics – the obesity discourse and body politics. *Social Theory Health*, **3**: 341–358.

Roberts, E. (1996) *A Woman's Place, an Oral History of Working Class Women, 1890–1940*. Blackwell Press, Oxford.

Seidell, J.C. (2000) Obesity, insulin resistance and diabetes – a worldwide epidemic. *British Journal of Nutrition*, **83** (Suppl s1): 5–8.

Sharpe, S. (1999) Bodily speaking: spaces and experiences of childbirth. In: Teather, E.K. (ed) *Embodied Geographies: Spaces, Bodies and Rites of Passage*. Routledge, London.

Shields, L., O'Callaghan, M., Williams, G.M., Najman, J.M. & Bor, W. (2006) Breastfeeding and obesity at 14 years: A cohort study. *Journal of Paediatrics and Child Health*, **42**: 289–296.

Silva, E. & Smart, C. (1999) (eds) *The New Family?* Sage, London.

Smart, C., Neale, B. & Wade, A. (eds) (2001) *The Changing Experience of Childhood. Families and Divorce*. Polity, Cambridge.

Soltani, H. & Fraser, R.B. (2000) A longitudinal study of maternal anthropometric changes in normal weight, overweight and obese women during pregnancy and postpartum. *British Journal of Nutrition*, **84**: 95–101.

Stamatakis, E., Primatesta, P., Chinn, S., Rona, R. & Falascheti, E. (2005) Overweight and obesity trends from 1974 to 2003 in English children: what is the role of socioeconomic factors? *Archives of Disease in Childhood*, **90**: 999–1004.

Stapleton, H. (2006) Doing sex, having the baby: young women and transitions to motherhood. Unpublished Ph.D. Thesis. University of Sheffield, Sheffield.

Stapleton, H. (2007) *I'm Not Pregnant, I'm Fat: The Experiences of Some Eating Disordered Childbearing Women and Mothers*. GRiP (Getting Research into Practice) Report. School of Nursing and Midwifery, University of Sheffield, Sheffield.

Stapleton, H., Kirkham, M., Thomas, G. & Curtis, P. (2002) Midwives in the middle: balance and vulnerability. *British Journal of Midwifery*, **10**: 607–611.

Tiggemann, M., Gardiner, M. & Slater, A. (2000) I would rather be a size 10 than have straight As: a focus group study of adolescent girls' wish to be thinner. *Journal of Adolescence*, **23**: 654–659.

Victora, C.G., Barros, F., Lima, R.C., Horta, B.L. & Wells, J. (2003) Anthropometry and body composition of 18 year old men according to duration of breast feeding: birth cohort study from Brazil. *British Medical Journal*, **327**: 901.

Villamor, E. & Cnattingus, S. (2006) Interpregnancy weight change and risk of adverse pregnancy outcomes: a population based study. *Lancet*, **368**: 1164–1170.

Walker, L.O., Sterling, B.S. & Timmerman, G.M. (2005) Retention of pregnancy-related weight in the early postpartum period: implications for women's health services. *Journal of Obstetric, Gynecologic, and Neonatal Nursing*, **34**: 418–427.

Walsh, J.M. & Murphy, D.J. (2007) Weight and pregnancy. *British Medical Journal*, **335**: 169.

Wanless, D. (2004) *Securing Good Health for the Health Population: Final Report*. Department of Health. At: http://www.hm-treasury.gov.uk/consultations_and_legislation/wanless/consult_wanless04_final.cfm (accessed 15 March 2008).

Wiles, R. (1994) I'm not fat, I'm pregnant: the impact of pregnancy on fat women's body image. In: Wilkinson, S. & Kitzinger, C. (eds) *Women and Health. Feminist Perspectives*. Taylor and Francis, London, pp. 33–48.

Willis, P. (1977) *Learning to Labour: How Working Class Kids Get Working Class Jobs*. Saxon House, Farnborough, England.

WHO (2003) *Infant and Young Child Nutrition: Global Strategy on Infant and Young Child Feeding*. WHO: Geneva. At: http://www.who.int/nutrition/publications/gs_infant_feeding_text_eng.pdf (accessed 13 April 2008).

WHO (2008) *Obesity and overweight*. At: http://www.who.int/dietphysicalactivity/publications/facts/obesity/en/ (accessed 13 April 2008).

8 Homeless Mothers and Their Children: Two Generations at Nutritional Risk

Anne Marie Coufopoulos and
Allan Frederick Hackett

8.1 Introduction

The importance of the role of nutrition in the prevention of disease and promotion of health throughout the life course has become increasingly recognised at a global and national level. Evidence strongly suggests that nutrition *in utero* and beyond is significantly correlated, not only with immediate risks, but also with disease risk in later life (Barker 1994; Davey-Smith 2007). The World Health Organization's *Global Strategy on Diet, Physical Activity and Health* (WHO 2004) emphasises the importance of the promotion and protection of health through healthy eating and physical activity. Similarly in England *Choosing a Better Diet: A Food and Health Action Plan* (Department of Health (DH) 2005) identifies redressing inequalities in health as the key priority with children and young people as a specific priority group in terms of improving nutrition. The document makes particular reference to the importance of the nutritional status of the mother in determining the long-term growth and development of her child. Consequently the British government has set out a number of actions to improve nutrition in the early years of a child's life, including improving diet in pregnancy and supporting breastfeeding (particularly among disadvantaged women). These actions reflect the goals of the *Global Strategy for Infant and Young Child Feeding* (WHO 2003) which clearly identifies feeding in exceptionally difficult circumstances as a key priority:

'Families *in* difficult situations *require special attention and practical support to be able to feed their children adequately*'.

WHO (2003, p. 10)

'Children *living in* special circumstances *also require extra attention, for example . . . mothers who are imprisoned or part of disadvantaged or other marginalized groups*'.

WHO (2003, p. 12)

Homeless mothers and their children are one such group that are in a 'difficult situation', living in accommodation that is often unattractive and having to adhere to restrictive rules and regulations during their period of stay. Furthermore the physical space (such as shared cooking and washing facilities) and social space (degree of supervision and privacy) in hostels can vary (Busch-Geertseema & Sahlin 2007), impacting on infant and young child feeding. Despite living in a wealthy industrialised society such as the UK, homeless mothers face considerable challenges. This causes disparity between WHO (2003) recommendations for infant and young child feeding and the practices of homeless mothers. In this respect this chapter focuses on homeless women with dependent children living in hostels. First, we provide an overview of homelessness in the UK and the use of temporary (hostel) accommodation. Second, we explore the structural constraints and psychological issues for women in this situation, drawing on a dietary study of homeless women in England (Coufopoulos 1998) and how these factors conflict with the recommendations of the *Global Strategy* (WHO 2003). Finally we make recommendations for bridging the gap between policy and practice. Policy development (international, national and local) and guidance for improving nutrition in homelessness is needed and must take into consideration the practical living situation and environmental constraints to ensure 'appropriate feeding of infants and young children in exceptionally difficult circumstances' (WHO 2003, p. 2).

8.2 Defining homelessness

There is no consensus in the UK or in Europe on what constitutes homelessness. Recently, a small number of international and European definitions have emerged such as the European Typology on Homelessness and Housing Exclusion (ETHOS) (European Federation of National Organisations Working with the Homeless (FEANTSA) 2007). In any discussion of homelessness it is important to point out that a home is more than simply having a 'roof over one's head', it must also be a place of privacy, safety and comfort. The word 'home' carries a meaning beyond the simple notion of shelter and suggests such images as personal warmth, stability and security. Moreover a 'home' is where social activities and relations take place (Watson 1984), such as feeding infants and young children and consequently if there is no 'home' these activities will be affected.

8.3 Homelessness in the UK and homeless mothers

Homelessness statistics in the UK clearly identify women (either pregnant or with dependent children) as a majority group (Self & Zealey 2007), that is they represent the largest proportion of the homeless population. This is largely a result of the so-called 'priority need' category in the housing legislation (Niner 1999), to whom local authorities in England have a statutory obligation to accommodate. Such groups include pregnant women and those who live with them, and people with dependent children (Office of Public Sector Information Housing/Housing Act 1996). The main reasons women with dependent children become homeless are complex and often the result of a culmination of experiences over a period of time, such as poverty, gendered violence and abuse and a shortage of low-cost housing (Williams 2000). As Calterone Williams (2000, p. 19) points out:

'The process of becoming homeless is often a long one; the causes of a woman's homelessness may have been building for a significant period before she actually has to enter a shelter. Moreover, multiple factors intersect to affect a woman's housing stability, such that it is impossible to find one reason explaining each woman's homelessness.'

The trauma which has often precipitated the loss of a home for a mother and her children (notably domestic violence) and the trauma of losing her home even if there is no violence and being placed in hostel/bed and breakfast accommodation will have far-reaching effects. Indeed Niner (1999) points out that a large number of children and their mothers are likely to have experienced a 'period of acute stress and disruption to family life before they were accepted as homeless' (Niner 1999, p. 107). Consequently this places a mother in a disadvantaged position in which to promote optimum nutrition for herself, her unborn child, or her children. The use of such a paradigm in which to explore the factors that can affect a mother and infant and child feeding is not new. Indeed it is similar to the unique set of experiences described by James (2003), who in her discussion of another marginalised group, refugee pregnant women, points to a 'unique set of experiences' (p. 96) which have affected a pregnant refugee prior to any engagement with healthcare professionals. These may include political repression at home, the traumatic events that resulted in leaving and exile itself (James 2003). Whilst recognising the differences in experience between pregnant refugees and homeless pregnant women/mothers, both often endure a gradual undermining process which can impact on their role as a mother and nurturer.

8.4   The use of temporary accommodation in the UK

There were 82 750 households in England in temporary accommodation at the end of September 2007 (representing a downward trend since 2005) of which 62 830 included dependent children and/or a pregnant woman (Communities and Local Government 2007). Although the majority of these households were in private sector/social landlord accommodation (86%), over 12 000 households (14%) were in accommodation with shared facilities, including hostels, women's refuges, and bed and breakfast accommodation (Communities and Local Government 2007). The length of time that homeless mothers and their children spend in temporary accommodation varies across the UK; from less than six months to up to two or more years (Communities and Local Government 2007). Hence the word 'temporary' does not necessarily mean homeless mothers and their children remaining in such accommodation for short periods of time. Such a period could embrace very significant nutritional physiological changes, for example a complete pregnancy, birth or a substantial period of infant, child and adolescent growth and development.

The hostel environment includes not only the physical structure, layout and facilities within it, but also the rules, regulations, 'gaoler' culture and surveillance that operate. Many homeless hostels have innumerable rules and regulations within which residents have to conform (Friedman 2000). These may include notifying hostel staff when they leave the premises, restricting the sex and/or number of visitors at any one time, or not being allowed to remain off the premises overnight. Such rules and regulations make up 'licence agreements' that are sometimes put forward by local authorities in England as 'maintaining safety'. It could be argued that such agreements erode autonomy thus diminishing self-esteem. In describing family shelters in America, Calterone Williams (2000) refers to curfews and caseworker surveillance that expect women to reveal very personal areas of their lives to staff. As Friedman (2000, p. 57) states:

> 'because of shelter rules and invasive staff practices, many homeless women exhaust other options before turning to a shelter as their last resort'

A range of uncomfortable questions concerning the shelter environment is put forward by Friedman (2000, p. 42) in her account of family shelters in the USA, including how comfortable should family shelters be and would families be tempted to stay longer in shelters that are warm, homely and comfortable? Such questions echo the concept of the 'undeserving poor' (i.e. homeless mothers should be supporting themselves) and the punitive nature of nineteenth-century workhouses.

In summary, women and children make up a considerable part of the homeless population in the UK and there are several pathways to becoming homeless. Temporary accommodation such as hostels may be unattractive and regulatory (even punitive) in their approach and women and children may spend substantial periods of time in them during crucial periods of nutritional and health development.

8.5   Homelessness and the health of mothers

To identify and explore the infant and child feeding practices of homeless mothers it is important to understand the psychosocial context in which homeless mothers live. The *Global Strategy* (WHO 2003) clearly identifies that the health and nutritional status of mother and child are inextricably linked:

> 'Improved infant and young child feeding begins with ensuring the health and nutritional status of women, in their own right, throughout all stages of life and continues with women as providers for their children and families'.
>
> WHO (2003, p. 5)

One of the protective factors against child hunger in low-income housed and homeless female-headed households is the mother's positive health (Wehler *et al*. 2004). Consequently the health of the mother is a major asset for the health and wellbeing of her children. A recent review of UK-based research found maternal depression and infant growth to be associated in mothers/infants experiencing socioeconomic disadvantage (Stewart 2007). Homeless mothers may have an additional risk of experiencing psychosocial problems with potential consequences on the health of their children. In a study of the mental health and health status of homeless mothers in Massachusetts in 1993–2003 (Weinreb *et al*. 2006), mental health deteriorated over time. Homeless households were poorer and female heads of households reported more physical health limitations, emotional distress and mental health disorders in 2003 than 1993. Furthermore there was a fourfold increase in depression rates over the 10-year period. The relationship between the mental health of homeless mothers and infant morbidity among homeless children has yet to be elucidated.

Previous studies have found depression and poor health among homeless women (Conway 1988). Such findings were reflected in research in Dublin, where homeless mothers living in temporary accommodation were often found to be highly stressed, to the point of being clinically significant, while caring for their children (Waldron *et al.* 2001). Whenever government intervention is required to provide for children's basic needs (usually provided by the parent), such as shelter, then a parent loses autonomy (Friedman 2000). Furthermore for women with dependent children, 'homelessness entails more than just the loss of a home; it almost inevitably disrupts the sense of identity and feelings of self-worth and self-efficacy' (Buckner *et al.* 1993, p. 385). Research has also shown that 'women bring their gender responsibilities with them into the homeless situation' (Burt & Cohen 1989, p. 510) and often neglect or compromise their own health needs in order to prioritise their children's needs. The condition of homelessness and the experience of living in temporary accommodation are extremely stressful:

> *'mothers are often depleted by the unrelenting demands of their young children. Many become anxious, guilty and depressed about raising children in such circumstances'*
>
> Bassuk (1993, p. 345)

Consequently the effects of being homeless will undoubtedly affect the psychological sense of wellbeing, which in turn is likely to affect food intake and hence the nutritional status of homeless mothers and their children.

8.6   Nutrition and homeless mothers

The impact on food choice and nutrition of homelessness cannot be separated from the impact of low income. There is a much larger literature on food intake and nutrition in low-income groups that clearly indicates that living on a low income often militates against following a healthy diet (Dobson *et al.* 1994; Dowler *et al.* 2001; Attree 2005; Nelson *et al.* 2007). Despite the studies of low income and diet there has been very little research undertaken in the UK into the nutritional intake of the homeless. Furthermore, no research in the UK has investigated breastfeeding among homeless mothers. Whereas the effects of low income on infant and child feeding are well documented in the UK, including differentials in breastfeeding rates between different socioeconomic groups (Bolling *et al.* 2007), there is neither reference to homeless households in the *National Diet and Nutrition Survey: Children Aged 1^1/$_2$ to 4^1/$_2$ Years* (Gregory *et al.* 1995) nor in the more recent *Low Income Diet and Nutrition Survey* (Nelson *et al.* 2007). Gregory *et al.* (1995) found clear disparities in the food intake of children from low-income households compared with those with higher incomes (for example, a lower consumption of wholegrains, fruit, vegetables and fish). Such differences are echoed in the *National Diet and Nutrition Survey: Young People Aged 4 to 18 Years* (Gregory & Lowe 2000). Findings of this survey showed that young people in households of lower socioeconomic status, particularly boys, had lower intakes of energy, fat and most micronutrients than those in households of higher socioeconomic status.

UK government recommendations on improving the nutrition of pregnant and breastfeeding mothers and children in low-income households (National Institute for Health and Clinical Excellence (NICE) 2008), make no specific reference to homeless mothers, but acknowledge that:

> *'dietary interventions which recognise the specific circumstances facing low-income families . . . or other disadvantaged groups are likely to be more effective than generic interventions'.*

NICE (2008, p. 19)

Although homeless mothers may be included as a 'disadvantaged group', this largely ignores the additional burden of not having a home over and above being on a low income.

The impact of being homeless on the health and nutrition of mothers living in the UK is illustrated by drawing on Coufopoulos' (1998) study. The discussion illuminates the structural constraints and psychological factors that impact on women in this situation and subsequent challenges for child feeding. Coufopoulos (1998) collected three-day estimated food diaries from a purposive sample of 66 homeless mothers living in hostel accommodation in north-west England. Thirty-six food diaries were completed by mothers on behalf of their children, who were aged between 1.5 and 4.5 years. This was the first study to estimate the dietary intake of homeless mothers and their children and compare their intake to government guidelines (Department of Health 1991) and to the intake of the low-income housed population (Gregory *et al.* 1995; Hoare & Henderson 2004). The study also carried out semi-structured, in-depth interviews with 15 homeless mothers to explore the lived experience of homelessness. As Dykes and Hall Moran (2006a, p. 303) suggest:

> *'Biomedical knowledge about maternal and infant nutrition generated through scientific methods is important. However, such knowledge should not be considered as more legitimate than women's embodied knowledge simply because it constitutes "evidenced-based" enquiry. Insights from biomedicine have a place, but their position must be alongside the knowledges generated through the experiences and accounts of women.'*

The dietary findings showed that the women had lower than recommended daily intakes of energy, protein, non-starch polysaccharide (NSP) (fibre), calcium, iron, vitamin C and folate. The mean intake of iron and folate failed to match the lower reference nutrient intake (LRNI) – indicating that some of the population would certainly be at high risk of deficiency (Dowler & Calvert 1995). When the results were compared with women in 'receipt of benefits' (i.e. low income) living in their own homes, from the UK National Diet and Nutrition Survey (Hoare & Henderson 2004), the homeless women had lower intakes of energy, protein, calcium, iron and folate. A group of homeless pregnant women (n = 10), were found to have mean intake of folate of 100 microgram/day (RNI of 300 microgram/day). A large proportion of the homeless comprises women of childbearing age, and their poor intake of folate is of concern as there is strong evidence linking low intakes of folic acid prior to conception with risk of neural tube defects (Department of Health 2000). For pregnant women, their intake and nutritional status will influence the growth and development of the fetus and the child's future health (Gluckman *et al.* 2005). Furthermore an adequate intake of folic acid may have long-term health benefits for mothers, for example a reduction in strokes (Scientific Advisory Committee on Nutrition (SACN) 2006).

Almost half of the women in the study did not regularly eat green vegetables while living in the hostel, with a quarter identifying poor cooking facilities and having to share cookers and pans (40%) as a key barrier. Shared cooking facilities that tended to be 'functional' rather than 'sociable', frequently located several floors away from bedrooms, are often a key feature of hostels. A large number of women (77%) shared kitchen facilities with six or more other families; 39% of the sample shared with 11 or more other families and 56% shared the use of a freezer, of which for 43% of families access was restricted. The consequences of limited/poor facilities also placed greater demands on the food budget:

> *'I can tell you what I've got in my cupboard without looking, tinned hamburgers in gravy, hot dogs, pot noodles. That's all we eat now in here, food that can be cooked in one pan as we have to share pans in here'*
>
> Lone mother, three children

> *'On this floor we are supposed to share a kitchen with only six families, but because the kitchen is locked upstairs all of those families come down here and use this one; so sometimes there can be about 13 families all wanting to use the cookers at the same time and there's only two of them'*
>
> Mother, partner and one child

> *'I find I can't budget my money in here like I could do in my own house, I get my money on a Wednesday and it's nearly all gone by Friday. It's because I'm buying food that I wouldn't usually buy, like convenience foods and biscuits for the kids'*
>
> Lone mother, two children

The quality of the women's food intake was also poor, as many of the women relied on 'snack foods'. For the majority of the women, their own diet, health and wellbeing was not a priority, maintaining that their children's diet and health took precedence:

'Most of the time all I can be bothered to make for myself is a butty [sandwich], because the kitchen is three floors away . . . but I always try and make sure the kids have proper meals, even if I don't feel like eating. I never miss meals for them'

Lone mother, two children

Living conditions in temporary accommodation are sometimes referred to in the literature as being similar those of the workhouses in the nineteenth century; for example Culhane (1996, p. 59) describes workhouses as being 'poorly constructed, crowded, noisy, filthy and foul smelling.' Many of the hostels included in Coufopoulos' study had pungent smells that often penetrated the whole building, deterring women from preparing meals for themselves or their family. Kitchens were sometimes only 'open' at certain times through the day, regulating when food could be prepared. The mothers spoke about the perceived monitoring of their own behaviour as a parent and worried that they were being watched by 'wardens' (a term in common use) in how they looked after their children:

'I feel like I've lost part of myself in here, you don't really have any control over your own life, you even feel like the staff are watching what you feed your children'

Lone mother, three children

Similar findings were echoed in a qualitative study exploring the lived experiences of homeless mothers in the USA, which found that 'some women expressed concerns that their behavior, particularly their parenting behavior, was being judged . . . that they were on guard' (Cosgrove & Flynn 2005, p. 134).

Women interviewed in Coufopoulos' study had to comply with the condition that 'in respect of food and cooking, they will be advised by, and under the supervision of, the warden'. The effects of such an infringement on women, who have previously managed their own homes and had control over their families' health and wellbeing, was associated with both physical and psychological problems. Sixty per cent of the women said they had missed meals since living in the hostel because 'they felt too depressed to eat' and several of the women also said they had lost weight since living in the hostel:

'Since I have been living in here, I have lost a stone, the whole place is so depressing, it gets me down. I don't eat anything some days, I just don't have any appetite. When I'm in here I just stay in my room and stare at the wall. It's like we're being punished.'

Lone mother, five children

'I just don't like eating in here, I know I've lost a lot of weight with all the stress of living in here. A lot of the time my stomach is in knots in here, especially if there is trouble with some of the women, I just stay in my room until the next day; so I just eat what I've got in the room like biscuits or crisps, but sometimes I don't eat anything'

Lone mother, one child

'I haven't eaten anything today, I've just been crying, I've got nowhere to go and I'm stuck in one room with a baby'

Lone mother, one infant

'I just can't cook a meal in here, the smell of the place makes me feel sick, I just make tea and toast in the room. My little girl won't eat in here either so we have to go out for most of our meals . . . I usually don't eat anything though, I couldn't afford for both of us to have something. As long as she eats then I don't mind as much'

Lone mother, one child

'Every morning when I wake up it hits me that I'm in here, I just feel sick, I couldn't face eating'

Lone mother, one infant and two children

The mothers in the study would take their children to fastfood outlets or 'buy them something' in order to compensate for their children having to live in the hostel, thus incurring greater demands upon their budget. Indulging in anything that benefited them was rarely admitted. Thus for homeless mothers the effects of not being able to provide food for their children are twofold: their already diminished self-esteem through being 'homeless' is further undermined by the fact that they are unable to control the types of foodstuff that they or their children eat (or even when they eat it), as a result of poor material circumstances; and their own nutritional and health status is compromised, through poor appetite, prioritising the needs of the children and the loss of motivation to cook and prepare food, thus resulting in low energy and nutrient intakes.

A systematic review of nutrition and health in low-income mothers (Attree 2005) found that lone mothers in poverty (in housed accommodation) were able to exert a greater degree of control over both household finances and their diet than women living with partners. However, this did not appear to be the case for homeless women living in temporary accommodation due to the loss of control and autonomy. When the physical environment and cooking facilities are dismal and unappealing, homeless households are forced to make food choices based upon satisfying a hunger within both financial and environmental constraints; for them the jeopardy is *twofold*.

In Coufopoulos' study women became passive about their own health, as coping with day-to-day survival in the hostel took precedence over focusing upon the future. Such findings have been reflected in an ethnographic study of homeless mothers in America, describing how homeless mothers living in shelters 'redefined instinct' and were on 'automatic pilot' (Connolly 2000, p. 83) in respect of caring for their children:

'In a life that has become chaotic and distressful, motherly activities are performed as lifeless routines, without thought or positive effect'

Connolly (2000, p. 83)

Research focusing on low income, diet and health, demonstrates that women often bear the brunt of poverty and sacrifice their own diet and health needs for the sake of their children (Dowler *et al.* 2001; Attree 2005). Yet for homeless women living in temporary accommodation the burden is even heavier and the sacrifice even greater, in terms of nutritional intake, potentially affecting their long-term health and that of any unborn children (Leather 1997). In addition, for women living in hostels, the frustration of not being able to cook for their family and themselves may further erode their identity of being a mother; thus their ability to nurture their family in terms of providing nutritious meals is weakened. As Thrasher and Mowbray (1995, p. 97) state:

'The absence of a home and residence in a shelter distorts the role of the mother, and thus she loses the opportunity to be primary nurturer, teacher and negotiator.'

In temporary accommodation there is the 'unravelling of the mother role' (Boxhill & Beaty 1990, p. 49); women are prevented from caring for their children as they would like to if they were in their own 'home'. A woman's identity and sense of self is often based on her ability to feed her family (van Esterik 1997), however in temporary accommodation this is commonly denied. The ability for food to act as a medium in which to convey love and affection is denied or distorted for homeless mothers. As Leather (1997, p. 23) states:

'Our feelings around food are clearly capable of engendering profoundly power-ful messages to us about our relationship with ourselves and others we love. It is an important key to self-esteem. So when someone is robbed of the means to provide food for themselves and others in the way they want, it is not just their immediate physical health which is damaged but their general sense of competence and autonomy.'

In summary, the health and nutrition of homeless mothers and their ability to nurture their children through feeding is largely determined by the lived experience of being homeless. As Cosgrove and Flynn (2005) assert, homeless women experience feelings of being humiliated and disrespected and confront 'dehumanizing stereotypes on a daily basis' (p. 135).

8.7 Homelessness and child feeding

Poor micronutrient and antioxidant intakes are the most likely dietary outcome of health inequalities (Davey-Smith & Brunner 1997). The children in Coufopoulos' study were found to have energy dense diets, similar to those in households 'receiving state benefits' (i.e. living in low-income households) (Gregory *et al.* 1995). However the actual quality of their diets was quite different in terms of total fat intake (higher) protein (lower), sodium (higher), calcium (lower) and vitamin C (lower). Homeless children tended to be with their mother most of the day and frequently ate savoury snacks or biscuits, perhaps because of boredom and the lack of play space. Many parents in the study sample stated that their children were bored in the hostel as they had nowhere to play and some of the mothers also believed that the children ate for comfort:

'All he [2-year-old son] seems to eat now is lollipops and crisps because he gets frustrated and bored in here and I feel guilty. When we get our own house he will have proper meals and more of a routine'

Lone mother, one young child

'I spend a lot more money on food in here because my daughter has crisps and snacks and things like that, more than she used to, but I think it's comfort food for her'

Lone mother, one child

A large number of the parents were aware that living in the hostel had affected their children's diet. Half of the sample stated that since living in the hostel their child 'ate more takeaway foods' and 60% of respondents said that the children 'ate more sweets and chocolate'. Parents always endeavoured to provide their children with 'proper meals', often at their own nutritional expense. Many of the parents expressed their concern for maintaining some stability in their children's lives while in temporary accommodation and ensuring that their children 'didn't go hungry', despite their adverse living conditions.

'My little girl won't eat in here so we have to go out to a café nearly everyday, at least that way I know she's eating, because when we first came in here she wouldn't hardly eat anything. I mean a lot of the time I don't have anything to eat when we go out, I can't afford to. When we're settled in our own home I know we'll get back into a routine again and be able to eat proper meals without having to hide from people'.

Lone mother, one child

The first few years of life constitute an important period when a child develops his or her own eating patterns, which may follow into adulthood. Indeed NICE (2008) highlights that this is an opportune time to develop a sound foundation for later life. Eating in a quiet, peaceful atmosphere, at a table with no distractions, helps to focus a child on the importance of meal times as a social occasion. Chaotic eating environments can create stress, thereby reducing children's appetites and opportunities for mealtime learning and social interaction (Albon & Mukherji 2008). Consequently homeless children are at greater risk of developing possibly lifelong eating habits detrimental to health, that is, the frequent consumption of low-nutrient fat-dense snack foods such as crisps and sweets (comfort eating), which may displace more nutritious foods.

8.8   The *Global Strategy for Infant and Child Feeding* and homeless mothers in the UK – bridging the gap between policy and practice

The *Global Strategy for Infant and Young Child Feeding* (WHO 2003) strongly urges the development of guidelines for infant and child feeding in 'exceptionally difficult circumstances' (p. 2). The strategy built on previous work aimed at actively promoting and encouraging breastfeeding (*International Code of Marketing of Breast-milk Substitutes*, WHO (1981) and the *Innocenti Declaration*, WHO (1990)). Central to the *Global Strategy* is the improvement of nutritional status and growth and development through optimal nutrition. However, the strategy also evokes a much stronger sense of urgency and is more ambitious from the outset stating:

'It should go further and emphasise the need for comprehensive national policies on infant and young child feeding, including guidelines on ensuring appropriate feeding of infants and young children in exceptionally difficult circumstances'

WHO (2003, p. 2)

Homeless mothers and their children, as illustrated in this chapter, are a group who are indeed living in *exceptionally difficult circumstances*. The *Global Strategy* sets a gold standard for infant feeding, i.e. 'infants should be exclusively breastfed for the first six months of life to achieve optimal growth, development and health' (WHO 2003, p. 8). However there are striking differences to the extent to which this is achieved in the UK. In 2005, the breastfeeding initiation rate (any breastfeeding) was 88% for mothers in managerial and professional occupations, compared with 65% of mothers in routine and manual occupations (Bolling *et al.* 2007, p. 27). At six weeks, the breastfeeding prevalence was 65% among mothers from managerial and professional occupations, compared with 32% of mothers in routine and manual occupations (Bolling *et al.* 2007, p. 33). The rates of exclusive breastfeeding are substantially lower. Thus the least affluent families, who are already at increased risk from ill health, are further jeopardised by not breastfeeding; this constitutes one aspect of the cycle of nutritional deprivation (Dykes & Hall Moran 2006b).

Homeless mothers are usually from lower socioeconomic households and have the added burden of not having a home. For this group of women, there is a cumulative effect of living in poverty, having no home and the stigma of being homeless and hence the experience of feelings of powerlessness (Walters & East 2001; Meadows-Oliver 2003). It is unlikely in these circumstances that breast feeding would be considered a priority.

There seems to be very little written about the experiences of mothers who become homeless in Europe. There is even less written about the experiences of homeless mothers and breastfeeding, even though most homeless women are of reproductive age (Haber & Toro 2004). A review of studies of interventions improving perinatal outcomes for disadvantaged women of childbearing age found no studies of interventions for homeless women (D'Souza & Garcia 2004). A study which may be relevant to homeless women focused upon supporting mothers to breastfeed in prison. This project provided breastfeeding support workshops for mothers and trained prison officers. The project resulted in an increase in breastfeeding initiation rate from 57% to 78% and an increased length of time of breastfeeding (Farrell cited by Dykes 2003). Moreover the project recognised the influence that breast-feeding can have on mother's feelings about themselves and on the mother–baby relationship. Given the geography of homeless hostels and 'public-mothering' that takes place (Boxhill & Beaty 1990, p. 49), such an approach could be transferable to homeless mothers living in temporary hostel accommodation.

Dykes (2005) identifies peer support programmes as having a significant impact on improving breastfeeding rates and duration in socially excluded communities. Furthermore the role of support from either peers or professionals in improving initiation and continuation of breastfeeding is now well established (Britton et al. 2007). Implementing peer support programmes in hostels may increase breast-feeding initiation and continuation rates and provide a buffer against mental health problems. Peer support groups could have a further effect of providing more general social support to this group of women. Tischler et al. (2007, p. 252) investigating support and social care needs of homeless mothers, found that:

'support from mothers is an important avenue by which the respondents coped with homelessness'

A recent meta-synthesis of barriers to antenatal care for marginalised women (including homeless women) in developed countries found that continuing access to care was influenced by a number of factors. These included the level of trust women had in healthcare providers, caregiver attitudes and fears of what might happen to them or their baby once they accessed 'the system' (Lavender et al. 2007; Downe et al. 2008). Conversely Little et al. (2007) suggested that ongoing support to young homeless pregnant women was crucial to enabling mothers to 'thrive in their new role' and prevent relapse into old coping mechanisms. They also stated that solutions had to be multifaceted and collaborative. Integral to these studies is the establishment of trust and continued support for homeless mothers. This may be quite a challenge to the hostel providers in the UK, where an authoritarian and surveillance approach prevails.

The *Global Strategy* recommendations that, for women and children living in exceptionally difficult circumstances, health workers should have accurate and up-to-date information about infant feeding policies and practices, and the specific knowledge and skills to support caregivers and children in all aspects of infant and young child feeding. This should apply to staff working in hostel accommodation, who could have a key part to play in the health of mothers and children. There is a need for training of staff in the area of nutrition and breastfeeding if they are to pro-vide appropriate and effective support. However this may be difficult to implement as there is often a high turnover of staff and agency staff tend to be employed in hostels. Yet this need should not be underestimated as such staff are often at the frontline of care. A study by Coufopoulos and Lowcock (2004) of hostel staff working with homeless families in Liverpool, UK, found that the perceived ambiguity of staff of their roles and poor interagency working were cited as barriers to quality services. Indeed the health of homeless families was often considered a low priority for staff.

The provision of a dedicated midwifery and health visiting service could be considered in areas where there are high levels of homeless families housed in hostel accommodation. Kirkpatrick et al. (2007) found that intensive home visiting of vulnerable women in pregnancy and during the first years of life, by health visitors trained to work in partnership with families, benefited the women in a number of ways. These included increased confidence, improved mental health, better parenting, improved relationships and changes in their attitudes toward professionals.

8.9   Conclusion

This chapter has provided insight into the experiences of homeless mothers and the factors affecting their own and their children's nutrition. The effects of being homeless and living in temporary accommodation negatively influence the feeding decisions of mothers. The physical conditions of hostels are often not conducive to breastfeeding or providing nutritious food for infants and young children. These conditions are further compounded by a lack of support in terms of nutrition and health. Despite some local authorities in the UK having some measures in place to support homeless families, nutrition and infant feeding has largely failed to receive the attention it deserves in homelessness policy and provision. In contrast guidelines for improving the nutritional status of homeless families living in shelters have been produced in America (Kourgialis et al. 2001). These guidelines include specific recommendations on developing nutrition policies and practices that meet the needs of homeless mothers and could be adopted within the UK.

The Homelessness Act (2002) requires all local authorities in England to publish homelessness strategies every five years by setting out an action plan for preventing and tackling homelessness. These strategies should explicitly address the nutritional needs of homeless mothers and their children and implement the recommendations of the Global Strategy for Infant and Young Child Feeding. However a long-term goal needs to be the eradication of the use of hostel accommodation for homeless mothers and their children. There needs to be the provision of good-quality temporary accommodation that facilitates and supports infant and child feeding.

Finally, there are many research needs in this area. First, research should explore experiences during pregnancy of homeless mothers in terms of antenatal care and their interaction with services. Second, in order to understand further the infant feeding decisions of homeless mothers, more in-depth qualitative research needs to be undertaken to investigate infant feeding decisions of homeless mothers. If effective interventions are to be designed to support infant and child feeding, then they must take account of the sociocultural context in relation to situation-specific determinants. By addressing these factors, the nutritional risk of two generations could be reduced.

References

Albon, D. & Mukherji, P. (2008) *Food and Health in Early Childhood*. Sage, London.

Attree, P. (2005) Low-income mothers, nutrition and health: a systematic review of qualitative evidence. *Maternal and Child Nutrition*, 1: 227–240.

Barker, D.J.P. (1994) *Mothers, Babies and Disease in Later Life*. British Medical Journal, London.

Bassuk, E.L. (1993) Social & economic hardships of homeless & other poor women. *American Journal of Orthopsychiatry*, 63: 340–347.

Bolling, K., Grant, C., Hamlyn, B. & Thornton, A. (2007) *Infant Feeding Survey 2005*. The Information Centre, London.

Boxhill, N. & Beaty, A. (1990) Mother/child interaction among homeless women & their children in a public night shelter in Atlanta, Georgia. In: Boxhill, N. (ed.) *Homeless Children: The Watchers & the Waiters*, pp. 49–64. Haworth Press, New York.

Britton, C., McCormick, F.M., Renfrew, M.J., Wade, A., King, S.E. (2007) Support for breastfeeding mothers. *Cochrane Database of Systematic Reviews*, 24: CD001141.

Buckner, J.C., Bassuk, E.L. & Zima, B.T. (1993) Mental health issues affecting homeless women. *American Journal of Orthopsychiatry*, 63: 385–399.

Burt, M.R. & Cohen, B.E. (1989) Differences among homeless single women, women with children & single men. *Social Problems*, 36: 508–522.

Busch-Geertsema, V. & Sahlin, S. (2007) The role of hostels and temporary accommodation. *European Journal of Homelessness*, 1: 67–93.

Calterone Williams, J. (2000) *A Roof Over My Head*. University Press of Colorado: Colorado.

Communities and Local Government (2007) *Statistical Release: Statutory Homelessness: 3rd quarter, 2007. England*. Communities and Local Government, London.

Connolly, D.R. (2000) *Homeless Mothers Face to Face with Women and Poverty*. University of Minnesota Press, Minneapolis.

Conway, J. (1988) *Prescription for Poor Health*. The Food Commission: London.

Cosgrove, L. & Flynn, C. (2005) Marginalized mothers: parenting without a home. *Analyses of Social Issues and Public Policy*, 5: 127–143.

Coufopoulos, A.M. (1998) *Homelessness, Diet and Health*. Unpublished Ph.D. thesis. Liverpool John Moores University, Liverpool.

Coufopoulos, A. & Lowcock, D. (2004) A homelessness strategy for Liverpool: An agenda for action to improve the health and well-being of homeless families. Proceedings of the 12th Annual Public Health Forum, Brighton, 19–22 April.

Culhane, D.P. (1996) The homeless shelter and the nineteenth century poorhouse: comparing notes from two eras of in-door relief. In: Lykes, B., Banuazizi, A., Liem, R. & Morris, W. (eds) *Myths about the Powerless*. Temple University Press, Philadelphia, pp. 50–71.

Davey-Smith, G. (2007) Life-course approaches to inequalities in adult chronic disease risk. *Proceedings of the Nutrition Society*, 66: 216–236.

Davey-Smith, G. & Brunner, E. (1997) Socio-economic differentials in health: symposium on nutrition & poverty in industrialised countries. *Proceedings of the Nutrition Society*, 56: 75–90.

Department of Health (1991) *Dietary Reference Values for Food Energy and Nutrients for the United Kingdom*. HMSO, London.

Department of Health (2000) *Folic Acid and the Prevention of Disease*. Report on health and social subjects 50. The Stationery Office, London.

Department of Health (2005) *Choosing a Better Diet: A Food and Health Action Plan*. Department of Health, London.

Dobson, B., Beardsworth, A., Keil, T. & Walker, R. (1994) *Diet, choice and poverty: Social, cultural and nutritional aspects of food consumption among low income families*. Family Policy Studies Centre for the Joseph Rowntree Foundation, London.

Dowler, E. & Calvert, C. (1995) *Nutrition and diet in lone-parent families in London*. Family Policy Studies Centre for the Joseph Rowntree Foundation, London.

Dowler, E., Turner, S. & Dobson, B. (2001) *Poverty Bites: Food, Health and Poor Families*. Child Poverty Action Group: London.

Downe, S., Finlayson, K., Walsh, D. & Lavender, T. (2009) 'Weighing up and balancing out': a meta-synthesis of barriers to antenatal care for marginalised women in high-income countries. *BJOG International Journal of Obstetrics and Gynaecology*, **116**: 518–529.

D'Souza, L. & Garcia, J. (2004) Improving services for disadvantaged childbearing women. *Child: Care, Health and Development*, **30**: 599–561.

Dykes, F. (2003) *Infant Feeding Initiative: A Report Evaluating the Breastfeeding Practice Projects 1999–2002*. Department of Health, London.

Dykes, F. (2005) Government funded breastfeeding peer support projects: implications for practice. *Maternal and Child Nutrition*, **1**: 21–31.

Dykes, F. & Hall Moran, V. (2006a) Nutrition and nurture: dualisms and synergies. In: Hall Moran, V. & Dykes, F. (eds) *Maternal and Infant Nutrition and Nurture: Controversies and Challenges*. Quay Books: London, pp. 299–306.

Dykes, F., Hall Moran, V. (2006b) Transmitted nutritional deprivation from mother to child: A socio-biological perspective. In: Hall Moran, V. & Dykes, F. (eds) *Maternal and Infant Nutrition & Nurture: Controversies and Challenges*. Quay Books, London.

FEANTSA (2007) *Child Homelessness in Europe – an Overview of Emerging Trends*. FEANTSA, Brussels.

Friedman, D.G. (2000) *Parenting in Public: Family Shelter and Public Assistance*. Columbia University Press, New York.

Gluckman, P.D., Hanson, M.A. & Pinal, C. (2005) The developmental origins of adult disease. *Maternal and Child Nutrition*, **1**: 130–141.

Gregory, J. & Lowe, S. (2000) *National Diet and Nutrition Survey: Young People Aged 4 to 18 Years, Volume 1. Report of the Diet and Nutrition Survey*. The Stationery Office, London.

Gregory, J., Collins, D., Davies, P., Hughes, J. & Clarke, P. (1995) *National Diet and Nutrition Survey: Children Aged 1$^1/_2$ to 4$^1/_2$ Years: Volume 1*. HMSO, London.

Haber, M. & Toro, P. (2004) Homelessness among families, children and adolescents: an ecological-developmental perspective. *Clinical Child and Family Psychology Review*, **7**: 123–164.

Hoare, J. & Henderson, L. (2004) *The National Diet and Nutrition Survey: Adults Aged 19 to 64 years*. Foods Standards Agency, London.

James, J. (2003) Refugee Women. In: Squire, C. (ed.) *The Social Context of Birth*. Radcliffe Medical Press, Oxford, pp. 93–106.

Kirkpatrick, S., Barlow, J., Stewart-Brown, S. & Davis, H. (2007) Working in partnership: user perceptions of intensive home visiting. *Child Abuse Review*, **16**, 32–46.

Kourgialis, N., Wendel, J., Darby, P., Grant, R., Kroy, W., Pruit, J. *et al.* (2001) *Improving the Nutrition Status of Homeless Children: Guidelines for Homeless Family Shelters*. The Children's Health Fund, New York.

Lavender, T., Downe, S., Finlayson, K. & Walsh, D. (2007) *Access to Antenatal Care: A Systematic Review*. At: http://www.cemach.org.uk/Publications/CEMACH-Publications/Maternal-and-Perinatal-Health.aspx (accessed 28 January 2009).

Leather, S. (1997) Food poverty: the making of modern malnutrition. *Health Visitor*, **70**: 21–24.

Little, M., Gorman, A., Dzendoletas, D. & Moravac, C. (2007) Caring for the most vulnerable. *Nursing for Women's Health*, **11**: 458–466.

Meadows-Oliver, M. (2002) Mothering in public: a meta-synthesis of homeless women with children living in shelters. *Journal for Specialists in Pediatric Nursing*, **8**: 130–136.

National Institute of Clinical Excellence (2008) *Improving the nutrition of pregnant and breast-feeding mothers and children in low-income households*. NICE public health guidance 11. NICE, London.

Nelson, M., Erens, B., Bates, B., Church, S. & Boshier, T. (2007) *Low Income Diet and Nutrition Survey, Volume 1. Background, Methods and Sample Characteristics*. The Stationery Office, London.

Niner, P. (1999) Effects of Changes in Housing Legislation. In: Vostanis, P. & Cumella, S. (eds) *Homeless Children: Problems and Needs*. Jessica Kingsley Publishers, London, pp. 97–111.

Office of Public Sector Information (2007) *Housing Act 1996 Chapter 52*. At: http://www.opsi.gov.uk/acts/acts1996/ukpga_19960052_en_1 (accessed 26 March 2009).

SACN (2006) *Folate and Disease Prevention*. The Stationery Office: London.

Self, A. & Zealey, L. (2007) *Social Trends No.37*. Palgrave Macmillan, Hampshire.

Stewart, R.C. (2007) Maternal depression and infant growth – a review of the recent evidence. *Maternal and Child Nutrition*, **3**: 94–107.

Thrasher, S.P. & Mowbray, C.T. (1995) A strengths perspective: an ethnographic study of homeless women with children. *Health & Social Work*, **20**: 93–101.

Tischler, V., Rademeyer, A. & Vostanis, P. (2007) Mothers experiencing homelessness: mental health, support and social care needs. *Health and Social Care in the Community*, **15**: 246–253.

van Esterik, P. (1997) Women and nurture in industrial societies. *Proceedings of the Nutrition Society*, **56**: 335–343.

Waldron, A.M., Tobin, G. & McQuaid, P. (2001) Mental health status of homeless children and their families. *Irish Journal of Psychiatric Medicine*, **18**: 11–15.

Walters, S. & East, L. (2001) The cycle of homelessness in the lives of young mothers: the diagnostic phase of an action research project. *Journal of Clinical Nursing*, **10**: 171–179.

Watson, S. (1984) Definitions of homelessness: a feminist perspective. *Critical Social Policy*, **4**: 60–73.

Wehler, C., Weinreb, L.F., Huntington, M.A., Scott, R.S., Hosmer, D., Fletcher, K. *et al.* (2004) Risk and protective factors for adult and child hunger among low-income housed and homeless female-headed families. *American Journal of Public Health*, **94**: 109–115.

Weinreb, L.F., Buckner, J.C., Williams, V. & Nicholson, J. (2006) A comparison of the health and mental health status of homeless mothers in Worcester, Mass: 1993 and 2003. *American Journal of Public Health*, **96**: 1444–1448.

WHO (1981) *International Code of Marketing of Breast-milk Substitutes*. WHO, Geneva.

WHO (1990) *Innocenti Declaration*. WHO, Florence, Italy.

WHO (2003) *Global Strategy for Infant and Young Child Feeding*. WHO, Geneva.

WHO (2004) *Global Strategy on Diet Physical Activity and Health*. WHO, Geneva.

9 Lifecycle Influences and Opportunities for Change

Anthony F. Williams

9.1 Introduction

Undernutrition accounts for about a third of all preventable deaths in young children, costing some three million lives each year. Most of these occur in poor countries, primarily in sub-Saharan Africa and South Asia. Deaths represent merely a fraction of the malnourished child population: in some African countries over a half of all young children are stunted and up to one in ten are severely wasted. Similar proportions are observed in South-central Asia. Substantial numbers of children are also deficient in micronutrients, most often zinc, iron, vitamin A and iodine (Black *et al.* 2008). Yet simultaneously many resource-poor countries are witnessing a rapid rise in adult diseases traditionally viewed as those of excess. For example a survey of six cities in India estimated that 12% of adults were diabetic, and 14% showed impaired glucose tolerance. The prevalence of diabetes is rising faster in India than in any other part of the world and it has been predicted that its diabetic population will approximate 57 million by 2025 (Yajnik *et al.* 2003). The economic consequences of such an explosion in morbidity are clear.

This apparent contrast in the fortunes of adults and children may at first seem paradoxical; food shortage seems rife in one sector of the population, yet the consequences of 'overnutrition' are prevalent in another. Effectively there is a 'double burden' of malnutrition (United Nations (UN) Standing Committee on Nutrition 2006). The *Global Strategy for Infant and Young Child Feeding* (World Health Organization (WHO) 2003) recognises in its opening paragraphs the challenges that these observations pose for policy makers. Among children of school age in Pakistan, particularly adolescents, there is an increasing prevalence of overweight and obesity despite the fact that about one in six remain stunted and one in three underweight during the earlier years (Jafar *et al.* 2008). At a societal level poverty is a root cause; in this context it is relevant to observe that the problem is not limited to poor countries. Even in the UK obesity and overweight coexist more commonly in poorer families than wealthier ones (Armstrong *et al.* 2003).

This chapter explores how events at different stages of the lifecycle cumulatively influence the individual's vulnerability to chronic disease. In particular it highlights how undernutrition during the earliest stages of development presages chronic adult illness, particularly cardiovascular disease and metabolic syndrome. It shows how intervening with women, children and young people through implementation of the *Global Strategy* (WHO 2003) can help to break the intergenerational cycle

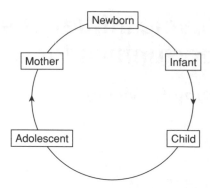

Figure 9.1   The lifecycle: potential stages for intervention. The mother's size, body composition and metabolic competence profoundly influence her physiological response to pregnancy. Intervention during early life through implementation of the WHO's *Global Strategy* offers opportunities for intergenerational change by promoting early growth and development.

(Figure 9.1). While the *Global Strategy* explicitly states that 'mothers and babies form an inseparable biological and social unit' (WHO 2003, p. 3) there is a need to appreciate that making preparation for the future health of a mother's children begins during the earliest phases of her own life, when her potential to grow and develop is greatest. The observation that 'the health and nutrition of one group cannot be divorced from the health and nutrition of the other' (WHO 2003, p. 3) has a longitudinal, intergenerational dimension just as important as a contemporary one.

9.2   Disease risk, genotype and phenotype

Over 40 years ago the geneticist J.V. Neel attempted to explain why the prevalence of diabetes mellitus was rising, 'as more and more people have come to enjoy the blessings of civilization' (Neel 1962, p. 357). He proposed the existence of 'a "thriftiness" genotype which is less of an asset now than in the feast-or-famine days of hunting and gathering cultures' (p. 360), arguing that such a genotype would have favoured survival in food shortage by promoting rapid deposition of body fat in times of plenty. Later he rejected this hypothesis, principally on the grounds that the timescale over which the prevalence of diabetes had increased was too short to be accounted for by evolutionary change at the population level.

Views on the leading role of genotype have been challenged over the past 20 years by the hypothesis that the organism's early environment interacts with genotype in such a way as to 'programme' it; that is, irreversible changes in form or function are induced by exposure to environmental stimuli at a critical stage of development. This 'developmental plasticity' permits variation in environmental conditions to give rise to a range of phenotypes sharing a common genotype. Examples of this phenomenon have been identified throughout the animal kingdom (Bateson *et al.* 2004). In humans, it has been proposed that fetal undernutrition induces lifelong change to metabolic function and body composition, favouring the later development of impaired glucose tolerance and other manifestations of the metabolic syndrome (Hales & Barker 1992). Since first proposed, this 'thrifty phenotype' hypothesis has undergone some conceptual refinement and in its current form proposes that the induction of nutritional phenotype by intrauterine events constitutes a 'predictive adaptive response'. In other words, nutritional signals operating on the fetus at the earliest stages of development 'forecast' the environment in which the offspring will grow and develop and programme the individual adaptively in such a way as to promote health (Bateson *et al.* 2004; Gluckman *et al.* 2005). A corollary is that when mismatch between the fetal and extrauterine environment occurs, 'adaptation' may fail and disease result.

9.3   Low birth weight

In general the hypotheses mentioned above link lower birth weight and smaller size at birth to poorer adult cardiovascular health. The public health importance of 'low birth weight', by definition birth at an attained weight of <2500 g, has been acknowledged for more than half a century. Historically it has had value as a marker of perinatal risk but there is growing appreciation of its contribution both to the pathogenesis of malnutrition in childhood and to adult non-communicable adult disease. Almost 11% of livebirths in developing countries globally are low birth weight at term, up to 30% in southern Asia. Term low birth weight is an acknowledged antecedent of stunting and low childhood weight, accounting together for about 2.1 million deaths annually, or a fifth of all child deaths under 5 years (Black *et al.* 2008).

'Low birth weight' is nevertheless a relatively poor descriptor of phenotype, particularly if the intention is to estimate medium or long-term nutritional risk. A baby may be low in weight either because of preterm birth (<37 weeks) or because weight is relatively low at a given gestational age. The term 'small-for-gestational age' (or 'light-for-dates') has been used to signify the latter but also is not straightforward: first, different birth weight references may be applied; second differing threshold definitions may be applied (for example the 2nd, 3rd or 10th centile); and third infants may arrive at smallness-for-gestation through a number of routes or different fetal growth trajectories. The last consideration has particular relevance to long-term chronic disease outcomes, yet only rarely can the fetal growth trajectory be specified with certainty, even in research studies. Many epidemiological studies have used body proportions (such as Ponderal index, PI) as a proxy for growth restriction at various stages of gestation, equating wasting with late growth restriction and proportionately small size with early growth restriction. Such binary distinction is probably inappropriate: in reality neonatal body proportions are normally, not bimodally, distributed within populations (Kramer *et al.* 1989) and not reliably related to nutrient restriction at particular stages of pregnancy. It must therefore be emphasised that from a nutritional standpoint the relationship between risk and birth weight is not so clear cut. There exists a gradation of risk across the range of weights encountered in the population, rather than a simple binary division into 'low' or 'normal' categories. From the point of view of intervening to improve health in childhood and later life there is a need to explore its broader relationship to birth weight throughout the range encountered in different populations, not merely to focus on reducing the number of individuals in the lower tail of birth weight distribution.

9.4   How strong is the link between birth size and chronic disease?

Despite widespread acceptance of the hypothesis linking birth weight to later health there remains controversy about the effect size. Clearly the length of the human lifespan significantly challenges direct empirical testing; consequently the human evidence is primarily epidemiological. However, it has raised a number of mechanistic hypotheses that have been explored principally in animal studies.

Although evidence of the relationship between birth weight and subsequent (adult) blood pressure has been described as 'substantial' (Leon 1999, p. 1313) estimates of actual effect size have varied markedly between epidemiological studies. A meta-analysis of the literature published to 2000 suggested that the impact of each 1 kg increment in birth weight on adult systolic blood pressure might be as small as -0.6 mmHg (Huxley et al. 2002). Huxley has pointed out that, even if such a major increment in average population birth weight was achievable, such a small reduction in population mean systolic pressure seems unlikely to confer important population health advantage. The yield of other interventions in this area such as reducing population daily salt intake from 9 g to 3 g per day (-06.7 mmHg) or reducing current weight by 2–4 kg (-02 mmHg) seem much greater (Huxley 2004). Similar reservations have been voiced about the inverse association between birthweight and serum cholesterol in adult life (Owen et al. 2003). A number of caveats need to be made about such statements, in relation both to the findings themselves and the conclusions drawn.

A striking finding in the blood pressure meta-analysis referred to above was that effect size varied with the size of study. The explanation proposed was that larger studies are less subject to publication bias. Similar inverse relationships between study size and effect size have also been observed in studies examining the effect of infant feeding on later body mass index (adiposity risk) and likelihood of publication bias has again been cited. However, an alternative explanation may be that the precision with which exposure and outcome are recorded is lower in larger studies involving numerous observers than in smaller ones. Such concerns may be particularly relevant to infant feeding data where lack of information about, for example, the exclusivity of breastfeeding and recollection of infant feeding history pose problems when attempting to define exposure accurately.

Most importantly, however, it is important to understand that demonstration of a small reduction in population mean blood pressure attributable to birth weight does not take into account the very limited value of birth weight as a descriptor of the individual's phenotype. Although birth weight is a readily available epidemiological measure of pregnancy outcome and neonatal risk ('an outcome of convenience') (Wilcox 2001) it has major limitations in explaining any causal relationship between maternal or fetal nutritional exposure and later offspring health outcomes. The fetus is at the end of a long supply line in which maternal body stores, the ability to mobilize these stores, and the preservation of optimal placental function can buffer relatively marked variability in dietary nutrient supply. Animal studies and some human epidemiological data show that nutritional exposures in pregnancy can alter body composition, structure and metabolism without necessarily affecting birth weight (Harding 2001).

The relatively weak effect of birth size on adult disease risk must not, therefore, be construed as an indicator that maternal or fetal nutrient supply is unimportant in the determination of fetal phenotype. The weakness of apparent effect may merely indicate the imprecision of birth weight as an outcome marker of the underlying processes.

9.5 Maternal nutritional influences on nutritional phenotype of the newborn

The nutritional status of a pregnant woman can be described in terms of her nutrient balance, body composition and metabolic capacity (Figure 9.2). Her nutrient balance will be largely determined by dietary intake, the size of her nutrient reserve by her body size and composition, and the availability of nutrients to the fetus by her metabolic competence both to mobilise nutrients from stores and to partition dietary supply between stores and the fetoplacental unit. All may change significantly during adaptation to pregnancy and interact in complex ways to cause variation in offspring phenotype. Pathological processes may also modify the efficacy of the fetal supply line, for example by affecting uterine or fetoplacental perfusion. In this context the growing global prevalence of chronic diseases related to diet and lifestyle (such as essential hypertension and diabetes) will in future compound the threat to successful pregnancy in resource-poor countries.

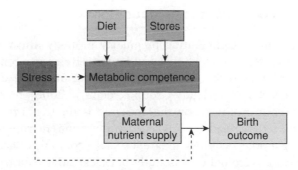

Figure 9.2 Maternal nutritional status in pregnancy. The maternal supply of nutrients to the fetus is regulated by the mother's ability to partition nutrients effectively from her diet and her body stores. Fetal uptake of nutrients to meet demand is governed by the size, early growth and effectiveness of the placenta. Stressors potentially act through the action of corticosteroids directly on the mother's metabolic function or at the interface with the fetoplacental unit. Epigenetic regulation of placental enzymes and fetal receptors has potential to modify the latter.

9.5.1   Maternal nutrient balance

The effect of energy supplementation during pregnancy on birth weight in poorly nourished populations has been generally modest; in one well-designed study conducted in a malnourished population targeted supplementation was associated with a 90–200 g seasonally influenced increase in birth weight at term, without any significant effect on length (Ceesay *et al.* 1997). However a meta-analytic review of balanced protein:energy supplementation of the maternal diet estimated the mean increase in birth weight attributable to dietary supplementation as only 37 g (Kramer & Kakuma 2003).

This finding apparently conflicts with a prevailing assumption about the importance of food supply during pregnancy, and a focus even in industrialised societies on linking to this stage the provision of welfare foods for less privileged sectors of society. Although it is important to recognise that these small changes in birth weight by no means preclude important underlying effects on other aspects of the offspring's phenotype, the disappointingly small average increment in weight needs explanation. One attractive hypothesis is that the fetal growth trajectory is set by the prevailing nutritional environment at a very early stage in pregnancy, before supplementation is commenced. In support of this, animal studies suggest that maternal dietary supply before pregnancy and at the stage of implantation influence placental size and, presumably thereby, the ability of the placenta to extract nutrients from the maternal circulation. In keeping with these observations a high carbohydrate diet in humans seems to be associated with decreased placental size (Godfrey *et al.* 1996), whereas macronutrient restriction around conception and the first trimester during the Dutch wartime famine was associated with a relative increase in placental size, unassociated with alteration in birth weight (Lumey 1998). Emerging evidence about the mechanism of phenotypic induction, in particular the role of micronutrients which affect methylation status of the mother, also suggests that the mother's periconceptional nutritional status is of high importance.

9.5.2   Maternal body size and composition

A mother's height and weight during pregnancy strongly affect the size of her offspring. Data from the WHO Multicentre Growth Reference Study, adopted as the global standard for postnatal growth monitoring of young children (WHO Multicentre Growth Reference Study Group & de Onis 2006), mark the extent of variation between countries and show that the effect is apparent even in pregnancies selected to offer the fetus a relatively privileged intrauterine environment (Table 9.1). Only non-smoking mothers without apparent social, economic or health constraints on fetal growth were recruited to this study but clear inter-country differences in offspring size at birth were very apparent. Differences in the mean birth weight of babies born to shorter mothers in India and Oman versus taller mothers in the USA and Norway approximated 300–400 g; mean infant length differed by approximately 0.5–1 cm. No data on maternal weight were cited.

Table 9.1 Mother's height and offspring size in selected centres from the WHO Multicentre Growth Study (WHO Multicentre Growth Reference Study Group & de Onis 2006)

Country	Mother's height (cm, SD)	Offspring weight (kg, SD)	Offspring length (cm, SD)
Oman	157 (6)	3.2 (0.4)	49.2 (1.7)
India	158 (5)	3.1 (0.4)	49.0 (1.8)
Norway	169 (7)	3.6 (0.5)	50.4 (1.9)
USA	165 (7)	3.6 (0.5)	49.7 (2.0)

The effect of indices of maternal body composition, such as height and mid-pregnancy weight, on birth size is marked even within individual countries. The Aberdeen survey of over 50 000 births between 1948 and 1964 attributed a >650 g difference in birth weight at term to variation in maternal height across the normal range (145–180 cm); when mid-pregnancy weight (range 35–80 kg) was also taken into account this differential increased to 1 kg (Thomson *et al.* 1968).

In most industrialised countries over the past 20 years there has been a secular trend to increasing birth weight, the pace of which suggests that it is likely to be more attributable to rising maternal weight than height. An opposing trend has been observed in Japan where a 40-year trend to declining body mass index (BMI), reflecting the cosmetic concerns of younger women, has been associated with a significant rise in the proportion of low birth weight babies born (Ohmi *et al.* 2001).

9.5.3   Maternal metabolic competence

A pregnant woman must also partition effectively the nutrient supply between her current dietary supply and body stores. This is a reflection of her metabolic capacity to sustain and support pregnancy. The nature of this process, the extent of variability and its consequences are clearly important but human experimental observations are very few. A small human study of protein turnover in mid-pregnancy and early third trimester showed that the fall in maternal amino acid oxidation at this stage accounted for 34% of the variance in birth weight, with heavier babies being born to mothers who showed the greatest fall (Duggleby & Jackson 2002). Similarly 25% of the variability in birth length was accountable to the rate of protein synthesis in mid-trimester. Yet, as might perhaps be expected in the context of a study conducted in the UK, no significant relationship between dietary protein intake and birth size was observed.

9.5.4   The mother's lifecycle and her offspring's birth weight

Box 9.1 lists maternal characteristics linked to offspring birth weight. As observed above, mothers who are taller and heavier have larger babies; thus the origins of

Box 9.1   Maternal characteristics affecting birthweight

- Own birthweight
- Age at menarche
- Current age
- Pre-pregnancy weight and height
- Pregnancy interval
- Parity
- Weight gain in pregnancy
- Ethnicity

offspring health potentially lie in the mother's own early years, particularly before two years of age when her growth potential is greatest.

These influences even antedate the mother's own birth. Infant birth weight is correlated with the mother's own birth weight, and with that of other female relatives. Analysis of human pedigrees shows that offspring birth weight is graded according to whether the mother herself was born relatively small, normal or relatively large in weight (Ounsted & Ounsted 1968). The mechanism that explains this is unlikely to be wholly genetic, since correlation with maternal birth weight is much stronger than with paternal birth weight (Coutinho *et al.* 1997). Indeed Ounsted *et al.* concluded in 1986 from their extensive analysis (re-published in 2008) that 'The set point of the constraining mechanism is adjusted *in utero* in female fetuses'. They further hypothesised that 'such a process would be adaptive, facilitating fairly fast changes in fetal growth rate as the conditions under which a population lives deteriorate or improve' (Ounsted *et al.* 2008, p. 245).

Whether, and if so how, maternal diet might play a part in setting the constraining mechanism remains to be understood, yet influences may be very subtle. For example, mothers in the second and third trimester subjected to undernutrition during the Dutch hunger winter showed a reduction in their own birth weight, yet this did not seem later to affect the birth weight of their offspring. The birth weight of babies born to women subjected to famine during the first trimester was not reduced (perhaps as the result of placental adaptation, see above). On the other hand the later offspring of the female babies among this group were of lower than expected birth weight and failed to show the normal increment in size associated with parity (Lumey & Stein 1997). These data are again consistent with a hypothesis that the phenotype, enabling a mother to fuel her fetus, is induced in very early pregnancy, perhaps through mechanisms which are considered below. They further illustrate the point made earlier that an individual's (in this case the mother's) nutritional phenotype can be altered in important ways – with intergenerational consequences – without evident effect on birth weight.

The importance of optimising the mother's nutrient supply around the time of her own conception and during the early childhood years has been stressed. It is equally important that later in her lifecycle the mother is able to complete her own growth before pregnancy occurs. It is well established that low birth weight is more common among teenage mothers, and that the mean birth weight of infants born to younger mothers is lower than that of women in their 20s or early 30s. Although this could partially be explained by a complex mix of social factors including poverty, smoking, drug and alcohol abuse, biological factors also operate. A study of American pregnant teenagers examined how mothers who are still growing themselves partition nutrients between themselves and their fetuses (Scholl *et al.* 1994). The mothers' pregnancy weight gain was acceptable during the last trimester but growing mothers continued to deposit upper body subcutaneous fat at a faster rate than non-growing controls of similar age. This was associated with a reduction in the weight of their offspring. Thus there was evidence of competition between the mother's own demands for nutrients to complete growth, and the concurrent needs of her fetus.

9.5.5   Relevance to interventions

A baby's nutritional phenotype at birth, indicated primarily by relative size, bears a much stronger relationship to the mother's physical characteristics (size, body composition and metabolic competence) than her diet in mid- or late pregnancy. The physical characteristics which equip a mother to balance effectively her own metabolic needs with those of her fetus are a consequence of her early childhood nutritional exposure, probably her exposure even in early fetal life. These observations challenge the long-standing practice of focusing dietary intervention in mid- or late-gestation. It is likely that early life interventions, including those around the time of the mother's own conception (which take account of powerful inter-generational influences) would offer greater health dividends. Interventions aimed at optimising her growth and development in early postnatal life, such as those set out in the *Global Strategy*, are therefore key.

9.6   Putative mechanism of phenotypic induction

Given the likelihood that the earliest nutritional exposures may exert the strongest influences it is useful to explore mechanisms. An understanding of these biological processes could yield insight both into both the specific nature of nutritional exposure and periods of peak susceptibility. A number have been envisaged as relevant. These include changes in the allocation of stem cell lineage, differential tissue mitotic rate during growth, variations in tissue apoptosis and altered gene expression. There is increasing interest in how nutrients might bring about the last through epigenetic change. It is the realisation that epigenetic change induced during a critical period of early development may exert lifelong consequences by propagation through the altered cell's progeny that is important (Waterland & Jirtle 2004; Burdge *et al.* 2007). The methylation of cytosine phosphate guanine dinucleotides (CpG; CpG islets) is of particular interest in this context because the methylation cycle may be prone to disturbance through disruption in the supply of methyl donors (such as choline, betaine and methionine), or intermediaries in methylation pathways such as folic acid, pyridoxine, vitamin B_{12} and riboflavin. The dietary supply of betaine, choline, folic acid and vitamin B_{12} in the Agouti mouse modifies the expression of coat colour through changing expression of the A^{vy} gene at a critical stage of hair follicle development (Wolff *et al.* 1998).

The induction of hypertension in the offspring of rats given a low protein diet during pregnancy can be similarly explained. There is evidence in rats and in sheep that the expression of both placental 11-β hydroxysteroid dehydrogenase and the fetal hepatic glucocorticoid receptor (Lillycrop *et al.* 2005) can be altered by dietary protein restriction during pregnancy. Similarly maternal nutrient restriction in sheep also reduces the placental expression of 11-β hydroxysteroid dehydrogenase in mid-gestation placenta and increases expression of the glucocorticoid receptor in liver and other tissues. Such changes offer a mechanism whereby both the placental transfer of maternal glucocorticoid to the fetus may be increased (reduced inactivation by placental 11-β hydroxysteroid dehydrogenase) and its effect on fetal tissue potentiated by enhanced receptor expression. Particularly interesting is the observation that folic acid supplementation in the pregnant rat reverses the changes in expression of glucocorticoid receptor brought about by a low protein diet (Lillycrop *et al.* 2005).

These and other changes in the metabolism of the offspring have implications for the response to postnatal diet and fasting. A number of key components of fuel homeostatic pathways are now known to be susceptible to epigenetic change. These include the peripheral peroxisomal activator receptor (PPAR) α and γ, acyl coA carboxylase, fatty acid synthase, glucokinase and phospho enol pyruvate carboxykinase (PEPCK). Protein restriction in the maternal diet of rats induces change in both the postnatal growth pattern and metabolic response of the offspring to fasting. These changes are modifiable by the dam's folic acid intake during pregnancy, and by the fat content of the post-weaning diet (Burdge *et al.* 2008).

Such experiments have a number of potential implications for intervention to improve the nutritional status of pregnant mothers. First, it should be noted that the process of demethylation and *de novo* remethylation of the fetal genome appears to occur just after fertilisation and before implantation. Thus, it is the micronutrient status of the mother *at conception* which might be most relevant. This accords with earlier remarks about the importance of the mother's nutritional status before conception and during early pregnancy in establishing the fetal growth trajectory. The *Global Strategy* makes particular mention of the importance of engagement with reproductive health and maternity services in order to increase access to antenatal care and promote good nutrition for pregnant women (WHO 2003, pp. 16–17). However it seems likely to be important also to disseminate this message among teenage girls and young women. Second, the observation that steps involved in regulation of the materno–fetal corticosteroid axis are sensitive to maternal nutrient supply opens the possibility that maternal nutritional status could determine the mother's response to mental or physical stress during pregnancy. For example low micronutrient status and stress of physical labour could act synergistically, the first amplifying the effect of the second. In this connection the *Global Strategy* importantly makes specific reference to the obligations of employers, trade unions and national governments to protect mothers' maternity entitlement. Third, animal evidence may help to explain why the apparent effects of macronutrient supplementation vary between populations. Just as micronutrient (folate) status altered the response to protein restriction in rats, it could affect the response to food supplements in human pregnancy. Of interest in this context is the observation that birth weight amongst a poorly nourished Indian population correlated positively with intake of green leafy vegetables and biochemical folate status of the mother (Rao *et al.* 2001). Dietary balance, particularly in relation to micronutrient intake, may be more important than the absolute amount of supplement provided. In this context there are further questions about the relative efficacy of pharmaceutical supplements and food in providing an adequate micronutrient supply, and the stage of pregnancy at which supplementation should be exhibited (Nestel & Jackson 2008). The *Global Strategy* alludes to the importance of 'access to suitable – including fortified – local foods, and when necessary micronutrient supplements' (WHO 2003, p. 17) specifically in relation to promoting adequate complementary feeding. However, there is a strong case for increasing the availability of such foods at a national level to widen access to all population groups, not merely young children. Such an approach offers a synergistic approach to improving the nutritional status of the young child by improving the nutritional status of the mother prior to conception and through pregnancy, thereby increasing nutrient reserves of the offspring at birth.

9.7 Nutritional status of the child: impact of early growth

The phenotype of the newborn, expressed in terms of body composition and metabolic capacity, alters with the normal processes of growth and development in a way that is also likely be modifiable by postnatal diet. This poses further key questions about the feasible extent of modification, the optimal timing and nature of dietary interventions, and potential for exacerbating rather than reducing risk of disease in later life. The pattern of early change in infant weight is complex: similar changes in infant weight may conceal differences in the type of tissue deposited, causing variation in body composition, metabolic competence and health. Understanding these changes requires recognition of the interaction between intrauterine nutritional exposure, timing of birth (term or preterm), phenotype at birth, genetic endowment and postnatal nutritional exposure.

International acceptance of the WHO growth standards, as captured in the *Global Strategy*, represents a clear consensus that the optimal pattern of postnatal growth is that shown by infants breastfed exclusively in the first half of infancy having been born to mothers who have experienced an uncomplicated and complete pregnancy without economic or social constraint. There is considerable evidence that such babies are less likely to experience ill health in the short term. Evidence from meta-analytic reviews also suggests that babies breastfed are at reduced risk of adiposity, expressed as BMI, in later life (Arenz *et al.* 2004; Owen *et al.* 2005). Infant feeding data in individual studies were of variable quality particularly in relation to the exclusivity and duration of breastfeeding; this is unfortunately a common feature of epidemiological studies relating early feeding outcomes to health in later childhood or adult life. Concern about the growing prevalence of obesity in the UK (among many industrialised countries) has nevertheless proved a key driver to implementation of the growth standards and of other measures which will implement the protection, promotion and support of breastfeeding: three synergistic policy areas identified by the *Global Strategy*.

Individual patterns of growth in infancy vary greatly. By and large infants who are born small grow relatively rapidly in early life, and infants who are born large grow more slowly. This tendency reflects both the statistical phenomenon of regression to the mean and the biological phenomenon of compensatory growth or 'canalisation' – identification of the infant's genetically determined trajectory when removed from the intrauterine environment. This creates a methodological difficulty with attribution of long-term consequence to patterns of early growth: the pattern of early growth is confounded by relative birth weight. Studies which adjust outcomes for current (adult) size effectively may simply be capturing this phenomenon (Lucas *et al.* 1999).

An associated issue is our current lack of understanding of factors that determine variation in the types of tissue deposited by babies showing different growth patterns. Studies have explored relationships between infant weight gain and later BMI (Stettler *et al.* 2002, 2003, 2005), or long term outcome (Barker *et al.* 1989) yet knowing the quality (or type of) of tissue deposited could be more informative than the quantity (amount measured by weight), whether or not weight is adjusted for length or height (i.e. BMI). This aspect of early infant development has not been widely explored, perhaps due to methodological limitations of body composition measurement in young infants and children. Although BMI is often used as a proxy for adiposity, it is not a precise reflection of fat mass across the normal range encountered. This can vary as much as twofold within children of the same BMI, age and gender (Wells 2000).

A small longitudinal study (n = 51) of small-for-gestational age infants (mean weight 2.1 kg at 39 weeks' gestation) and controls of appropriate weight for gestation (mean birth weight 3.3 kg at 39 weeks) illustrates well the importance of this point. Despite highly significant differences in birth weight, postnatal weight catch-up in the small-for-gestational age group resulted in both groups showing similar BMI and body weight at 2, 3 and 4 years of age. More detailed studies of body composition (dual energy x-ray densitometry) nevertheless revealed very different patterns of fat deposition. Small-for-gestational age infants were more likely to show central adiposity and showed a lower lean mass at 4 years of age, the amount of total and abdominal fat correlating more strongly with weight gain in the first two years than later. In keeping with these differences in the distribution and relative amount of body fat, the small-for-gestational age infants showed significantly lower plasma insulin growth factor-1 concentration in the early years, and greater fasting insulin concentrations at 4 years, indicative of relative insulin resistance (Ibanez *et al.* 2006).

A retrospective study conducted among older men also supports the proposition that changes during fetal life and the early years have lifelong influences on body composition. Amongst Hertfordshire men who were born with a weight in the bottom quartile (mean 2.76 kg) or top quartile (mean 4.23 kg) those in the lower birth weight group had relatively higher fat mass and lower muscle-fat ratio even in their seventh decade. For men of equivalent adult BMI, the relative amount of body fat was higher among men from the lower birth weight group (Kensara *et al.* 2005).

It is therefore crucial when considering compensatory growth not merely to consider the amount of tissue deposited but its type and distribution. It is likely that the latter has greater bearing upon metabolic capacity, disease risk and (in the context of this chapter) a girl's later metabolic competence to fuel fetal growth. These observations emphasise the limitations of body mass index as an indicator of body composition, despite its widespread application in large epidemiological studies. Although at the population level it may indicate adiposity *risk*, at the individual level it is not necessarily a precise indicator either of the amount or distribution of fat.

From the point of view of promoting growth optimal for later health, important questions relate to the timing of intervention and to the qualities of diet that might be important in promoting compensatory growth of the lean tissue compartment at the expense of fat. In relation to timing there is particular controversy. A large systematic review suggested that high weight or rapid weight gain in infancy are important precursors of later obesity (Baird *et al.* 2005), but two reservations need to be expressed about this conclusion. First, 'obesity' was defined in almost all studies using anthropometric criteria (BMI or W/H) and thus did not necessarily measure adiposity, which as we have observed is likely to more closely equate to disease risk. Studies that have correlated metabolic or disease outcomes – such as coronary events in Finnish men and women (Barker *et al.* 2005) or glucose tolerance in young Indian men and women (Bhargava *et al.* 2004) – have instead associated risk with a pattern of early (or infant) underweight and thinness followed by upwards crossing of BMI centiles after the age of 2. Second, almost all the studies included in the systematic review (Baird *et al.* 2005) were conducted in developed countries, most of which would have exhibited low prevalence of breastfeeding and little exclusive breastfeeding during the first six months. The few available studies to quantify accurately body fat suggest that this may be important. Early infant weight or BMI gain in poorer countries seems to be associated with deposition of lean tissue rather than fat, in contrast with the situation in industrialised countries where fat deposition seems more common (Wells *et al.* 2007). Among formula-fed infants weight gain in the early weeks could well be an important precursor of later adiposity (Stettler *et al.* 2005), but it is important not to generalise such a conclusion to breastfed infants; breastfed infants grow more quickly in the first few months of life than those formula fed, yet are of lower weight and BMI towards the end of infancy. These differences in the tempo of infant ponderal growth are potentially relevant to later body composition, and by implication metabolic risk. Indeed this is the implicit justification underlying adoption of the WHO multicentre growth standard in the UK (Scientific Advisory Committee on Nutrition 2007). The *Global Strategy* also alludes to importance of international application for the new growth standard (WHO 2003, p. 13).

Studies of *preterm* infants randomly allocated to diets of very divergent nutrient density (banked donor breast milk (DBM) or preterm formula (PF)) have also shown that relatively brief differences in early nutrient exposure have longlasting effects. The linear and ponderal growth of these infants was very different during the first few weeks of life yet no differences were apparent in any anthropometric parameter at school age (mean 7.5 years) (Morley & Lucas 2000). Despite physical catch-up the DBM group showed reduced cardiovascular risk profile in terms of blood pressure (Singhal *et al.* 2001), glucose tolerance (Singhal *et al.* 2003) and lipo-protein profile (Singhal *et al.* 2004) as adolescents. These studies show that, at least in preterm infants, longlasting metabolic effects may be attributable to relatively brief differences (over a few weeks in the neonatal unit) in early life nutritional exposure. Their relevance to term infants, including those who have suffered intrauterine growth restriction, needs qualification. The body composition of preterm infants at birth is very different to that of term infants, raising the possibility that growth of the adipose organ could be disrupted by premature birth (Wells *et al.* 2007). This hypothesis is supported by the observation that children who were prematurely born have a reduced fat mass but not a reduced lean mass when both are adjusted for current body size (Fewtrell *et al.* 2004).

In the case of low birth weight infants born at term, the period of complementary feeding, extending through the second half of infancy and into the second year of life, is likely to be crucial to the promotion of lean tissue growth. Low iron and zinc intake is prevalent at this age, and deficiency of either may limit lean tissue growth. The importance of promoting a nutritionally adequate, micronutrient-rich weaning diet in this context is widely accepted and emphasised at several points in the *Global Strategy*. It makes specific reference to the importance of education, the provision of food supplements (including fortified foods and micronutrient supplements), and the appropriate treatment of severe malnutrition using therapeutic foods. All have been shown to increase height-for-age z-score (Bhutta *et al.* 2008). Controversy remains about the routine use of iron supplements in iron-replete individuals, however. They have been associated with a reduction in both ponderal and linear growth in some studies (Idradjinata *et al.* 1994; Dewey *et al.* 2002; Lind *et al.* 2008). Pre-school children in malarial areas receiving iron supplements were also at increased risk of death (Sazawal *et al.* 2006).

9.8 Conclusion

This chapter has examined the complex intergenerational relationships between a mother's nutritional status, the phenotype of her newborn, the nutritional status of her young child and his or her later health. There is strengthening evidence that the current epidemic of adult non-communicable disease has its roots in the earliest years of life, and that nutrient supply through the continuum from conception to the pre-school years is a key determinant. Much discussion has focused on the link between birth weight, particularly low birth weight, and later adult disease. Yet birth weight is not a causal determinant in this process; it is merely a marker, and probably a relatively weak one. Experimental animal evidence shows that nutrient restriction in fetal life can bring about important changes in form and function, without necessarily affecting size at birth. Similarly the human offspring's body composition and metabolic competence may be stronger determinants of later outcome than birth weight.

Understanding how early life experience and diet determines later body composition and metabolic competence has special relevance for girl children and women because it may later influence their nutritional response to pregnancy. Achieving a pattern of body composition and metabolic competence that will best support long-term outcome of their offspring – 'optimising' fetal development – requires additional understanding of how these factors determine fetal nutrient supply, and when in pregnancy interventions might achieve most effect. Although historically much effort has been directed at interventions delivered during mid or late gestation (particularly food or micronutrient supplementation), there is a growing realisation that the mother's nutritional status around the time of conception exerts strong effects.

These considerations help to place the *Global Strategy* in a lifecycle context. Promoting growth during the early years of childhood when the potential rate is greatest presents an opportunity for lifelong health dividend, not just for the individual but for her offspring too. Preventing intrauterine growth restriction and preterm delivery, promoting exclusive breastfeeding, and supporting timely, adequate and safe dietary diversification after the first six months are complementary strategies which together can achieve intergenerational change. On the other hand the prevention of excessive adipose growth during the pre-school years is also of fundamental importance. Achieving a balance in feeding of the infant and young child that successfully steers this course will require much greater understanding of how the newborn's nutritional phenotype, set before birth, determines the variation in response to postnatal diet with respect to the rate, type and amount of tissue deposited.

References

Arenz, S., Ruckerl, R., Koletzko, B. & von Kries, R. (2004) Breast-feeding and childhood obesity – a systematic review. *International Journal of Obesity and Related Metabolic Disorders*, 28: 1247–1256.

Armstrong, J., Dorosty, A.R., Reilly, J.J., Child Health Information Team & Emmett, P.M. (2003) Coexistence of social inequalities in undernutrition and obesity in preschool children: population based cross sectional study. *Archives of Disease in Childhood*, 88: 671–675.

Baird, J., Fisher, D., Lucas, P., Kleijnen, J., Roberts, H. & Law, C. (2005) Being big or growing fast: systematic review of size and growth in infancy and later obesity. *British Medical Journal*, 331: 929–931.

Barker, D.J., Winter, P.D., Osmond, C., Margetts, B. & Simmonds, S.J. (1989) Weight in infancy and death from ischaemic heart disease. *Lancet*, 2: 577–580.

Barker, D.J., Osmond, C., Forsen, T.J., Kajantie, E. & Eriksson, J.G. (2005) Trajectories of growth among children who have coronary events as adults. *New England Journal of Medicine*, 353: 1802–1809.

Bateson, P., Barker, D., Clutton-Brock, T., Deb, D., D'Udine, B., Foley, R.A., *et al.* (2004) Developmental plasticity and human health. *Nature*, 430: 419–421.

Bhargava, S.K., Sachdev, H.S., Fall, C.H.D., Osmond, C., Lakshmy, R., Barker, D.J.P., *et al.* (2004) Relation of serial changes in childhood body-mass index to impaired glucose tolerance in young adulthood. *New England Journal of Medicine*, 350: 865–875.

Bhutta, Z.A., Ahmed, T., Black, R.E., Cousens, S., Dewey, K., Giugliani, E., *et al.* (2008) What works? Interventions for maternal and child undernutrition and survival. *Lancet*, 371: 417–440.

Black, R.E., Allen, L.H., Bhutta, Z.A., Caulfield, L.E., de Onis, M., Ezzati, M., *et al.* (2008) Maternal and child undernutrition: global and regional exposures and health consequences. *Lancet*, 371: 243–260.

Burdge, G.C., Hanson, M.A., Slater-Jefferies, J.L. & Lillycrop, K.A. (2007) Epigenetic regulation of transcription: a mechanism for inducing variations in phenotype (fetal programming) by differences in nutrition during early life? *British Journal of Nutrition*, 97: 1036–1046.

Burdge, G.C., Lillycrop, K.A., Jackson, A.A., Gluckman, P.D. & Hanson, M.A. (2008) The nature of the growth pattern and of the metabolic response to fasting in the rat are dependent upon the dietary protein and folic acid intakes of their pregnant dams and post-weaning fat consumption. *British Journal of Nutrition*, 99: 540–549.

Ceesay, S.M., Prentice, A.M., Cole, T.J., Foord, F., Weaver, L.T., Poskitt, E.M., *et al.* (1997) Effects on birth weight and perinatal mortality of maternal dietary supplements in rural Gambia: 5 year randomised controlled trial. *British Medical Journal*, 315: 786–790. (Erratum appears in *British Medical Journal* (1997), 315: 1141.)

Coutinho, R., David, R.J. & Collins, J.W.Jr. (1997) Relation of parental birth weights to infant birth weight among African Americans and whites in Illinois: a transgenerational study. *American Journal of Epidemiology*, 146: 804–809.

Dewey, K.G., Domellof, M., Cohen, R.J., Landa, R.L., Hernell, O. & Lonnerdal, B. (2002) Iron supplementation affects growth and morbidity of breast-fed infants: results of a randomized trial in Sweden and Honduras. *Journal of Nutrition*, 132: 3249–3255.

Duggleby, S.L. & Jackson, A.A. (2002) Higher weight at birth is related to decreased maternal amino acid oxidation during pregnancy. *American Journal of Clinical Nutrition*, 76: 852–857.

Fewtrell, M.S., Lucas, A., Cole, T.J. & Wells, J.C. (2004) Prematurity and reduced body fatness at 8–12 y of age. *American Journal of Clinical Nutrition*, 80: 436–440.

Gluckman, P.D., Hanson, M.A. & Pinal, C. (2005) The developmental origins of adult disease. *Maternal and Child Nutrition*, 1: 130–141.

Godfrey, K., Robinson, S., Barker, D., Osmond, C. & Cox, V. (1996) Maternal nutrition in early and late pregnancy in relation to placental and fetal growth. *British Medical Journal*, 312: 410.

Hales, C.N. & Barker, D.J. (1992) Type 2 (non-insulin-dependent) diabetes mellitus: the thrifty phenotype hypothesis. *Diabetologia*, 35: 595–601.

Harding, J.E. (2001) The nutritional basis of the fetal origins of adult disease. *International Journal of Epidemiology*, 30: 15–23.

Huxley, R. (2004) Early life origins of adult disease: is there really an association between birthweight and current disease risk? In: Langley-Evans, S.C. (ed). *Fetal Nutrition and Adult Disease*. CABI Publishing, Oxford, UK, pp. 105–128.

Huxley, R., Neil, A. & Collins, R. (2002) Unravelling the fetal origins hypothesis: is there really an inverse association between birthweight and subsequent blood pressure? *Lancet*, 360: 659–665.

Ibanez, L., Ong, K., Dunger, D.B. & de Zegher, F. (2006) Early development of adiposity and insulin resistance after catch-up weight gain in small-for-gestational-age children. *Journal of Clinical Endocrinology and Metabolism*, 91: 2153–2158.

Idradjinata, P., Watkins, W.E. & Pollitt, E. (1994) Adverse effects of iron supplementation on weight gain of iron-replete young children. *Lancet*, 343: 1252–1254.

Jafar, T.H., Qadri, Z., Islam, M., Hatcher, J., Bhutta, Z.A. & Chaturvedi, N. (2008) Rise in childhood obesity with persistently high rates of undernutrition among urban school-aged Indo-Asian children. *Archives of Disease in Childhood*, 93: 373–378.

Kensara, O.A., Wootton, S.A., Phillips, D.I., Patel, M., Jackson, A.A. & Elia, M. (2005) Fetal programming of body composition: relationship between birthweight and body composition using DXA and anthropometry in older Englishmen. *American Journal of Clinical Nutrition*, 82: 980–987.

Kramer, M.S. & Kakuma, R. (2003) Energy and protein intake in pregnancy. *Cochrane Database of Systematic Reviews*, (4): CD000032.

Kramer, M.S., McLean, F.H., Olivier, M., Willis, D.M. & Usher, R.H. (1989) Body proportionality and head and length 'sparing' in growth-retarded neonates: a critical reappraisal. *Pediatrics*, **84**: 717–723.

Leon, D.A. (1999) Twins and fetal programming of blood pressure. Questioning the role of genes and maternal nutrition. *British Medical Journal*, **319**: 1313–1314.

Lillycrop, K.A., Phillips, E.S., Jackson, A.A., Hanson, M.A. & Burdge, G.C. (2005) Dietary protein restriction of pregnant rats induces and folic acid supplementation prevents epigenetic modification of hepatic gene expression in the offspring. *Journal of Nutrition*, **135**: 1382–1386.

Lind, T., Seswandhana, R., Persson, L.A. & Lonnerdal, B. (2008) Iron supplementation of iron-replete Indonesian infants is associated with reduced weight-for-age. *Acta Paediatrica*, **97**: 770–775.

Lucas, A., Fewtrell, M.S. & Cole, T.J. (1999) Fetal origins of adult disease – the hypothesis revisited. *British Medical Journal*, **319**: 245–249.

Lumey, L.H. (1998) Compensatory placental growth after restricted maternal nutrition in early pregnancy. *Placenta*, **19**: 105–111.

Lumey, L.H. & Stein, A.D. (1997) Offspring birth weights after maternal intrauterine undernutrition: a comparison within sibships. *American Journal of Epidemiology*, **146**: 810–819.

Morley, R. & Lucas, A. (2000) Randomised diet in the neonatal period and growth performance until 7.5–8 y of age in preterm children. *American Journal of Clinical Nutrition*, **71**: 822–828.

Neel, J.V. (1962) Diabetes mellitus: a 'thrifty' genotype rendered detrimental by 'progress'? *American Journal of Human Genetics*, **14**: 353–362.

Nestel, P.S. & Jackson, A.A. (2008) The impact of maternal micronutrient supplementation on early neonatal morbidity. *Archives of Disease in Childhood*, **93**: 647–649.

Ohmi, H., Hirooka, K., Hata, A. & Mochizuki, Y. (2001) Recent trend of increase in proportion of low birthweight infants in Japan. *International Journal of Epidemiology*, **30**: 1269–1271.

Ounsted, M. & Ounsted, C. (1968) Rate of intra-uterine growth. *Nature*, **220**: 599–600.

Ounsted, M., Scott, A. & Ounsted, C. (2008) Transmission through the female line of a mechanism constraining human fetal growth. *International Journal of Epidemiology*, **37**: 245–250.

Owen, C.G., Whincup, P.H., Odoki, K., Gilg, J.A. & Cook, D.G. (2003) Birth weight and blood cholesterol level: a study in adolescents and systematic review. *Pediatrics*, **111**: 1081–1089.

Owen, C.G., Martin, R.M., Whincup, P.H., Smith, G.D. & Cook, D.G. (2005) Effect of infant feeding on the risk of obesity across the life course: a quantitative review of published evidence. *Pediatrics*, **115**: 1367–1377.

Rao, S., Yajnik, C.S., Kanade, A., Fall, C.H., Margetts, B.M., Jackson, A.A., *et al.* (2001) Intake of micronutrient-rich foods in rural Indian mothers is associated with the size of their babies at birth: Pune Maternal Nutrition Study. *Journal of Nutrition*, **131**: 1217–1224.

Sazawal, S., Black, R.E., Ramsan, M., Chwaya, H.M., Stoltzfus, R.J., Dutta, A., *et al.* (2006) Effects of routine prophylactic supplementation with iron and folic acid on admission to hospital and mortality in preschool children in a high malaria transmission setting: community-based, randomised, placebo-controlled trial. *Lancet*, **367**: 133–143.

Scholl, T.O., Hediger, M.L., Schall, J.I., Khoo, C.S. & Fischer, R.L. (1994) Maternal growth during pregnancy and the competition for nutrients. *American Journal of Clinical Nutrition*, **60**: 183–188.

Scientific Advisory Committee on Nutrition (2007) *Application of WHO Growth Standards in the UK*. The Stationery Office, London.

Singhal, A., Cole, T.J. & Lucas, A. (2001) Early nutrition in preterm infants and later blood pressure: two cohorts after randomised trials. *Lancet*, **357**: 413–419.

Singhal, A., Fewtrell, M., Cole, T.J. & Lucas, A. (2003) Low nutrient intake and early growth for later insulin resistance in adolescents born preterm. *Lancet*, **361**: 1089–1097.

Singhal, A., Cole, T.J., Fewtrell, M. & Lucas, A. (2004) Breastmilk feeding and lipoprotein profile in adolescents born preterm: follow-up of a prospective randomised study. *Lancet*, **363**: 1589–1597.

Stettler, N., Zemel, B.S., Kumanyika, S. & Stallings, V.A. (2002) Infant weight gain and childhood overweight status in a multicenter cohort study. *Pediatrics*, **109**: 194–199.

Stettler, N., Kumanyika, S.K., Katz, S.H., Zemel, B.S. & Stallings, V.A. (2003) Rapid weight gain during infancy and obesity in young adulthood in a cohort of African Americans. *American Journal of Clinical Nutrition*, 77: 1374–1378.

Stettler, N., Stallings, V.A., Troxel, A.B., Zhao, J., Schinnar, R., *et al.* (2005) Weight gain in the first week of life and overweight in adulthood: a cohort study of European American subjects fed infant formula. *Circulation*, 111: 1897–1903.

Thomson, A.M., Billewicz, W.Z. & Hytten, F.E. (1968) The assessment of fetal growth. *Journal of Obstetrics and Gynaecology of the British Commonwealth*, 75: 903–916.

UN Standing Committee on Nutrition (2006) *Double Burden of Malnutrition – a Common Agenda*. UN, Geneva.

Waterland, R.A. & Jirtle, R.L. (2004) Early nutrition, epigenetic changes at transposons and imprinted genes, and enhanced susceptibility to adult chronic diseases. *Nutrition*, 20: 63–68.

Wells, J.C. (2000) A Hattori chart analysis of body mass index in infants and children. *International Journal of Obesity & Related Metabolic Disorders*, 24: 325–329.

Wells, J.C.K., Chomtho, S. & Fewtrell, M.S. (2007) Programming of body composition by early growth and nutrition. *Proceedings of the Nutrition Society*, 66: 412–422.

WHO (2003) *Global Strategy for Infant and Young Child Feeding*. WHO, Geneva.

WHO Multicentre Growth Reference Study Group & de Onis, M. (2006) Enrolment and baseline characteristics in the WHO Multicentre Growth Reference Study. *Acta Paediatrica*, Suppl 450: 7–16.

Wilcox, A.J. (2001) On the importance – and the unimportance – of birthweight. *International Journal of Epidemiology*, 30: 1233–1241.

Wolff, G.L., Kodell, R.L., Moore, S.R. & Cooney, C.A. (1998) Maternal epigenetics and methyl supplements affect agouti gene expression in Avy/a mice. *FASEB Journal: Official Publication of the Federation of American Societies for Experimental Biology*, 12: 949–957.

Yajnik, C.S., Fall, C.H., Coyaji, K.J., Hirve, S.S., Rao, S., Barker, D.J., *et al.* (2003) Neonatal anthropometry: the thin-fat Indian baby. The Pune Maternal Nutrition Study. *International Journal of Obesity and Related Metabolic Disorders*, 27: 173–180.

10 Use of Economics to Analyse Policies to Promote Breastfeeding

Kevin D. Frick

10.1 Introduction

The introduction to the *Global Strategy for Infant and Young Child Feeding* (WHO 2003) states that two principles guided the development of the *Global Strategy*. The first principle was that it 'should be grounded on the best available scientific and epidemiological evidence' (p. 2). The second principle was that 'it should be as participatory as possible' (p. 2). No one would deny that these are laudable principles to follow when developing guidelines for a topic as important as infant and young child feeding.

One aspect noticeably missing from the guiding principles is economic consideration. Economic considerations include:

- The budgetary feasibility of initiating a strategy
- The budgetary feasibility of sustaining a strategy
- Any incentives over which policy makers have control that can be used to enhance the likelihood that providers, mothers, families and employers will support the behaviours that are implied by the recommendations for infant feeding
- The cost-effectiveness of the set of policies and interventions that flow from the strategic recommendations.

Integrating these considerations into the process of making strategic recommendations could lead to more realistic recommendations for strategies to promote infant and young child nutrition within a broader societal public health context. The considerations reflect the most basic notion within economics, i.e. that all decision makers ultimately face trade-offs when they are making resource allocation decisions.

10.2 Economic considerations

10.2.1 Budgetary feasibility

An example of budgetary feasibility may be illustrated by the situation in which any government or private for-profit or not-for-profit agency or organisation that is responsible for promoting infant and young child nutrition may not have resources available to dedicate to a new strategy. To consider a new strategy, an old strategy to achieve the same objective may need to be set aside, another objective may need to be set aside, or additional resources may need to be procured. Obtaining additional resources will require taxpayers or donors to make trade-offs when they are required to or make a choice to provide more resources to the government or not-for-profit organisation.

10.2.2   Sustaining a strategy

Government and not-for-profit organisation decision makers understand that the resources necessary to initiate a strategy may be considerably different from the resources that are necessary to sustain a strategy over time. An example of this type of difference is the difference between paying for the change in infrastructure needed to begin implementing a strategy and paying for the recurring costs once the infrastructure is in place. While the costs of building the infrastructure are likely to be higher than the one year recurrent costs, this does not change the fact that the recurrent costs will need to be supported year after year while the infrastructure costs essentially be paid once.

10.2.3   Incentives

Any new policy brings changes in the economics of the decisions that mothers, fathers, families in general, and the remainder of the society make about infant and young child nutrition. The economics of decisions refer to the incentives that individuals, families and society face when making decisions about how to provide nutrition for infants and young children. In other words: how much money is required, how much time is required, what else could be done with the time and money that are being used to provide infant and young child nutrition, and how much the mother, father, the remainder of the family and the remainder of the society value the wellbeing of infants and young children.

10.2.4   Cost-effectiveness

The final consideration is the economics of policy making. Government and private policy makers have a number of criteria for making policy – many of which are political rather than economic and may seem to defy logic. However, economics will usually play at least some role in the decision-making process. For infant and young child nutrition, policy makers will need to compare the money being spent on an intervention with the changes in infant and young child nutrition, health and development that are brought about by the intervention. Decision makers must determine whether the value of the results of the resource reallocation to change the incentives to provide different types of infant nutrition is sufficient to warrant the spending; the value is determined by the behavioural, health and developmental changes that result from the new resource allocation.

The remainder of this chapter has the following objectives: to provide definitions of economic terminology with examples relevant to infant nutrition; to outline an economic framework for the general evaluation of policy related to infant and young child nutrition; and to apply the outlined framework to the *Global Strategy* to improve infant and young child nutrition.

10.3   Economic terminology

10.3.1   What is economics?

Economics can be defined simply as the study of how individuals, organisations and governments make decisions about the allocation of scarce resources. Readers who are familiar with economic concepts will recognise the phrasing above because nearly every economics textbook begins with a similar phrase. Readers who are unfamiliar with economic concepts should understand that referring to resources as 'scarce' is almost redundant because all resources are scarce. In some cases that scarcity is more apparent than in others. Each person has only 24 hours available in a day to dedicate to earning income, improving health and improving their children's health. Even the richest person has only a finite amount of money to spend on goods that they and their children will consume and goods that are particularly intended to improve health and nutrition. The world has a finite amount of arable land; thus there is a finite amount of food to provide nutrition for all the members of society.

10.3.2   Individual objective optimisation

Given the limits on resources, individuals must ascertain what satisfies their desires in life and make decisions about how to spend their money, how to use the goods they already possess, and how to spend their time in order to maximise their satisfaction. Individuals live within families that require joint decision making which incorporates compromises made among the individuals in a family who may have different priorities. With respect to nutrition, people make a decision as to how to use their time and money to obtain nutrition for themselves and for their children. More money can be spent on purchasing prepared food, or more time can be spent on preparing one's own food. Time and money can be spent on healthier or less healthy foods to achieve the number of calories a person desires per day with the foods that a person enjoys. Individuals may be willing to spend time and money obtaining and preparing more healthy foods for which they prefer the flavour less in order to obtain health benefits. However, not all individuals will make these choices and they are ultimately choices rather than something that can be legislated.

10.3.3   Government and organisation objective optimisation

Individual decision making is sometimes easier to conceptualise than organisational or government decision making. Individual decision making is inherently variable because individuals have their own ideas about what maximises their happiness. In contrast, organisations and governments are expected to follow objectives set by social norms or mandates. A government or organisation must define or identify its objectives (e.g. private firms are expected to seek to maximise profits and a not-for-profit health facility may seek to maximise the health of a population in a catchment area it serves), find ways to procure resources, and find ways to use the resources to achieve the maximum amount of the objective that it can. A key link between individual and organisational behaviour is that economics supposes that individuals, governments and organisations all use resources to maximise their objectives.

10.3.4   Economics is about more than spending the least amount of money

There is a general impression that economics focuses only on monetary costs – particularly on minimising such costs. While economists are interested in cost minimisation, this term must be used with an understanding of a nuance in its interpretation. Specifically, the economic paradigm implies that what society produces should be produced at the minimum possible cost. In other words, the production of goods and services should be technically efficient. However, economics does not unambiguously imply that costs should be minimised when limiting costs results in producing less output. Taken to an extreme, costs of providing nutrition are minimised when no nutrition is provided, but that would be an extremely negative outcome. Economics could focus instead on how to produce and distribute sufficient caloric content for all children and adults in the world population.

With respect to infant and young child nutrition specifically, cost minimisation does not imply that society should spend the least possible on infant nutrition. Rather cost minimisation with respect to infant and young child nutrition suggests that if there are multiple interventions that can be used to achieve excellent nutrition for all children, the least expensive method should be chosen. Further, if there are multiple options for improving infant nutrition and they do not all achieve the same outcome, the alternatives should be compared based on the following criterion: if an intervention achieves better nutrition at a higher price, is the higher price worth while? If society finds that improving infant nutrition has a very high value and that such improvements can occur at a relatively low cost, then an economist would suggest that society should allocate more resources to efforts to improve infant nutrition. When determining the cost of nutrition it should include both the cost of goods used to produce nutrition, the time used to produce nutrition, and the cost of risks associated with various ways of providing nutrition. This may lead to different conclusions about the breastfeeding/formula feeding mix in different cases.

10.3.5   Economics for health policy is similar to economics in our daily lives

Sometimes economic considerations are overlooked because individuals find it at least somewhat distasteful to have to decide whether health benefits are valued at a level that is greater than what must be spent to achieve them. While individuals may find this distasteful or difficult for healthcare, each person makes decisions about whether certain items are worth the resources required in daily life. Is a person willing to pay the price for a dozen eggs or a litre of milk? Alternatively, for the person who would certainly purchase the eggs or milk, is it worth spending the extra money to buy an organic product?

Although these are not 'life and death' decisions, the logic of economic decision making can be extended to other individual decisions that are more directly about life and death in ways similar to infant and young child nutrition. For example, each person must decide whether to lead an active or sedentary lifestyle. This decision must be balanced against family, professional and community responsibilities. There is a cliché about a person not having enough hours in the day to do everything he or she would like. Sometimes, exercise does not fit into a person's schedule despite the fact that they know that their health would improve if they were more active. That person has inherently placed a value on their health. The value may be monetary if by not exercising a person spends more time working; some individuals may find this to be necessary to have sufficient income to purchase food to provide nutrition for themselves and their children. These decisions also may limit a person's choices about how to provide nutrition for an infant or child. These examples demonstrate that people make health related decisions guided by economics in their everyday life and that this concept should be acceptable to apply to health policy decisions for society. Complexities arise from having to make decisions in a society with heterogeneous preferences for different outcomes and the distributions of those outcomes. Even the concept that those who are most disadvantaged within society should be the primary focus of the help that can be provided by a government is not a universally agreed upon proposition.

10.3.6 Economic policy evaluation methods and tools

An economist performing a policy evaluation of a new infant and young child nutrition programme would:

- Identify the resources that are needed to implement the intervention
- Place a monetary value on all those resources
- Assess the changes in infant nutrition and ultimately infant and later life health that would result from the new intervention
- Place a value (monetary or otherwise) on the outcomes
- Compare the costs with the benefits to determine whether the value of the monetary benefits is larger or to determine whether the improvements in health are worth what must be spent to achieve them.

Economists sometimes assign a dollar value to the benefits of health interventions. This can be easy in the case of medical care expenses that are avoided because of fewer infections that a breastfed child is likely to experience. On the other hand, it is difficult to value improved child development. An analysis in which monetary values are assigned to all benefits is referred to as a *cost-benefit analysis*. In a purely economic sense, no policy for which the value of the costs exceeds the value of the benefits should be adopted.

In some cases economists will use non-monetised clinical, quality of life or length of life outcomes in their analyses of whether spending more money for more health is worth the cost. This type of analysis is referred to as a *cost-effectiveness analysis*. For infant nutrition, if an intervention could increase the exclusive breastfeeding duration of many women to the recommended 6 months, a policy maker will need to decide how much it is worth spending for each 1% increase in the proportion of women who breastfeed to the target duration.

Another economic evaluation tool critical for infant nutrition and breastfeeding is *cost-consequence analysis*. This type of analysis simply describes the costs and the benefits. In many ways, this is little more than a list of pros (the benefits) and cons (the extra costs). This type of study is important when it is difficult to devise a summary measure for the effects of an intervention or health outcome. Because breastfeeding has multiple effects on the child and mother that are difficult to summarise in a single measure, providing a description of how much money is spent on an intervention to encourage breastfeeding and juxtaposing it with a list of the increase in breastfeeding duration, decrease in infections, improvements in development, decrease in the risk of early childhood obesity for the children, decrease in time to return to pre-pregnancy weight for the mother, and decreased risk of breast cancer for the mother would be one way to present a cost consequence analysis related to breastfeeding.

A final economic tool related to infant nutrition and breastfeeding is a *cost of illness study*. Cost of illness studies describe the lifetime costs associated with a condition. If improved breastfeeding relative to other means of providing infant nutrition can reduce the risk of chronic conditions for the children and their mothers, then cost of illness studies can help analysts to understand the value of improved breastfeeding and this value can be compared with the costs of achieving improved breastfeeding.

10.4 Economic framework for assessing infant and young child nutrition and feeding strategies

The definitions above can be used to formulate a framework for assessing infant and young child nutrition strategies – particularly for assessing when a government should not leave decisions to individuals and organisations in a private market. This section will review: the degree of economic urgency for infant and child nutrition interventions; the justification for infant and young child nutrition being a high priority for the use of public resources; the unit of analysis for economic evaluation; the evidence that would be useful to support any proposed programme; and the incentives to develop political commitment to obtain the resources necessary to implement a strategy.

10.4.1   Degree of urgency

Even without reviewing all the recommendations made in the *Global Strategy* to promote infant and young child nutrition, those who developed the strategy clearly consider that there is a high degree of urgency associated with this topic. An economist would assign a high degree of urgency to government intervention when the market is said to experience 'market failure'. The following is not a comprehensive list of potential market failures, but is a list of market failures related to infant and young child nutrition generally and to breastfeeding specifically: production involving a relatively high fixed cost but a low marginal cost; a small number of producers of non-breast milk infant nutrition options; information that is understood by some but not all; and effects of an intervention or behaviour that affect individuals other than those who are directly involved in the transaction.

10.4.1.1   Production of health with high fixed costs

Breastfeeding itself is part of a process of 'producing child health'. This process involves a variety of start-up costs that may be perceived as relatively high compared with formula feeding such as nursing clothes, learning about breastfeeding, and overcoming family and society objections (Chatterji & Frick 2005). Breastfeeding also includes marginal costs that may be considered as relatively low compared with formula feeding, i.e. the ease of feeding any time, anywhere with no preparation or storage. Economists model decision making as a process of comparing marginal costs and marginal benefits, or the costs and benefits of more breastfeeding. The initiation costs are not generally part of the decision model. A government or not-for-profit organisation may be interested in providing incentives to overcome high start-up costs so that mothers and families can focus on the marginal decisions when deciding on whether to invest in the initiation of breastfeeding.

10.4.1.2   Limited non-breast milk alternative producers

The market for infant and young child nutrition is also characterised by a limited number of major producers of formula. The resulting market can be referred to as monopolistic competition rather than perfect competition. A market characterised by perfect competition would result in a uniformly nutritious formula product being manufactured at a minimum cost and sold to consumers at a similar cost regardless of the manufacturer. A monopolistically competitive market yields much different results. Formula manufacturers use substantial resources to differentiate themselves from other manufacturers (marketing) and compete on quality rather than competing only on price. As a result, the market does not operate efficiently, producing goods at a minimum cost. The value of product differentiation leading to many formula alternatives available for mothers who do not breastfeed is not clear.

10.4.1.3 Poor information

The benefits and costs of different types of infant nutrition production are not necessarily understood by all adults who need to provide nutrition for infants and young children. Markets can only operate efficiently if everyone has the same information and understands that information. Thus, the government may find it necessary to provide information, either through public service announcements or through other types of educational and behavioural change campaigns, to ensure that individuals are making decisions about nutrition for infants with full information.

10.4.1.4 Externalities

A final market failure is the inability to realise the effects of one's behaviour on others' wellbeing. The most obvious case of this issue with respect to breastfeeding is the mother making a decision on how to provide nutrition that affects her child. The mother and child are often seen as an inseparable biological and social unit, as is pointed out in the *Global Strategy*. The perception is that a mother will take full account of how her actions will affect her child and take only actions that will maximise the benefits to her child. However, mothers must balance their own needs, the needs of other children and family members, and the needs of a new infant when making infant nutrition decisions so that the decision may not always be to the benefit the new infant. Finally, there may be other factors, for example pressure from significant others.

A second obvious example of some individual/organisational choices that affect others is employers' policies about the maximum amount of time that a mother may be absent from work or provision of opportunities and space for expressing breast milk while in the workplace (Galtry 2003). The policies and allocation of time and space does not affect only the employer and employees but also affects other members of the families of the employees. The government can provide incentives for employers to take actions that favour employees who are trying to provide optimum nutrition for infants and young children. There are several counter-arguments to this as some employers would find it difficult to provide time off or the space to express breast milk with privacy and the space to store expressed breast milk and the cost to the business would be very high. Society would need to decide when the cost to businesses would be too high to mandate this type of change. Alternatively, employers may find that providing women with the opportunity to express breast milk privately and store the expressed milk will produce happier employees and healthier children so that employees are more productive and need to miss less work. Governments would need to determine which of these alternatives holds and decide when it would be acceptable to counsel and suggest rather than to mandate. A third example is institutional (hospital) policy and healthcare practices that encourage or fail to support breastfeeding. Again, this affects not just the provider and a single mother but the provider and a combination of individuals.

All of these market failures suggest that a government may take some interest in providing incentives for or mandating behaviours that facilitate breastfeeding. These are further supported by the magnitude of the cost of illness and burden of diseases that affect infants and young children who are undernourished. Malnutrition leads to a series of specific conditions that can affect long-term development and even lead to mortality.

10.4.2   Justifying intervention

The results of cost-benefit, cost-effectiveness, and cost-consequence analyses can be used to justify interventions to reallocate resources. In markets (particularly healthcare markets) that fail to operate in an economically efficient manner, it is often simple to justify interventions. However, even when markets operate inefficiently and result in a high burden of disease, economic evaluation is still useful. Policy analysts and policy makers must determine how using resources to change the market for infant and young child nutrition ranks in comparison with other potential health-related and non-health related uses of the resources to benefit society.

Governments and not-for-profit organisations in many countries have many demands for their resources. Another important realisation is that unless breastfeeding is mandated or formula is made available only by prescription, an economist would still argue that the ultimate choice of how to provide nutrition for an infant or young child is ultimately best left to the mother and family who have to consider the many uses of money and time that a family faces. The *Global Strategy* document suggests that infants fed with formula be treated as a risk group for policy analysis; this is only likely to be accepted in more developed economies if a study of formula-fed children shows that they are sufficiently at risk to justify any expenditure of resources.

There are a number of ways in which governments and not-for-profit organisations can attempt to change the market failures in the market for infant and young child nutrition and limit the burden of disease associated with poor results for the children in this market. When making policy or recommendations the government must provide evidence of the need for change, must clearly state its objectives and must justify the importance of these objectives. Policy is often made with very little attention to the economic considerations of the actual magnitude of the problem or burden of the disease expressed in monetary terms or a clear realisation of a comparison of the costs and the benefits of an intervention.

10.4.3   Unit of analysis

When formulating an objective related to infant and young child nutrition and justifying its inclusion as an item high on the list of uses of public resources, a government or not-for-profit organisation must consider the appropriate unit of analysis and perspective for the analysis. The perspective of an analysis defines the boundaries of the analysis, in other words whose costs and whose benefits matter to the decision maker. Some governments may see their own bottom line as the ultimate perspective for decision making. This is less likely to lead to a high priority being placed on the intervention than if a so-called societal perspective is used. When conducting an analysis from a societal perspective, all costs and all benefits to everyone affected by a market over the lifetime of the individuals affected by the policy should be considered. This is the perspective recommended by economic theory (Gold *et al.* 1996; Tan-Torres Edejer *et al.* 2003). It does not necessarily guarantee that there will not be economic winners and losers associated with a policy related to infant and young child nutrition, but it does ensure a greater consideration of a wider set of the benefits (and costs) associated with this market. The government may consider applying a new policy to all individuals or applying a policy to only individuals and families who are at high risk for malnutrition. This reflects not only a consideration of whether to focus on the government or society but also on whether to focus only on all families with infants and young children, only high risk individuals with infants and young children, or all of society. A key result when considering all members of society is that there are real costs to some members of society that must be considered in addition to realising the benefits to the infants and their families. Ultimately, a mother's perspective must be considered as the mothers are the individuals who must make a choice to breastfeed.

10.4.4   Evidence

Health policy making is influenced by epidemiological data and may be influenced by economic data. For epidemiological data, particularly when there are new interventions or treatments, there are specific and well-defined criteria that charac-terise the quality of evidence. Some studies are stronger than others and this can be characterised in ways that are understood by researchers and policy makers. The same is not true in economic evaluation, although there are many sets of standards in existence (Tarn & Dix Smith 2004).

10.4.5   Political coalitions

Finally, as noted above, even policies that result in a benefit for society as a whole are likely to lead to benefits for some members of society and costs for others. Thus, any policy that is developed will likely require a process of building a political coali-tion. Those making recommendations about infant and young child nutrition must then consider whether specific advocates for infant nutrition have the resources and an incentive to build coalitions to bring about change. This is an additional use of resources that may ultimately benefit society but that clearly represents a true cost to society in the short-term.

10.5   Economic analysis of global breastfeeding strategy

The description of economics and the economic framework that have been dis-cussed can now be used to analyse the specific recommendations in the *Global Strategy for Infant and Young Child Feeding*. In some cases, consideration is given to very specific elements of what has been recommended. In other cases, the general approach of the document will be the focus of the analysis.

The *Global Strategy* document mentions renewing a commitment to promoting infant and young child health and nutrition. Those considering the economic arguments for promoting breastfeeding for infant and young child nutrition must realise that there are many aspects of infant and young child health that extend beyond nutrition and that assuring child health is just part of the overall goal of assuring the general health of society. Resources must be divided among all these needs. As the epidemiological situation in a country changes, the usefulness and cost of promoting breastfeeding relative to other methods of improving infant and young child nutrition and health may change. There are excellent reasons to consider it appropriate to provide all women everywhere with the opportunity to undertake the natural and child health producing activity of breastfeeding. However, the economics of health in a country result in a trade-off between the promotion of breastfeeding and the promotion of other child health producing activities. In addition, the *Global Strategy* document gives consideration to children with the most difficult situations; for some infants, providing breast milk may be very difficult and a society may ultimately decide to use relatively scarce resources in another way.

The *Global Strategy* document describes malnutrition and the associated morbidity and mortality in a way that paints an appropriately bleak picture of the results of infants and young children having insufficient or inappropriate nutrition. This should be sufficient to draw attention to the problem of malnutrition. However, the description is presented in only epidemiological terms. While decision makers are interested in this type of data, the same decision makers are faced with a large variety of claims on the resources that they have at their disposal and a large variety of claims for new resources that must be procured. Advocates for dealing with many other conditions can present summary measures such as the economic cost per year of all the problems associated with a particular condition or the lifetime costs of all that is lost in a year because of a condition, or the number of disability-adjusted life years associated with a condition. The *Global Strategy* document mentions the need for resources and at least indirectly addresses the need to consider the incentives that different parties face for taking actions that are suggested by the strategy. However, the *Global Strategy* document does not provide any summary measure of what treating malnutrition is likely to cost per year, or the lifetime productivity loss of all incident cases of malnutrition in a year, or the disability-adjusted life years associated with the malnutrition and its effects on morbidity and mortality. In addition to having information on the current burden of disease to draw attention to the problem, the ultimate economic evaluation will require evidence regarding the change in burden that might be brought about by a new intervention. This will require even more information about the cost and effectiveness of interventions in addition to providing data on the costs related to the conditions themselves.

The ultimate objective of the *Global Strategy* document is identified at many points within the document. The ultimate objective could be summarised as a programme aimed at the entire family to ensure appropriate feeding practices to maximise the probability of appropriate infant and young child development; the expected result is the maximisation of the opportunity for positive economic outcomes for the individual, the family, and the society. This is a clear objective, although it focuses only on infant and young child nutrition as an input into the child's, family's and society's wellbeing rather than noting that infant and young child nutrition is just one input into infant and young child health and development that contribute to the wellbeing of the individual, family and society. Other inputs and the resources needed for the entire set of inputs must be considered relative to one another when choosing how to advocate for and to implement new policies.

We can use the stated aim to suggest the type of economic evaluation that would be useful to conduct to make decisions about resource allocation related to infant and young child nutrition. One statement of the aim is to improve nutritional status. In this case, a key question is how to compare the nutritional status of the population achieved by different potential interventions. Any economic evaluation would need to compare the costs of alternative strategies for improving nutritional status and compare the value of the gains with the cost of the different strategies. While this would suggest a more traditional type of cost-effectiveness analysis rather than a cost-minimisation analysis (asking which alternative achieves a goal at the lowest cost), there is an important constraint on the decision-making process that must be acknowledged. The *Global Strategy* refers to the optimal nutrition for each child. This does not allow for a trade-off between perhaps having somewhat less than optimal nutrition at the individual level but being able to help more children, or achieving only optimal nutrition for those for whom nutrition is improved but possibly being able to help fewer children. Paragraph seven in the document lists specific objectives that could be used as the 'pros' in a cost-consequence analysis (WHO 2003, pp. 6–7).

The *Global Strategy* document provides a clear description of specific roles for specific parties among all those who might influence whether a strategy is likely to succeed. Although the *Global Strategy* document does not claim that it should be implemented at any cost with no recognition of the trade-offs that result, it does suggest optimising nutrition for children without mentioning how much it will cost. If infant and young child nutrition is viewed as a right within society, then the only relevant economic question is 'what is the least costly way to satisfy that right'? However, a complete analysis of the question would have to ask whether enforcing a right to infant nutrition would, in some way, impinge on other rights of other citizens and how to rank one right relative to another.

One type of intervention that the *Global Strategy* document mentions is the provision of appropriate information for individuals to use in their decision-making process. Economists treat information as a resource that shapes decisions that are being made. Individuals with more complete and more accurate information are better able to decide how to efficiently allocate resources to achieve their objectives. Information is always important as long as the ultimate decision on feeding practices is going to be left to the mother and her family and not dictated. The likelihood that individuals will make decisions that are consistent with the decisions that infant nutrition experts consider to be the most appropriate will increase if individuals have information that is similar to that which the experts have and in a format that is understandable.

The many links in the process from promoting breastfeeding and better infant and young child nutrition to better health, development and economic outcomes need to be considered. First, poor infant nutrition can lead to costs for an economic system through the loss of lives and reduced morbidity that would potentially help an economy to develop. Second, on average, more developed economies have lower rates of infant malnutrition. However, the *Global Strategy* document does not spell out whether poor infant and young child nutrition is a cause of limited development or an effect of limited development. The argument is presented that a decrease in infant malnutrition will contribute to development. Notably, even if all infants in a country avoid malnutrition it does not guarantee development. This fact again draws attention to the need to examine a comprehensive set of activities and alternatives that play a role in infant and young child nutrition, health and development as they contribute to economic development rather than focusing only on infant and young child nutrition. A government must decide whether its objective is only to maximise infant and young child nutrition or whether its objective is to maximise the wellbeing and development of all of society.

To make an even stronger argument of the need for government interest in this issue, one could glean from the *Global Strategy* some of the improvements in health that could occur as a result of choosing to provide infant nutrition through breast-feeding rather than formula. The argument could be refined by further linkages to health and development and by providing recognition of the competing alternatives to providing infant nutrition and their costs and benefits. Recall, the economic question is not whether allocating resources to breastfeeding could improve population health and productivity holding everything else equal. Instead, the question is whether allocating resources to breastfeeding is going to improve population health and productivity in a relatively short time period (as policy makers rarely focus on the future as much as analysts might prefer) given that resources will have to be taken away either from other medical/public health areas, from non-health governmental programmes, or from taxpayers to be used by the government. Each of these choices means that there will be benefits taken away from other parts of the healthcare system or economy at large. To make a convincing economic argument, the benefits of improving breastfeeding must exceed the costs of increasing breast-feeding, i.e. it must yield a positive net benefit. In addition, the positive net benefit must be larger the money spent than the positive net benefit of other intervention that could use the same resources.

Once a goal has been set and a particular policy option has been shown to be economically favourable, policy makers and programme managers can consider how programmes can be implemented most efficiently. At several points, the *Global Strategy* document describes the type of personnel who would be best suited to provide relevant services. Using the information on the personnel would be a first step in the cost calculations. The cost calculations should also consider the *Global Strategy* suggestion for a comprehensive and integrated approach to infant nutrition programmes. While having an integrated and comprehensive approach may seem intuitively appealing, making a programme integrated and comprehensive does not necessarily guarantee that it will be produced at a minimum cost. To determine whether there are economies to be gained from integrating programs, planners must understand the process and cost of implementing each programme individually, the ways in which the programmes might be combined to take advantage of shared resources, and the degree to which resources could be shared so the resources could be economised. In reality, the economics of all possible individual interventions have not been evaluated, and the economics of multiple interventions together have almost never been investigated. As a result, planners have essentially no knowledge of whether an integrated and comprehensive approach is actually a more efficient way to produce infant nutrition. Despite the intuitive appeal of the potential for shared resources, a comprehensive programme may, in fact, be difficult to integrate and additional layers of administrative infrastructure may need to be developed. As such, an integrated programme may be more expensive to operate than a series of smaller and less integrated programmes. To summarise, the costs of alternative methods of implementing individual programmes or combinations of programmes need to be assessed to understand the trade-offs that must be made in the process of allocating resources.

One way to minimise costs is to follow a suggestion from the *Global Strategy* document that focuses on proper and, as appropriate, local foods. The idea of using local agricultural products is critical for minimising the cost of food transport, although it may not minimise the total costs of the programme. However, it is important to remember that if a national government makes the *Global Strategy* part of its policy it will have implications for agricultural policy and this will have potentially even larger economic consequences. The *Global Strategy* document clearly recognises the potential for trade-offs in cost and nutritional value between locally produced and prepared foods and processed foods that are not necessarily local. The document also mentions fortification and supplementation that would each have cost implications.

When setting policy, the government must consider not only how much can be spent and how the resources that are used can change outcomes, but they also must consider other constraints. Paragraph five of the document (p. 6) discusses constraints that planners face when trying to implement a strategy to improve infant nutrition. The possibility of vertical human immunodeficiency virus (HIV) transmission places constraints on options for some mothers providing infant nutrition. The emergencies mentioned in this paragraph place other constraints on the options that are available.

Programme implementation that is economically favourable for society as a whole may still involve winners and losers. The *Global Strategy* document refers to the formation of alliances to achieve optimum infant nutrition on principles that avoid conflict of interest. This reflects that organisations will respond to incentives. If the incentives are to provide items to improve infant nutrition in ways that will create a conflict of interest, this will serve as an additional constraint to alternatives that can be chosen.

In addition to combining resources among interventions, programmes managers can consider what the *Global Strategy* document recommended – the use of existing infrastructure. This is one of the few points at which the document directly addressed an economic issue. Obviously, if a new programme or policy is built on existing infrastructure, this will conserve resources and possibly allow for the least cost implementation of a programme or policy to encourage breastfeeding.

Besides the policy level uses of economics, the economics of individual and family decision making should also be considered. Regardless of whether the mother and child are actually seen as a single unit for decision making or whether it is thought that the mother makes decisions for her own wellbeing with some recognition of how she affects the child's health and development, the mother will respond to economic incentives. The *Global Strategy* document demonstrates a recognition that mothers face a number of economic incentives not to spend a large amount of time providing nutrition to their infant and young children. Researchers in economics have spent some time studying how decisions are made at the family level and how parents make decisions that affect their children, although the quantity of economics research focusing directly on breastfeeding behaviour is quite limited. The incentives and disincentives that mothers face when making decisions about infant nutrition are not completely understood. Further, as noted earlier, the decisions made regarding breastfeeding affect and are affected by more than just the mother and her child. The father, other family members, an employer, co-workers, and others in the community can all be affected and have an effect on infant nutrition decisions. How to provide incentives rather than mandates for all interested parties to consider the wellbeing of infants and young children is a clear policy challenge that is not addressed by the *Global Strategy* document that primarily takes as given the worthiness of the goal to improve infant and young child nutrition. In short, in order to formulate better policies and interventions in the future that help to promote breastfeeding and to achieve infant nutrition goals, the economics of breastfeeding itself must be understood better.

10.6   Conclusion

Although the *Global Strategy* sends a fairly consistent message about the need for optimal infant and young child nutrition through breastfeeding and appropriate complementary feeding, it is important to note that the 'aims and objectives section' ends with two paragraphs that describe the strategy as a guide that will need to be updated over time and that cannot be fulfilled by a single intervention from a single group. Similar to economic reasoning, this allows for the fact that heterogeneous populations will require different interventions to achieve goals and that the best science for one area will not necessarily be the best science for all areas. The fact that infant nutrition interventions cannot be planned using a 'one size fits all' approach is critical for different planners around the world using this information. All interventions might share the same objectives that are put forward by the document, in particular ensuring optimal infant and early childhood nutrition, but this does not imply that all countries/places/settings should use the same policies or programmes.

The choice of new programmes or policies will be a function of what is effective in different settings, what helps to bring fairness and justice in different contexts, and what is shown to be economically feasible and economically efficient in different settings.

Using economics to guide the discussion forces decision makers to focus on the decisions that individuals and communities make in terms of the trade-offs that are required. Obviously, if programmes can be found that ultimately make everyone better off without costing anyone, these are 'low hanging fruit' for policy that should be adopted. However, most decisions do involve trade-offs. Optimising infant nutrition through the protection, promotion and support of breastfeeding and ensuring that it is an option for all mothers is an important goal, but it still needs to be considered in light of the cost of implementing such policies and the benefits of other health interventions that must be given up.

In summary, there is a need for additional information on the effectiveness and cost-effectiveness of breastfeeding policy and interventions. The *Global Strategy* document mentions a research agenda but does not list economic evaluation as a research need. Of course, the developers of the *Global Strategy* never suggested that economics be the basis of implementing the strategy. Further, some consider assessments of effectiveness to be science and the process of placing values on resources and benefits to be a 'valuation process' that relies on the science undertaken by others. It is important to remember that there is a science to economics that supplements the science that it relies on in building models to evaluate. As a result, a scientific research agenda must be developed that will answer questions about the resources that are needed to implement a variety of breastfeeding programmes. Research must also be undertaken to address how each of the potential policies and interventions influences mothers' and families' behaviours. All of this information can be taken together to make the best possible policies to promote breastfeeding, to ensure optimal infant nutrition and development, and to ensure optimal health and wellbeing of the population as a whole.

References

Chatterji, P. & Frick, K.D. (2005) Does returning to work after childbirth affect breastfeeding practices? *Review of Economics of the Household*, 3: 315–335.

Galtry, J. (2003) The impact on breastfeeding of labour market policy and practice in Ireland, Sweden and the USA. *Social Science and Medicine*, 57: 167–177.

Gold, M.R., Siegel, J.E., Russell, L.B. & Weinstein, M.C. (eds) (1996) *Cost-Effectiveness in Health and Medicine*. Oxford University Press, New York.

Tan-Torres Edejer, T., Baltussen, R., Adam, T., Hutubessy, R., Acharya, A., Evans, D.B., *et al.* (eds) (2003) *Making Choices in Health: WHO Guide to Cost-Effectiveness Analysis*. WHO, Geneva.

Tarn, T.Y.H. & Dix Smith, M. (2004) Pharmacoeconomic guidelines around the world. *ISPOR Connections*, 10, 5–15.

WHO (2003) *Global Strategy for Infant and Young Child Feeding*. WHO, Geneva.

11 Complex Challenges to Implementing the *Global Strategy for Infant and Young Child Feeding*

Victoria Hall Moran and Fiona Dykes

The chapters in this book powerfully illuminate the need to address the political, sociocultural and economic influences on eating, feeding and nutrition in infant and young children. In this short concluding chapter we re-emphasise the global significance of optimising practices in this area and we highlight the rhetoric–reality gap between policy and practice.

Almost a third of children globally are malnourished. It is also suggested that as many as 55% of infant deaths from diarrhoeal disease and acute respiratory infections may be the result of inappropriate feeding practices. As less than 35% of infants worldwide are exclusively breastfed for even the first four months of life (World Health Organization (WHO) 2003), the imperative to improve maternal and infant nutritional status has never been greater. This urgency has been re-emphasised through the United Nations Millennium Development Goals[i] (MDG) to (by 2015):

1. Eradicate extreme poverty
2. Achieve universal primary education
3. Promote gender equality and empower women
4. Reduce child mortality
5. Improve maternal health
6. Combat human immunodeficiency virus (HIV)/acquired immune deficiency syndrome (AIDS), malaria and other diseases
7. Ensure environmental sustainability
8. Develop a global partnership for development.

We cannot disconnect maternal health from that of the child as emphasised by the WHO, which states that:

'*The health and nutritional status of mothers and children are intimately linked. Improved infant and young child feeding begins with ensuring the health and*

[i] See http://www.un.org/millenniumgoals/ (accessed 22 June 2009).

nutritional status of women, in their own right, throughout all stages of life and continues with women as providers for their children and families. Mothers and infants form a biological and social unit; they also share problems of malnutrition and ill-health. Whatever is done to solve these problems concerns both mothers and children together.'

WHO (2003, p. 5)

So taking this intimate mother-child connection into account, improving maternal and infant nutritional status can have a significant impact upon MDGs 3, 4, 5 and 6. This is particularly the case with the protection, promotion and support of breastfeeding, which has a significant impact on MDGs 4 and 5 and some impact on 1, 3, 6 and 7.

The *Global Strategy for Infant and Young Child Feeding* (WHO 2003) emphasises the scientific and epidemiological basis for the protection, promotion and support of breastfeeding and optimising infant and young child nutrition and feeding practices. Furthermore, the *Global Strategy* refers to the broader socio-political implications of failing to achieve appropriate infant and young child feeding practices. Inappropriate feeding practices and their consequences are major obstacles to sustainable socioeconomic development and poverty reduction. Governments will be unsuccessful in their efforts to accelerate economic development in any significant long-term sense until optimal child growth and development, especially through appropriate feeding practices, are ensured (WHO 2003, p. 3). Thus the attainment of appropriate feeding practices, which in turn will help to reduce child mortality and improve maternal health, is a central consideration in progress towards eradicating extreme poverty (MDG 1).

The *Global Strategy* not only considers the implications of failing to optimise infant and young child feeding practices but it also recognises the social, political and economic constraints upon women and families in securing the optimum nutritional standards. There is a growing body of research by anthropologists and health and social care researchers that illuminates the ways in which maternal dietary and infant feeding practices relate substantially to local cultural norms and constraints (Sellen 2001; Dykes 2005a,b, 2006; Spiro 2006; Scavenius 2007; Bhutta *et al.* 2008). One example of cultural difference is seen in the primary emphasis on the nutritional aspects in some industrialised cultures, particularly in Europe, USA and Australia. In other more traditional, rural communities, around the world, breastfeeding is seen as primarily relationally orientated with absence of any dichotomy between the baby's nutritional and emotional needs (Maher 1992; Dykes 2005a). This reflects the contrast made between the Western biomedical conceptualisation of breast milk as a product important for its nutritional components and breastfeeding seen as a holistic and integrated activity within some less industrialised cultures (Van Esterik 1989; Dykes 2005a). Relationality and breastfeeding may also be influenced by institutional settings such as neonatal units, as described by Flacking in Chapter 3.

The chapters in this book illustrate a wide range of barriers to achievement of optimum feeding and nutrition, include structural issues such as poverty, gender inequality, limited access to appropriate foods, cultural taboos and beliefs, negative attitudes towards the body and breastfeeding and lack of community based knowledge. Living in poverty, for example, perpetuates the cycle of nutritional deprivation and its association with chronic disease, as discussed by Williams in Chapter 9. Poverty is not confined to resource-poor communities, as illustrated by Groleau and Rodriguez in Chapter 5. It is distributed in pockets throughout the world and in some countries it is the extensive norm; it stems from and manifests in a range of circumstances. Refugees, for example, constitute a displaced, disempowered group who may be living in poverty that is worse than that experienced by the indigenous people. The homeless mothers, referred to by Coufopolous and Hackett in Chapter 8, serve as an example of a vulnerable group, often living in poverty, in a resource-rich country and the HIV-positive women referred to by Thairu in Chapter 6 serve as an example of a highly vulnerable group in a resource-poor country. All are examples of those classified by the WHO as being in 'exceptionally difficult circumstances' (WHO 2003, p. 10).

Some of the key areas in which there is a clear rhetoric–reality gap are exclusive breastfeeding and complementary feeding, as discussed by Akre in Chapter 1. The *Global Strategy* recommends that 'infants should be exclusively breastfed for the first six months of life' (p. 8). Exclusive breastfeeding is defined as giving the baby only breast milk and no other liquids or foods. However, despite overwhelming scientific and epidemiological evidence for the importance of this practice, only 35% of infants worldwide are exclusively breastfed during the first four months of life (WHO 2003). Yet, as Bhandari *et al.* (2008) notes, interventions to promote exclusive breastfeeding have the potential to prevent an estimated 13% of all under-5 deaths in developing countries and, as such, are the single most important preventive interventions to protect against childhood mortality.

The *Global Strategy* also recommends that complementary feeding (commencement of weaning foods) should be 'timely', 'adequate' and 'safe'. However, women may be impeded in this by, for example availability of appropriate foods due to a very limited budget. Also, as the *Global Strategy* states (WHO 2003, p. 9):

'Appropriate complementary feeding depends on accurate information and skilled support from the family, community and health care system. Inadequate knowledge about appropriate foods and feeding practices is often a greater determinant of malnutrition than the lack of food.'

Infant feeding practices have undergone enormous changes over the past century and these relate to a complex combination of factors such as medicalisation of infant feeding, development of infant formulae, associated commercial activities and changing lives of women. There are many reasons why women do not breastfeed at all, prefer to partially breastfeed, discontinue breastfeeding early and/or introduce complementary foods before 6 months. In some countries and communities breastfeeding tends to be portrayed in the media and experienced by many women, particularly in socially deprived communities, as a marginal activity, rarely seen and barely spoken about (Hoddinott & Pill 1999; Henderson *et al.* 2000;

Mahon-Daly & Andrews 2002). Women are always in the process of negotiating any embodied experience within their own perceptions of their body and bodily activities as discussed by Stapleton and Keenan in Chapter 7. In some countries and communities, there is a culture in which breastfeeding combined with formula feeding has become normalised, for example in Japan, as described in Chapter 4 by Hashimoto and McCourt. Women may lack knowledge of appropriate complementary foods and feeding and in situations of perceived insufficient milk the babies may be being given solid food earlier than 6 months (see Chapter 6 for example). Finally, there is a wide range of cultural factors that influence women in giving other foods and drinks to babies under 6 months of age.

The MDGs and, more specifically, the *Global Strategy* provide us with unique drivers to make strategic change at national and local community levels to improve infant and young child nutrition and feeding practices. However, we cannot simply recommend programmes for change without thoroughly exploring the sociocultural context and constraints that operate within a given community or cultural setting (see Chapter 2). In addition there are complex economic considerations to be made at every level, as illuminated by Frick in Chapter 10. Without in-depth sociocultural knowledge and culturally sensitive management of change any intervention may well 'fall at the first hurdle' due to contradictory cultural beliefs and/or constraints on families in taking up or implementing designated changes. We hope and trust that this book will help those with responsibility to make a difference to understand some of the complexities and challenges involved in supporting individuals and communities in optimising infant and young child feeding and nutrition.

References

Bhandari, N., Kabir, A.K.M.I. & Salam, M.A. (2008) mainstreaming nutrition into maternal and child health programmes: scaling up of exclusive breastfeeding. *Maternal and Child Nutrition*, 4: 5–23.

Bhutta, Z.A., Shekar, M. & Ahmed, T. (2008) Mainstreaming interventions in the health sector to address maternal and child under-nutrition. *Maternal and Child Nutrition*, 4: 1–4.

Dykes, F. (2005a) Supply and demand: breastfeeding as labour. *Social Science and Medicine*, 60: 2283–2293.

Dykes, F. (2005b) Government funded breastfeeding peer support projects: Implications for practice. *Maternal and Child Nutrition*, 1: 21–31.

Dykes, F. (2006) *Breastfeeding in Hospital: Midwives, Mothers and the Production Line.* Routledge, London.

Henderson, L., Kitzinger, J. & Green, J. (2000) Representing infant feeding: content analysis of British media portrayals of bottle feeding and breast feeding. *British Medical Journal*, 321: 1196–1198.

Hoddinott, P. & Pill, R. (1999) Qualitative study of decisions about infant feeding among women in east end of London. *British Medical Journal*, 318: 30–34.

Maher, V. (1992) *The Anthropology of Breastfeeding. Natural Law or Social Construct.* Berg Publishers, Oxford.

Mahon-Daly, P. & Andrews, G.J. (2002) Liminality and breastfeeding: women negotiating space and two bodies. *Health and Place*, 8: 61–76.

Scavenius, M., van Hulsel, L., Meijer, J., Wendte, H. & Gurgel, R. (2007) In practice, the theory is different: a processual analysis of breastfeeding in north east Brazil. *Social Science and Medicine*, 64: 676–688.

Sellen, D.W. (2001) Weaning, complementary feeding, and maternal decision making in a rural East African pastoral population. *Journal of Human Lactation*, **17**: 233–244.

Spiro, A. (2006) Gujarati Women and Infant Feeding Decisions. In: Hall Moran, V. & Dykes, F. (eds) *Maternal and Infant Nutrition & Nurture: Controversies and Challenges*. Quay Books, London, 2006.

Van Esterik, P. (1989) *Motherpower and Infant Feeding*. London: Zed Books.

WHO (2003) *Global Strategy for Infant and Young Child Feeding*. WHO, Geneva.

Index